Marathon in Hong Kong

Marathon in Hong Kong: Challenges and Health

edited by

Dr. Ben FONG

Dr. WAI Heung On

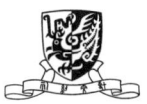

The Chinese University Press

Marathon in Hong Kong: Challenges and Health

Chief Editor: Dr. Ben FONG
Assistant Editor: Dr. WAI Heung On

© **The Chinese University of Hong Kong**, 2010

ISBN: 978-962-996-430-6

THE CHINESE UNIVERSITY PRESS
The Chinese University of Hong Kong
SHA TIN, N.T., HONG KONG
Fax: +852 2603 6692
       +852 2603 7355
E-mail: cup@cuhk.edu.hk
Web-site: www.chineseupress.com

Printed in Hong Kong

Contents

Preface

Marathon running has always been considered to be the ultimate test of human performance in sports. It is also ironic that the first man to "run the marathon", millenia ago, died at the finish line.

In the modern marathon, we have seen a great deal of growth with regard to participation and popularity, emphasis on scientific disciplines to enhance performance, and, certainly, the continuous drive to exceed personal limits.

Marathon running has now come into all walks of life as a symbol of exercise for health. We have witnessed an overwhelming enthusiasm for mass participation in different formats, including 10 km "fun runs" and half-marathons. It is also enlightening to see that marathons have become city icons by staging them in city streets, thereby arousing public awareness.

People participating in marathons engage in considerable preparations and place a strong emphasis on its scientific aspects, including pre-season training, attention to hydration and nutrition, and awareness of over-use injuries.

I am delighted that this book can include such diversified expertise, talent, and experience from professionals in different disciplines. It is presented in a very systematic way that affords readers both a wide perspective and a depth of understanding. I recommend this book to all runners, and I wish them the greatest fun in running and exercising for their health.

Professor CHAN Kai Ming
Chair Professor
Department of Orthopaedics & Traumatology
The Chinese University of Hong Kong

Foreword

The annual international Hong Kong Marathon, held in February or March every year, has gained worldwide attention and importance over the last decade. It has continued to attract world-class marathon runners from many countries, as well as local participants from all walks of life.

With the wide spectrum of participation and the ever-growing number of runners, this annual sports event has developed some festival components to accompany the physically and mentally demanding endurance competition. Sixty percent of participants join the 10 km event and, hence, they are not as likely professional as the marathon and half-marathon runners. Most of these nonprofessional participants have a good time on the open road and enjoy the festival atmosphere and the companionship of their friends and the crowd.

The Auxiliary Medical Service (AMS) is pleased to provide first-aid and medical support to this demanding sports event. Over 400 members and officers are deployed each year. Although most of the cases managed are of a relatively minor nature, some serious, and often unexpected, cases would have been managed by the doctors on duty during the race. Over the years, the AMS has gained considerable field experience and has applied it to the improvement and betterment of our services not only in this event, but in other major activities as well.

This book records the first decade of the Hong Kong Marathon. It is comprehensive and includes topics of importance and interest to anyone interested in the marathon. The contents also serve as a good reference for all potential runners and students pursuing knowledge in sports medicine.

Dr. CHAN Yiu-Wing
Chief Staff Officer
Auxiliary Medical Service

Biography of Contributors

Professor CHAN, Kai-Ming 陳啟明教授
MBBS (HK), FRCS (Edin), FRCS (Glas), M.Ch. Orthopaedic (Liverpool), FRCS Ortho-paedic (Edin), FACS, FHKAM (Orthopaedics), FHKCOS, FCSHK

- Chair Professor, Department of Orthopaedics & Traumatology, Faculty of Medicine, The Chinese University of Hong Kong
- Chief of Service, Orthopaedics & Traumatology, Prince of Wales Hospital, Hospital Authority
- Director, WHO Collaborating Centre for Sports Medicine & Health Promotion, Faculty of Medicine, The Chinese University of Hong Kong
- Co-Director, The Hong Kong Jockey Club Sports Medicine & Health Sciences Centre, Faculty of Medicine, The Chinese University of Hong Kong
- President, Asia-Pacific Orthopaedic Society for Sports Medicine (APOSSM)
- Co-Editor In Chief, Journal of Orthopaedic Surgery and Research (JOSR)
- Co-Editor In Chief, Journal of Sport Medicine, Arthroscopy, Rehabilitation, Therapy & Technology (SMARTT)

Dr. CHAN, Kwok-Ki 陳國基醫生
MBBS, FRCS (Edin), FCSHK, MScSEM (Bath), DPD (Wales), FHKAM (Surgery)

- Member, Anti-doping Disciplinary Panel, Hong Kong Anti-doping Committee, Sports Federation & Olympic Committee of Hong Kong, China
- Advisor on Aquatic Rescue, Ruttonjee Hospital & Tang Shiu Kin Hospital Accident & Emergency Training Centre, Hospital Authority
- Part-time Lecturer, Department of Physical Education, Hong Kong Baptist University
- Assistant Commandant, Training Institute, Auxiliary Medical Service, Hong Kong SAR Government
- Manager, Jockey Club Ti-I College

Dr. CHAN, Man-Chung 陳文仲醫生
MBBS (HK), MSc (PH), FHKCCM, FHKAM (Community Medicine)

- Specialist in Community Medicine
- Assistant Commissioner, Unit Commander, Health Protection Unit, Auxiliary Medical Service, Hong Kong SAR Government
- Vice-Chairman, Hong Kong Disaster Medicine Association
- Member, Scientific Committee on Vector-Borne Diseases, Centre for Health Protection, Hong Kong SAR Government
- Member, Scientific Committee on Vaccine Preventable Diseases, Centre for Health Protection, Hong Kong SAR Government

Dr. CHAN, Yiu-Wing 陳耀榮博士
BSocSc (HKU), MSocSc (HKU), MA (HKU), MA (CUHK), MBuddhStud (HKU), DBA [PolyU(HK)]

- Chief Staff Officer, Auxiliary Medical Service, Hong Kong SAR Government
- Vice President, Hong Kong Disaster Medicine Association
- Technical Adviser, The Hong Kong Life Saving Society

Dr. FONG, Ben Yuk-Fai 方玉輝醫生
MBBS (Syd), MPH (Syd), DFM (CUHK), DOM (CUHK), FRACMA, FHKCCM, FH-KAM (Community Medicine)

- Clinical Associate Professor (Honorary) in Family Medicine, The Chinese University of Hong Kong
- Adjunct Associate Professor, School of Chinese Medicine, The Chinese University of Hong Kong
- Senior Assistant Commissioner (Medical), Auxiliary Medical Service, Hong Kong SAR Government
- Chairman, Hong Kong Disaster Medicine Association

Professor FUNG, Anthony Ying-Him 馮應謙教授
MA; PhD (University of Minnesota)

- Associate professor in the School of Journalism and Communication, the Chinese University of Hong Kong
- Research interests: political economy of popular music and culture, gender and

youth identity, cultural studies, and new media technologies

- Publications: *New Television Globalisation and the East Asian Cultural Imaginations* (coauthored with Keane and Moran, 2007), *Global Capital, Local Culture: Transnational Media Corporations in China* (2008), *Riding a Melodic Tide: The Development of Cantopop in Hong Kong* (edited Chinese volume 2009), and *Policies for the Sustainable Development of the Hong Kong Film Industry* (2010) (coauthored with Chan and Ng).

Dr. FUNG, Ho-Tak Marcus 馮浩德醫生
BDS (HK), MPH (CUHK), MSc (London), MFGDP (UK), FRACDS

- Basic Life Support Instructor, American Heart Association
- First-aid Instructor, Auxiliary Medical Service, Hong Kong SAR Government

Dr. HO, Chung-Ping 何仲平醫生
MBBS (HK), MRCP (UK), FRCP (Glas), FRCP (Edin), FHKCP, FHKAM (Medicine)

- Medical Officer I, Health Protection Unit, Grade VI officer, Auxiliary Medical Service, Hong Kong SAR Government
- Council member, Hong Kong Medical Association
- Associate Clinical Professor, Department of Family Medicine, The Chinese University of Hong Kong

Dr. LAM, Kin-Kwan 林建群醫生
MBchB (CUHK), MRCP (UK), FRCS Ed., DCH (Ire.), DPD (Cardiff), FHKEM, FHKAM (Emergency Medicine)

- Senior Medical Officer, Accident and Emergency Department, United Christian Hospital
- Honorary Consultant, Accident and Emergency Department, Conde S. Januário General Hospital, Região Administrativa Especial de Macau
- Member, Pre-Hospital Care Subcommittee, Hong Kong College of Emergency Medicine
- Medical Officer I, Kowloon City District, Auxiliary Medical Service, Hong Kong SAR Government
- Vice-Chairman, Executive Committee, Building Healthy Kowloon City Association

Dr. LI, Ching-Fan Carina 李靜芬醫生

MBBS, FANZCA, FHKCA, FHKAM (Anaes), Dip.Pain Mgt

- Specialist Anaesthesiologist and Honorary Consultant, Pain Management Clinic, Hong Kong Sanatorium and Hospital
- Mobilization Officer (Medical), Auxiliary Medical Service, Hong Kong SAR Government
- Honorary Clinical Assistant Professor, Department of Anaesthesiology, University of Hong Kong
- Clinical Assistant Professor (Honorary), Department of Anaesthesia and Intensive Care, The Chinese of University of Hong Kong
- Honorary Medical Advisor, Hong Kong Multisports Association

Dr. LIT, Chau-Hung Albert 列就雄醫生

MBBS (HK), MRCP (UK), FRCS (Edin), FHKCEM, FHKAM (Emergency Medicine), FFAEM (UK), MHA (NSW)

- Specialist in Emergency Medicine
- Assistant Force Commander, Emergency Response Task Force, Auxiliary Medical Service, Hong Kong SAR Government

Dr. LONSDALE, Chris 梁啓思博士

MA (Victoria), PhD (Otago)

- Lecturer, School of Physiotherapy and Performance Science, University College Dublin, Ireland
- Sport Psychology Consultant, Irish Rugby Football Union

Mr. NG, Elton Chun-Ting 吳俊霆運動物理治療師

MSc Sports Physio (HKPU), Exercise Specialist® (ACSM), BSc Physio (HKPU), Dip Acu & Moxi (GUTCM), CPT (NASM)

- Principal Physiotherapist, Centre Of Rehabilitation & Exercising Specialist (CORES)
- Vice-chairman, Sports Specialty Group, Hong Kong Physiotherapy Association Limited
- Grade IV Officer, Auxiliary Medical Service, Hong Kong SAR Government
- Champions in Hong Kong Multi-sports Events

Mr. NG, Johan Yau-Yin 吳又言先生
BSc (CUHK), MPhil (CUHK)

- PhD Candidate, School of Sport and Exercise Sciences, University of Birmingham

Mr. O'REILLY, John 何禮樂先生
BA (Waterford), BSc (Dublin)

- Research Assistant and MSc student, Department of Sports Science and Physical Education, The Chinese University of Hong Kong

Mr. SHUM, James Kai-Yan 岑啓欣先生
MArch (HK)

- Disaster Medical Assistant Instructor, Auxiliary Medical Service, Hong Kong SAR Government
- Member, Emergency Response Task Force, Auxiliary Medical Service, Hong Kong SAR Government
- First-Aid Lecturer, Hong Kong St. John Ambulance Association

Dr. SIA, Yin-Shan Jacky 謝賢山醫生
MBBS (HK), MRCS (Edin), FHKCEM, FHKAM (Emerg Medicine), PG Dip SEM (Bath)

- Private practice, Town Health Centre.

Dr. SZETO, King-Ho 司徒敬豪醫生
BMedSc(CUHK), MBChB(CUHK), MRCS(Edin), FHKCEM, FHKAM (Emergency Medicine)

- Health Informatics Manager in Infectious Disease Control Training Centre, Hospital Authority and Infection Control Branch of Centre for Health Protection
- Specialist in Emergency Medicine, Department of Accident & Emergency, Ruttonjee and Tang Shiu Kin Hospital
- Field Physician in UBS Hong Kong Open (Golf Tournament)
- District Medical Officer, Auxiliary Medical Service, Hong Kong SAR Government

Dr. WAI, Heung-On Jonathan 衛向安醫生

MBBS (HK), DLO (RCS Eng), DFM (CUHK), MSc in Sports Medicine & Health Science (CUHK)

- Honorary Consultant in Ear, Nose and Throat Surgery, Precious Blood Hospital
- Clinical Associate Professor (Honorary), Department of Otorhinolaryngology, Head and Neck Surgery, The Chinese University of Hong Kong
- Clinical Associate Professor (Honorary), School of Public Health and Primary Care, The Chinese University of Hong Kong
- Part-time Lecturer, Department of Orthopaedics and Traumatology, The Chinese University of Hong Kong
- Deputy Regional Commander of New Territories West Region and Medical Advisor to the First Aid Bicycle Team, Auxiliary Medical Service, Hong Kong SAR Government

Professor WONG, Stephen Heung-Sang 王香生教授

BEd (Hons) (Liverpool), MSc, PhD (Loughborough), FACSM, R. Nutr.

- Professor, Department of Sports Science and Physical Education, The Chinese University of Hong Kong
- Associate Dean, Faculty of Education, The Chinese University of Hong Kong
- Dean of Students, United College, The Chinese University of Hong Kong
- Chairman, Hong Kong Physical Fitness Association (PFA)
- Council Member, Hong Kong Association of Sports Medicine and Sports Science
- Honorary Professor, South China Normal University

Dr. WONG, John T. 王泰鴻醫生

MBBS Hons (Monash), MRCP (UK), FHKCP, FHKAM (Medicine)

- Deputy Associate Consultant (Cardiology), Department of Medicine and Geriatrics, United Christian Hospital
- Honorary Adjunct Tutor, Department of Medicine and Therapeutics, The Chinese University of Hong Kong
- Honorary Aide-De-Camp to the Chief Executive, the Honourable Donald Tsang Yam Kuen, Hong Kong SAR Government
- Medical Officer I and Director of Community CPR program, Auxiliary Medical Service, Hong Kong SAR Government
- BLS and ACLS Instructor, American Heart Association

Ms. WU, Daphne Mei-Yi 胡美怡小姐

BSc (Hons) (HK), Postgrad Dip (UK), MSc (UK), SRD (UK), Grad Dip Sports Nutr (IOC)

- Registered Dietitian in Private Practice
- Panel Member, Hong Kong Primary Care Foundation
- PhD Candidate, School of Sport and Health Sciences, University of Exeter

Dr. YEUNG, Sai-Mo Simon 楊世模博士

PDPT (PolyU), Grad Dip Ergonomics (La Trobe), MPhil (CUHK), PhD (CUHK)

- Associate Professor, Department of Rehabilitation Sciences, The Hong Kong Polytechnic University

Dr. YUNG, Shu-Hang Patrick 容樹恒醫生

MBChB, FCSHK, FRCSEd, FHKCOS, FRCSEd (Orth), FHKAM (Orthopaedics Surgery)

- Orthopaedic Specialist
- President, Hong Kong Association of Sports Medicine & Sports Science (HKASMSS)
- Consultant, Department of Sports Medicine, Hong Kong Sports Institute
- Deputy Director, The Hong Kong Jockey Club Sports Medicine and Health Sciences Centre
- Chairman, Liaison Commission, International Federation of Sports Medicine (FIMS)

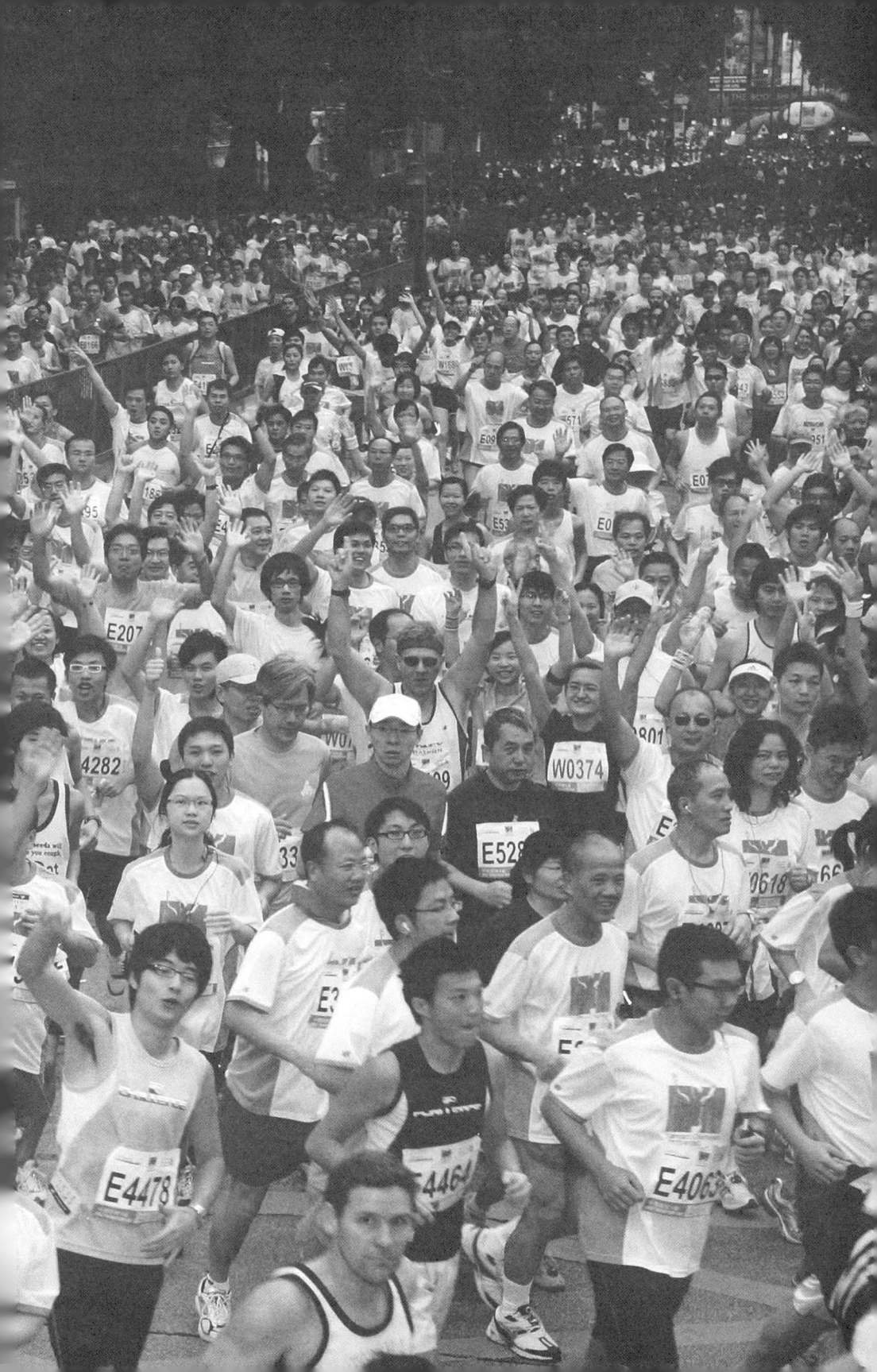

SECTION I

Introduction

History of the Marathon

Dr. CHAN Man Chung

The Greek Legend

There is a general belief that marathons started in ancient Greece because of the trained messenger Phidippides. This account was first recorded by the second century writer Lucian.

In 490 BC, King Darius of Persia sent twenty thousand men to the Greek city of Marathon. He wanted to punish the citizens there because they had helped the Ionians, Persia's enemy in western Asia Minor. General Miltiades, the defending Greek general, was in command of a much smaller army and, therefore, was greatly outnumbered by the Persians. He sought help from Athens, which was forty kilometers to the southwest, and sent Phidippides on mission with this objective. Spartans were the dominant military force in Greece at that time, so the messenger had to run on foot to Athens and Sparta to request troops for reinforcement. Miltiades defeated Darius before any support arrived, so Phidippides, a member of the *hemerodromoi*—the class of Greek runners trained as messengers—had to run back to Athens with news of the victory. The errand took several days and Phidippides traveled almost six hundred kilometers. The exact distance was never known, and Phidippides collapsed and died soon after he finally arrived in Athens and uttered the phrase "We have won!" The death of Phidippides, then, was the first sudden death reported in sports medicine. The legend was subsequently recorded in poetry and folktales.

The Olympics and the Marathon

The Ancient Greek Olympic Games can be dated to well before 400 BC. The competition was a celebration for the Greek god Zeus who lived in his sanctuary, Mount Olympus. Interestingly, there is no record of a specific distance run whatsoever in the ancient games. However, the revival of the games as a global sports competition in 1896 rekindled interest in Phidippides's distance run. Organizers of the Olympic Games favored the inclusion of a unique event relevant to Greek history. Therefore, the legendary run from Marathon to Athens was adopted. The first event was a long-distance run from the Marathon battlefield where Miltiades had defeated the Persians. The finishing line was at the specially built Panathenaikon stadium. The total distance was approximately forty kilometers.

The first six modern Olympic Games each had different lengths for the marathon. The first 42.195 km marathon was held in London in 1908. Because the starting line was moved to Windsor Castle from Windsor Park, this added an additional 385 yards, almost a lap around the stadium, so it was not a round figure of 26 miles (approximately 40 km). The race would end inside the studium, allowing Queen Alexandra and the entire stadium packed with spectators to see the grand finale. Such an arrangement gratified both the spectators and the athletes. The International Amateur Athletic Federation (IAAF) adopted this distance in its Fifth IAAF Congress in Geneva. There was no explanation given as to why the distance was chosen.

The Modern Marathon

The modern Olympic Games, now more than one hundred years old, gave birth to the marathon as a sporting event, no longer merely a battlefield in northern Greece. General Miltiades slowly faded into history, and the newly coined word was given life as a challenging physical event. The race is also unique in that it is conducted not on a track but on the road.

The 1970s was a watershed era for the modern marathon. The 1972 Olympic marathon champion, American Frank Shorter, said that there is no such thing as an "easy" marathon. Perhaps it is fair to say that the modern marathon only started after his victory because there was extensive media coverage and the race was widely televised around the world. Shorter's second victory came during the 1976 Montreal Olympic Games, which was again televised live. From then on, the modern marathon became a participatory sport. The New York Marathon further escalated its status by moving the route out of Central Park and onto the bridges and city streets. It further developed into a visible and interactive sport on the street level. From 1970 to 1975, the number of marathons raced in the United States increased five fold.

Marathon tourism has become a unique, new movement for international travelers. There are currently almost two thousand marathons held around the world each year, and the Big Five are Boston, New York, Chicago, London, and Berlin. They attract tens of thousands of running enthusiasts, and many travel around the world to join the elite runners. They are like golf aficionados, travelling with their bags and teeing off at every prestigious course. Unfortunately, none of them would be offered a handicap.

The ING New York City Marathon has more than eighty thousand runners and many world-class professional athletes. The prize money is more than USD $500,000. Over two million spectators usually line the streets, and another 260 million watch on television. It is one of the largest single-day sporting events in the world.

The common concept of world record does not apply to marathon. Given the different courses, course elevations, climate conditions, and other factors, there are only records for the best time on specific courses. The most an athlete can claim is the world's best time on a specific course.

References

1. Martin, David. 2001. "Marathon running as a social and athletic phenomenon: historical and current trends." In Dan Tunstall Pedoe (Ed.), *Marathon Medicine*. London: RSM Press.

2. Wallechinsky, David. 2004. *The complete book of the summer Olympics: Athens 2004 edition*. Toronto: Sportclassic Books.

3. Young, David C. 1966. *The modern Olympics: A struggle for revival*. Baltimore: Johns Hopkins University Press.

Issues of the Marathon: A Review

Dr. Ben FONG

Introduction

The first marathon runner, Phidippides, collapsed and died after running 39 km from the plain of Marathon to Athens to deliver news of the Greek victory over Persia in 490 BC. Legend has it that this was the beginning of the marathon race. Fortunately, death has not been a frequent concern for marathon runners.[1] The marathon is a physical and mental endurance test for the human body; yet it is human nature to take the challenge. Over time, the marathon has gained worldwide acceptance and popularity, and it is now a regular international event.[2]

Individual runners often have different goals. A runner's first marathon may be the only one in his or her life. Many people enjoy running and receiving medals, while others aim to improve their health through lifestyle changes that occur as a result of training. However, there was a controversy over marathon immunity (the impact on body immunity in acute exercise such as in the marathon) suggested by Dr. Thomas J. Bassler, a pathologist, in the mid 1970s.[2]

The first official marathon was held in 1896 at the first modern Olympic Games in Athens, and the course stretched roughly 25 miles from the plains of Marathon on the eastern coast of Greece to the Olympic Stadium in downtown Athens. The standard distance—26 miles and 385 yards (or 42.195 kilometres)—was adopted during the 1908 London Olympic Games when the race stretched from Windsor Castle to the Olympic Stadium in order to let the Royal Family watch the race.[2]

The five most famous and prestigious marathons are held in Chicago, New York, Boston, London and Berlin, and more than thirty thousand runners compete in each event. One of the most experienced marathon runners was Norm Frank of New York, who ran forty marathons a year and had competed in 870 different races by the end of 2004, when he was 73 years old! In addition, more women are also running marathons now.[2]

Various aspects of the marathon have been investigated. This chapter aims to introduce and present some of the significant and relevant findings related to several issues of concern. Experience and observations from Beijing, Singapore, Macau, and Kawaguchi are illustrated in a separate chapter.

Limits

An average time of 3.75 hours has been estimated for the full marathon.[3] Individual runners' experiences of running in a marathon may influence running habits. For example, people who dropped out of races often report more injuries and less training.[4]

Endurance training, such as that required for the marathon, may lead to enlargement of the heart, slower heart rates, and some electrocardiographic changes, which is commonly known as athlete's heart syndrome. Professor K. M. Chan's group followed the cardiac symptoms in a 43-year-old British amateur athlete who ran the super-marathon run from Beijing to Hong Kong in 1983 to study the importance of team approach in sports medicine. This run covers about three thousand kilometres over fifty-five days from October to December, and the subject did not have any cardiac symptoms before, during, or after the run. Hence, careful planning for the total care of the athlete should take place before, during, and after any endurance sport so that the maximum capability of the athlete can safely and confidently be realised. Most of all, prevention of injuries is always the first priority.[5]

Chan et al. (1985) suggests that we should strive to achieve the ultimate goal of "sports for all."[5] Thompson (1997) remarks that a protective effect of exercise, such as a reduction in blood pressure and an improved lipid profile, leads to a lesser possibility of heart attacks. The American College of Sports Medicine recommends that every adult should participate in at least thirty minutes of moderately intense physical activity every day.[3] Marathon training, and its associated healthy lifestyle, has led to positive health changes in many runners. Those athletes who do not have the proper prepa-ration or who have not sufficiently trained may require medical attention or experience problems during and after the race.[6]

According to the International Olympic Committee, it is the responsibility of the sports medicine profession to care for the health and welfare of Olympic athletes, treat and prevent them from injuries, conduct medical examinations, evaluate performance capacity, provide nutritional advice, prescribe and supervise training programs, and monitor substance use.[7]

To achieve the objectives of the Olympic motto of becoming faster, higher, and stronger, some speculate that performance records will continue to improve because more scientifically valid sports medicine information will be available to athletes.[7] Nevertheless, there is a performance limit, and age has proven to be the single best predictor of endurance running performance. This results from a beneficial effect of habitual physical activity arising from the retention of functional capacity with aging.[8] Physical activity is believed to slow down the natural aging process in older people, and elite masters have continued to improve running times at a greater rate than younger athletes, whose performance levels have plateaued.[9]

Endurance performance is also influenced by neural drive and biomechanical factors (e.g., cardiovascular capacity, metabolic characteristics of skeletal muscles) and environmental factors, such as altitude and temperature.[10,11] Physiologically, the runner's glycogen storage will be used up and fat will be used to fuel the muscles at twenty miles or two hours, which is less efficient. The runner will then "hit the wall" for the remaining six miles, which is when the race becomes significantly more mental, and the mind games begin. At this point, the mind must push the body to extremes to continue.[2]

Annually, there is only one estimated death for every fifteen thousand to eighteen thousand healthy joggers. Increased risk factors include an age greater than 35, a history of smoking and drinking, hypertension, high cholesterol, a fast-food diet, a family history of heart attack, and no regular exercise.[2]

The Gender Issue

Roberta Gibb became the first woman to run the marathon at the 1966 Boston Marathon. However, this was not regarded as an official entry until several years later. The marathon was only sanctioned by the International

Amateur Athletics Federation in 1980. Amazingly, by 2003, 37% of all marathon finishers were women, a statistic that doubled over the previous ten years.[2,3]

During the last two decades, dramatic improvements for women runners have leveled off, and women's times in the marathon have now reached a plateau similar to that observed for men.[12] It has been suggested that gender differences should disappear as distances increase, but the average time difference indicates a 12.4% faster pace for men.[13] The gender difference in performance will remain fairly constant and is unlikely to narrow naturally. This is the case because of biological differences between men and women that give men a larger aerobic capacity and greater muscular strength.[12,14] On the other hand, women runners have greater fatigue resistance than do men of comparable training, and they often have stronger motivations for participating in athletic competition.[15,16]

Environment, Climate and Altitude

Environmental stress such as heat, humidity, air pollution, altitude, and geographical features of the race course can severely affect even a well-trained athlete's thermal balance and performance so that he or she must reduce speed to prevent heat-related injuries. Fluid balance is important for thermoregulation because dehydration can compromise heat loss and increase thermal strain. There is therefore a direct relationship between heat casualties and ambient temperatures.[17,18,19]

At times, environmental stress arises from poor timing and organisation of events, especially in highly variable temperate climate zones. Hence, it is recommended that a race should be cancelled or postponed if the weather forecast is not favourable.[17,18,20]

Medical Problems

A number of medical problems, in addition to injuries, may arise during a marathon. Although cardiac events are rare, gastrointestinal complaints are common. Symptomatic hyponatraemia is a serious but mostly preventable problem.[21] Musculoskeletal and respiratory problems have also been reported.[22] Exercise-induced muscle cramps are very common and may not be associated with gross disturbances of fluid and electrolyte balance.[23] Headaches and migraines are also common for marathon runners.[24]

As competitors become more experienced, they will hopefully seek medical assistance earlier and ultimately experience fewer problems overall, and those problems that they do experience will be less serious at the finish.[25]

Sudden Death in Sports

Epidemiology studies suggest that long-term exercise may protect against coronary heart disease and reduce the risk of sudden death. However, this may not always hold true after strenuous physical exertion. Up to and including 1993, there were two reported deaths from coronary heart disease out of an estimated total of 275,000 runners who competed in fourteen London marathons.[3,26] Higdon (2005) opines that, "An occasional cardiac death in a race was considered no more or less alarming than someone's dying while attending a symphony concert."[2]

Sudden death, mainly caused by cardiovascular conditions during athletic activities such as the marathon that require extreme exertion, is highly visible and attracts controversy regarding the true risks associated with sports.[27] The risk of sudden cardiac death in such events is exceedingly small with an incidence of 1 in 50,000 subject years. Death in younger athletes is rare. The victims are often regarded as being very fit and may have competitive personalities. The deceased runners may not have documented history of heart disease or related symptoms, and may well have previously completed other marathons.[28]

Education should be emphasised to increase awareness of the warning symptoms and risk factors including smoking, a family history of myocardial infarction before 55 years of age, hypertension, and hypercholesterolaemia. Runners experiencing dizziness, syncope, pre-syncope, palpitations, chest pain, or undue dyspnoea should have a detailed medical examination to assess their functional capacity, and they should be considered for cardiological investigation, if appropriate.[26,29]

Considerable controversy exists regarding the cost and effectiveness of screening young people by examination before participation in a marathon. Moreover, the low risk for sudden death in these events suggests that routine screening of runners for cardiovascular disease may not be justifiable.[28]

Fluid and Electrolytes

During a marathon, changes associated with fluid and electrolyte balance significantly increase levels of serum sodium, potassium, blood urea nitrogen, creatinine, uric acid, creatine phosphokinase, protein, plasma renin, vasopressin, and urinary potassium. Significant decreases are also noted in body weight, blood pressure, and urinary sodium in marathon runners who compete under warmer conditions.[30]

During endurance exercise, approximately 75% of the energy produced from metabolism is in the form of heat, which cannot accumulate. Sweat evaporation provides the primary cooling mechanism for the body, so athletes are encouraged to drink plenty of fluids to ensure continued fluid availability for evaporation and circulatory flow to the tissues. Runners might be in danger of heat illness if they race too quickly in hot or humid conditions, and they might even collapse at the end of their event. Elite athletes are often urged to drink "as much as tolerable" or "according to thirst" and to manage adequate hydration by ingesting 200–800 ml per hour.[31]

Excessive drinking, however, can lead to hyponatraemia severe enough to cause life-threatening illnesses and fatalities. Hyponatraemia, which is associated with substantial weight gain, occurs in a substantial fraction of marathon runners. The incidence of hyponatraemia requiring medical treatment has been found to be 5.6%–13%.[32] There is no correlation between running time and serum sodium level. Therefore, presentation of exercise-associated hyponatraemia may be delayed. Some runners who finished their race with a normal mental state soon became confused, a symptom associated with hyponatraemia.[34]

Efforts to prevent hyponatraemia should focus on minimising over-drinking.[33] Individual runners vary considerably in size, degree of training, heat acclimatisation, rate of perspiration, rate of water and sodium loss, etc. Therefore, a global recommendation for fluid replacement is not possible. Thirst or individual perspiration rates have been suggested as a primary guide. Optimal treatment is also controversial, but the early use of hypertonic fluids and potassium solutions in symptomatic patients has been recommended.[34,35]

Psychology

Training for and running a marathon exerts significant influence on the emotional, cognitive, and behavioral aspects of the participants. It also connects their past experence to present and future marathon events.[36] A lifetime of regular physical activity is associated with desirable physical and mental health.[37] Most runners have reported that during the race their thoughts are internally associative; internally dissociative thoughts, as reported, are the least prevalent.[38]

Injuries

Marathon running is a relatively safe sport as long as runners train intelligently, behave rationally, and take proper precautions. Despite this, the physical exertion required to complete a marathon, coupled with exposure to often harsh environmental conditions and an increase in the number of novice participants, makes injuries inevitable. The three general categories of injuries encountered in marathons are medical conditions, musculoskeletal injuries, and dermatologic complaints. To avoid such injuries, it is important to have thorough pre-race planning and preparedness.[1]

Acute musculoskeletal injuries are common, but running does not result in increased rates of musculoskeletal disability.[21] The clinical and social consequences of the injuries seem to be relatively mild.[39]

The most common injuries that occur in marathon runners are minor and include corns, calluses, blisters, muscle cramps, acute knee and ankle injuries, plantar fasciitis, and metatarsalgia, predominantly involving the lower limbs.[40,41]

First Aid and Medical Services

The medical team's main goal is to implement strategies that prevent serious injury and illness through pre-event planning, race-day preparedness, and post-event evaluations.[1] Mild injuries and illnesses account for 90% of finish-line medical encounters, and more than 99.9% of runners leave the finish area without hospital or emergency room care. The mean hospital contact rate has been estimated to be 1.6 per 1,000 entrants, and this is not related to the total number of runners in a race, density of first-aid posts, or sophistication of the first aid offered.[42]

In Hong Kong, the Auxiliary Medical Service (AMS) is a government department under the authority of the Security Bureau. The AMS comprises 4,400 volunteers, predominantly lay persons, who provide first aid and disaster medical services to the public. Among the volunteers, there are about 150 doctors. These doctors come from all backgrounds within the public and private sectors. Medical volunteers play a rather unique role in the AMS and are well positioned to share their knowledge, skills, and experience with other volunteers to enhance the standards of the entire service. In recent years, volunteers' responsibilities have included more duties involving major sporting events like the marathon. Doctors are assigned to strategic posts to help members and to perform more complicated resuscitations. It has been demonstrated that this involvement of doctors in the marathon has reduced the percentage of runners transferred to the Accident and Emergency Departments of hospitals.[43]

The Hong Kong Standard Chartered Marathon is a major international event that had 54,272 runners in 2009. It attracts both professional athletes and also amateur and fun runners. With the help of the Auxiliary Medical Service, Hong Kong benefits from more advanced medical support and a lower injury rate, when compared to other major marathon events. Staffed by four hundred trained volunteers, there are twenty first-aid posts along the route, and they are all well equipped with Automated External Defibrillators (AEDs) and emergency medical kits. In addition, the AMS First Aid Bicycle Team patrols the route with AEDs and other equipment.

In 2006, there were about 4,800 cases of cramps or minor sprains, while 232 required further attention. Of the twenty-two people taken to the hospital, one died of asthma and heart failure. This number of medical cases is very normal considering the large number of participants. Sports physiotherapy is also provided to marathon runners on a volunteer basis by professional physiotherapists.[44]

Mobile first aid arrangements are commonly employed to prevent dehydration and treat collapsed runners, but they do not replace static posts. The inadequacy of such medical precautions at some marathon events suggests that marathon organisers should be required to apply consistent and high standards to the prevention and treatment of medical problems.[45] An injury and illness profile can be used to tailor medical care at the finish area of marathons.[42] There should be flexibility when planning the provision of such services.[44] A Taiwan team has expressed support for the use of the triage-based Personal Digital Assistant (PDA) at mass gatherings such as marathons to cover pre-hospital emergency medical services and onsite evaluation.[46,47]

Spectators who also happen to be doctors may potentially find themselves in a difficult position at major sports events. In 1998, two junior doctors who went to the aid of a marathon runner, who collapsed and died at the finish line of a half-marathon in Bath. They later found themselves answering a battery of questions from the victim's lawyer, which ultimately resulted in a verdict of natural causes.[48] The parents of the deceased runner launched a campaign requiring organisers to provide advanced life support at strenuous events. They also made the point that emergency medical assistance should remain the responsibility of race organisers and those hired to provide emergency medical care because competitors pay for medical assistance as part of their entrance fee. Moreover, in France, medical rules introduced in 1992 require highly trained doctors skilled in resuscitation, paramedic ambulances, and an effective means of radio communication in major sport events.[49]

Elite Runners

High-energy output seems to be the discriminating factor for top-class male marathon runners who train at higher relative intensities.[50] Most elite runners have a healthly lifestyle: they are slim, fit non-smokers who rarely suffer from serious injuries. Most try to optimise their performance by changing their diet in the days before a run. These runners train between 90–150 km per week and are generally careful about stretching and warming up and down to avoid injuries. Like most runners, their major medical problems include gastrointestinal disturbances, skin lesions, and pain or cramps in the lower extremities. The most common reasons for not completing a race are exhaustion and injuries to the lower extremities.[51,52,53]

The dominance of East-African athletes in distance running remains largely unexplaint. Some proposed reasons include favourable physiological characteristics, favourable genetic endowment, and optimal environmental conditions. Elite endurance athletes come from distinct environmental backgrounds in terms of geographical distribution, ethnicity, and a history of travelling farther to school, often by running. These findings highlight the importance of genetic, environmental, and social factors in the success of East-African (notably Kenyan) endurance runners.[54,55]

Training Programmes

Training profiles are a useful predictor of success in a marathon. Mileage covered per training session is the best predictor for a successful completion of a race. In the 1998 Hong Kong Standard Chartered Marathon, non-finishers were found to be poorly prepared.[56]

In general, training influences runners' maximal oxygen uptake and running economy, which appears to be limited by genetic factors.[57,58] Many people enjoy health-orientated training programs that focus primarily on the prevention of injuries and diseases, provided that they simultaneously offer a high enjoyment factor.[59]

References

1. Jaworski CA. 2005. Medical concerns of marathons. *Curr Sports Med Rep* 4 (3): 137–43.
2. Higdon, Hal. 2005. *Marathon: The ultimate training guide.* 3ed. PA: Rodale.
3. Thompson GR. 1997. Grand Rounds—Hammersmith Hospital: Hazards of running a marathon. Creatine Kinase MB can be raised without myocardial infarction. *BMJ* 314 (5 April): 1023.
4. Clough P J, Shepherd J, Maughan R J. 1989. Marathon finishers and pre-race drop-outs. *Br J Sports Med* 23 (2): 97–101.
5. Chan KM, Diamond P, Law CK, Hsu S, Leung PC, So SY, et al. 1985. Beijing to Hong Kong super-marathon—sports medicine research. *Br J Sports Med* 19 (3): 145–47.
6. Kretsch A, Grogan R, Duras P, Allen F, Sumner J, Gillam I. 1984. 1980 Melbourne marathon study. *Med J Aust*141 (12–13): 809–14.
7. Tipton CM. 1997. Sports medicine: a century of progress. *J Nutr* 127 (5 Suppl): 878S–885S.
8. Takeshima N, Tanaka K. 1995. Prediction of endurance running performance for middle-aged and older runners. *Br J Sports Med* 29 (1): 20–23.

9. Jokl P, Sethi PM, Cooper AJ. 2004. Master's performance in the New York City Marathon 1983–1999. *Br J Sports Med* 38 (4): 408–12.

10. Maud P J, Pollock ML, Foster C, Anholm JD, Guten G, Al-Nouri, et al. 1981. Fifty years of training and competition in the marathon: Wally Hayward, age 70—a physiological profile. *S Afr Med J* 59 (5): 153–57.

11. Maughan RJ. 2005. The limits of human athletic performance. *Ann Transplant* 10 (4): 52–54.

12. Cheuvront SN, Carter R, Deruisseau KC, Moffatt RJ. 2005. Running performance differences between men and women: an update. *Sports Med* 35 (12): 1017–24.

13. Coast JR, Blevins JS, Wilson BA. 2004. Do gender differences in running performance disappear with distance? *Can J Appl Physiol* 29 (2): 139–45.

14. Sparling PB, O'Donnell EM, Snow TK. 1998. The gender difference in distance running performance has plateaued: an analysis of world rankings from 1980 to 1996. *Med Sci Sports Exerc* 30 (12): 1725–29.

15. Bam J, Noakes TD, Juritz J, Dennis SC. 1997. Could women outrun men in ultramarathon races? *Med Sci Sports Exerc* 29 (2): 244–47.

16. Pierce EF, Rohaly KA, Fritchley B. 1997. Sex differences on exercise dependence for men and women in a marathon road race. *Percept Mot Skills* 84 (3 Pt 1): 991–94.

17. Peiser B, Reilly T. 2004. Environmental factors in the summer Olympics in historical perspective. *J Sports Sci* 22 (10): 981–1001; discussion 1001–02.

18. Nielsen B. 1996. Olympics in Atlanta: a fight against physics. *Med Sci Sports Exerc* 28 (6): 665–68.

19. Cheuvront SN, Haymes EM. 2001. Thermoregulation and marathon running: biological and environmental influences. *Sports Med* 31 (10): 743–62.

20. Porter AM. 1984. Marathon running and adverse weather conditions: a miscellany. *Br J Sports Med* 18 (4): 261–64.

21. Sanchez LD, Corwell B, Berkoff D. 2006. Medical problems of marathon runners. *Am J Emerg Med* 24 (5): 608–15.

22. Macera CA, Pate RR, Woods J, Davis DR, Jackson KL. 1991. Post-race morbidity among runners. *Am J Prev Med* 7 (4): 194–98.

23. Maughan RJ. 1986. Exercise-induced muscle cramp: a prospective biochemical study in marathon runners. *J Sports Sci* 4 (1): 31–34.

24. Swain R, Rosencrance G. 1999. Headache occurrence and classification among distance runners. *W V Med J* 95 (2): 76–79.

25. Ridley SA, Rogers PN, Wright IH. 1990. Glasgow marathons 1982–1987. A review of medical problems. *Scott Med J* 35 (1): 9–11.

26. Hillis W S, McIntyre P D, Maclean J, Goodwin J F, McKenna W J. 1994. ABC of Sports Medicine: Sudden death in sport. *BMJ* 309:657–60.

27. Hanzlick RL, Stivers RR. 1983. Sudden death due to anomalous right coronary artery in a 26-year-old marathon runner. *Am J Forensic Med Pathol* 4 (3): 265–68.

28. Maron BJ, Poliac LC, Roberts WO. 1996. Risk for sudden cardiac death associated with marathon running. *J Am Coll Cardiol* 28 (2): 428–31.

29. Parsons MA, Anderson PB, Williams BT. 1984. An "unavoidable" death in a people's marathon. *Br J Sports Med* 18 (1): 38–39.

30. Nelson PB, Ellis D, Fu F, Bloom MD, O'Malley J. 1989. Fluid and electrolyte balance during a cool weather marathon. *Am J Sports Med* 17 (6): 770–72.

31. Noakes T. 2003. Fluid replacement during marathon running. *Clin J Sport Med* 13 (5): 309–18.

32. Hsieh M, Roth R, Davis DL, Larrabee H, Callaway CW. 2002. Hyponatremia in runners requiring on-site medical treatment at a single marathon. *Med Sci Sports Exerc* 34 (2): 185–89.

33. Montain SJ, Cheuvront SN, Sawka MN. 2006. Exercise associated hyponatraemia: quantitative analysis to understand the aetiology. *Br J Sports Med* 40 (2): 98–105.

34. Goudie AM, Tunstall-Pedoe DS, Kerins M, Terris J. 2006. Exercise-associated hyponatraemia after a marathon: case series. *J R Soc Med* 99 (7): 363–67.

35. Kavanagh T, Shephard RJ. 1977. On the choice of fluid for the hydration of middle-aged marathon runners. *Br J Sports Med* 11 (1): 26–35.

36. Hoag J, Gissen M. 1984. Marathon: a life-and-death experience. *J Psychoactive Drugs* 16 (1): 47–50.

37. Morgan WP, Costill DL. 1996. Selected psychological characteristics and health behaviors of aging marathon runners: a longitudinal study. *Int J Sports Med* 17 (4): 305–12.

38. Stevinson CD, Biddle SJ. 1998. Cognitive orientations in marathon running and "hitting the wall". *Br J Sports Med* 32:229–34; discussion 234–35.

39. van Middelkoop M, Kolkman J, van Ochten J, Bierma-Zeinstra SM, Koes BW. 2007. Course and predicting factors of lower-extremity injuries after running a marathon. *Clin J Sport Med* 17 (1): 25–30.

40. Caselli MA, Longobardi SJ. 1997. Lower extremity injuries at the New York City

Marathon. *J Am Podiatr Med Assoc* 87 (1): 34–37.

41. Satterthwaite P, Larmer P, Gardiner J, Norton R. 1996. Incidence of injuries and other health problems in the Auckland Citibank marathon, 1993. *Br J Sports Med* 30 (4): 324–26.

42. Roberts WO. 2000. A 12-yr profile of medical injury and illness for the Twin Cities Marathon. *Med Sci Sports Exerc* 32 (9): 1549–55.

43. Fong B. 2006. Doctors and voluntary service. *HK Med J* 12 (3): 245–46.

44. Yeung SS, Yeung EW, Wong TW. 1998. Provision of physiotherapy at the Tsing Ma Bridge international marathon and 10 km race in Hong Kong. *Br J Sports Med* 32 (4): 336–37.

45. Williams BT, Nicholl JP. 1984. Medical arrangements in 108 open-entry Britain marathons, 1983. *Health Trends* 16 (3): 68–70.

46. Chang P, Hsu YS, Tzeng YM, Sang YY, Hou IC, Kao WF. 2004. The development of intelligent, triage-based, mass-gathering emergency medical service PDA support systems. *J Nurs Res* 12 (3): 227–36.

47. Chang P, Hsu YS, Tzeng YM, Hou IC, Sang YY. 2004. Development and pilot evaluation of user acceptance of advanced mass-gathering emergency medical services PDA support systems. *Medinfo* 11 (Pt 2): 1421–25.

48. Dyer Clare. 1998. "Good Samaritans" face grilling. *BMJ* 317:1100.

49. Loyley P, Loyley P. 1999. Medical rules are needed in marathons in the United Kingdom. *BMJ* 318:1285.

50. Billat VL, Demarle A, Slawinski J, Paiva M, Koralsztein JP. 2001. Physical and training characteristics of top-class marathon runners. *Med Sci Sports Exerc* 33 (12): 2089–97.

51. Hölmich P, Darre E, Jahnsen F, Hartvig-Jensen T. 1988. The elite marathon runner: problems during and after competition. *Br J Sports Med* 22 (1): 19–21.

52. Hölmich P, Christensen SW, Darre E, Jahnsen F, Hartvig-Jensen T. 1989. Non-elite marathon runners: health, training and injuries. *Br J Sports Med* 23 (3): 177–78.

53. Tokudome S, et al. 2004. Anthropometric, lifestyle and biomarker assessment of Japanese non-professional ultra-marathon runners. *J Epidemiol* 14 (5): 161–67.

54. Scott RA, Georgiades E, Wilson RH, Goodwin WH, Wolde B, Pitsiladis YP. 2003. Demographic characteristics of elite Ethiopian endurance runners. *Med Sci Sports Exerc* 35 (10): 1727–32.

55. Onywera VO, Scott RA, Boit MK, Pitsiladis YP. 2006. Demographic

characteristics of elite Kenyan endurance runners. *J Sports Sci* 24 (4): 415–22.

56. Yeung SS, Yeung EW, Wong TW.2001. Marathon finishers and non-finishers characteristics. A preamble to success. *J Sports Med Phys Fitness* 41 (2): 170–76.

57. Maldonado S, Mujika I, Padilla S. 2002. Influence of body mass and height on the energy cost of running in highly trained middle- and long-distance runners. *Int J Sports Med* 23 (4): 268–72.

58. Sjödin B, Svedenhag J. 1985. Applied physiology of marathon running. *Sports Med* 2 (2): 83–99.

59. Platen P, Schaar B. 2003. How to carry out a health-orientated marathon training programme for running and inline skating. *Eur J Cardiovasc Prev Rehabil* 10 (4): 304–12.

Marathon Races Across Asia

Dr. CHAN Man Chung & Dr. Ben FONG

Singapore

The Singapore International Marathon is quite a challenge to the runners as well as to the organizing committee, since the race has developed to be such an international event. Not only does the hot weather compromise runners, but race organizers and volunteers have also found their working environment so hot and humid that extra effort is required to complete the task.

About eighteen thousand runners join the race each year, and the city practically shuts down as the race spans across the heart of the metropolis. Singapore is located near the equator, so hot weather and heavy perspiration are guaranteed for every marathon competitor and tourist.

On 4 December 2005, the full marathon started at 6 am to minimize the searing heat that the city would experience at noon. Races of other lengths started at different times in order to ease the congestion on the city streets. It started at Esplanade Drive and ended at the nearby Padang, the old English parade ground. The course wrapped around the Singapore River, Marina South, the Central Business District, East Coast Park, and City Hall. The abundance of greenery along the Singapore route provided an enjoyable view for runners, and the tame environment along the East Coast Parkway provided a tranquil trot for every participant. The route was carefully designed to allow runners the opportunity to view this scenic city. Singapore weather is tropical, and running in temperatures higher than 26°C is extremely demanding on the cooling physiology of the human body. The race is almost entirely on level ground, at a minimum elevation, and has no tunnels.

Prior to 2008, medical facilities and aid were contracted to Alexandra

Hospital. Paramedics and consultants from the hospital were on site at the marathon, and a strategically located medical post with senior medical staff was deployed at the finish line. All medical personnel were positioned at the finish line with an adequately lit, powered, and ventilated marquee. Along the route, there were members of St. John Ambulance Brigade. They were deployed to attend to the first-aid needs of the runners. There were only a handful of first-aid posts scattered along the route, but motorbikes with mobile Automated External Defibrillators (AEDs) were allowed to patrol the course.

Medical evacuation was meticulously planned and executed at the finish line. This allowed the medical team, equipped with ambulatory aid, access to victims who collapsed after their final sprint to the finish. The ambulance loading area was next to the marquee, and it was facilitated with a gentle ramp. Special arrangements were also made to allow emergency vehicles with sirens sounding to exit the compound easily.

Beijing

The Beijing International Marathon has been organized by the Chinese Athletics Association annually since 1981. The course is almost entirely flat, and it encompasses the old city like maple syrup spreading over a pancake. Elevations are slight, and the few hills along the course are modest and bearable. The race typically starts very early in the morning at 8 am. It starts at Tiananmen Square and then continues along the winding city roads. The race is also conducted almost exclusively outdoors, unlike the Standard Chartered Marathon in Hong Kong which passes through two tunnels.

The 2006 Beijing International Marathon began with a temperature of 15°C and with light winds. Humidity was moderate, and the balmy weather eased some of the tensions of the runners. Pollution, however, was a worrysome factor to both the athletes and the organizing committee.

The event was sponsored by the ANA, a Japanese enterprise, and the prize money was relatively modest when compared to other international marathons. However, it was well supported by universities, institutes, and individuals. A handbook was distributed to each runner with tips and advice. Athletes participating in the half and full marathons were required to submit their own medical report to prove the state of their health. They were also required to prepare themselves with a pair of comfortable running shoes, thick socks, breathable shorts, a rain jacket, and a small tube of Vaseline.

Runners assembled at Tiananmen Square, near the Chairman Mao Memorial Hall. More than twenty-one thousand runners participated in the events, which included 5 km, 10 km, half marathon, and full marathon races. The full marathon ended at the Olympic Center at the outskirts of the city. Almost all runners began at the same time; elite runners, though, were allowed to start fifteen minutes before the rest.

In order to help full marathon runners keep pace with their targeted finishing times, organizers provided pace markers—veteran runners bearing colored balloons that indicate specific finishing times.

Finish lines for the full marathon, half marathon, 8 km, and mini marathon were located at different places. First-aid posts were manned by the "120" emergency centers (120 is the emergency telephone number in Beijing) as well as ambulances from different centers and hospitals. These posts were strategically positioned at each 5 km point, and signs was placed fifty meters ahead of each station. A total of five ambulances were dedicated for evacuation purposes. Hospitals along the route were notified and ready to receive any casualties.

Along the route, young volunteers from the Sports Institute were positioned every one hundred meters. These young men and women were trained with basic life-support skills, and they had gone through two rounds of refresher training during the previous year. Therefore, almost four hundred volunteers were scattered along the route, but they were not equipped with advanced resuscitation instruments. A specific ambulance was also assigned to follow the elite group of runners.

Storage for runners' personal items was well organized with the help from the University Sports Federation. The organizing committee provided buses, and each bus was responsible for the storage of a large number of bags, according to the runners' bib numbers. This facilitated the logistics of moving bags and belongings to the finishing point.

Water stations were crucial to all runners. They were provided almost every 2.5 km along the route. At the finish line there was a first-aid post manned by paramedics. An ambulance with paramedics from the city's emergency center was deployed there. It was placed at a strategic point next to the evacuation route. Stretchers, AEDs, and resuscitation equipment were available. Observation showed that those who finally reached the finish line seldom needed the help of the paramedics. Five hours were allowed for the final runner to cross the finish line.

31st Lake Kawaguchi Marathon, Japan

A meeting with Professor Hidedaru Tanada, of the Department of Emergency Medical System Trauma, Burn and Critical Care Medicine, Kokushikan University, was arranged the day before the marathon to clarify and provide first-hand understanding of the medical and first-aid support that would be available. The department had been involved in the event for four years and their team was funded by the university.

The medical team consisted of sixty members—all volunteers from the university—and included five doctors. The rest were nurses, paramedics, and students. There were sixteen mobile AEDs carried on bicycles and handled by the paramedics. Two ambulances were available on site and were manned by doctors. One was actually driven by Professor Tanada himself. There were five moving first-aid stations that moved along with the runners. About one thousand cases were managed each year in the past. Two local hospitals were informed about the race, and they used mobile phones for communication.

Observations were made during the marathon on 26 November 2006. Runners had to follow the scenic course along the side of the lake twice to complete the full marathon. The starting line was the same as the finish line. The first-aid station at the starting line was not easily accessible from the track, and vice versa, thereby making

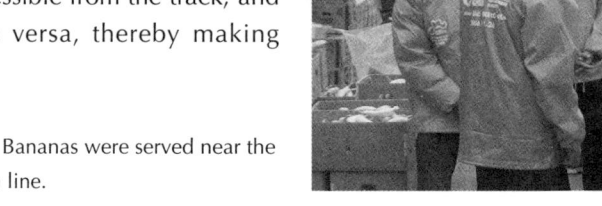

Fig 1 Bananas were served near the finish line.

transfer of cases a problem. Fortunately, crowd control was not a problem. Bystanders were very disciplined and ready to give way. Only one paramedic and four students were stationed at the finish line, and there was no stretcher available there. The students were not readily identified as rescuers, and they did not carry any supplies or equipment.

A special and unique provision was the stalls in an open area (a car park), fifty meters away from the finish line, where hot soup, tea, water, and bananas were served. Another interesting matter was the handling of the runners' personal belongings and tents that they spent the night in. They were scattered on the lawns along the side of the road, and no one seemed concerned about their belongings getting stolen.

25th Macau Galaxy Entertainment International Marathon

A group of six doctors went to Macau in the early morning on Sunday, 3 December 2006 and were greeted by the secretary of the organizing committee. VIP permits were issued to the team so that they could wander around and observe the event.

Members met the director of the sports medicine unit of the sports centre and were shown to the treatment room in the Sports Centre. There were two rooms and a waiting area. Bags with first-aid supplies, dressings, and common medicines were seen in the treatment room. An AED was kept inside a cupboard, though was not carried by the first-aid teams along the race course.

Race-day medical deployment consisted of five doctors, five nurses, forty Red Cross first-aid assistants, paramedics from the fire service, and the staff of the Sports Centre's Sports Medicine Unit. Red

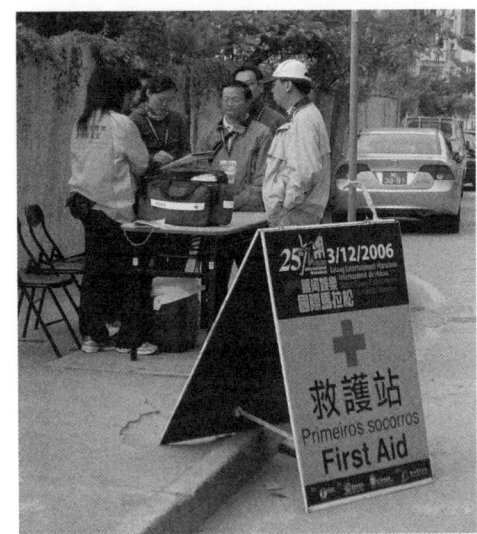

Fig 2 A first-aid post along the course.

Cross and fire service staff were also stationed at the starting and finish line. Ambulances were manned by the Sports Medicine Unit, the fire service, and the Red Cross.

Five first-aid posts were set up. One was inside the Sports Centre near the starting and finish line with four beds and a large open tent with mattresses. A stretcher from the fire service was also available on standby. The other four posts were positioned along the course, entirely uncovered and with a long table and two chairs. Each was manned by a doctor and nurse, equipped with simple first-aid supplies. They did not have an AED or a stretcher. They treated more than fifty minor cases, mostly cramps and minor injuries, during the entire event which lasted a little more than five hours. The ambulance was called when necessary.

There were also five water stations staffed by many volunteer helpers. At the finish line, a towel, water bottle, and bananas were given to all runners in an orderly manner.

SECTION II

Hong Kong Experience:
1997–2009

The Hong Kong Experience: 1997–2009

Dr. WAI Heung On & Dr. CHAN Man Chung

First-Aid Support

After only holding marathons for barely a decade (beginning in 1997), Hong Kong has joined the ranks of other prestigious marathon cities such as New York, London, and Boston. The city provides our local running community and international runners with a friendly atmosphere and a scenic backdrop along two bridges, two tunnels, and the world-famous Victoria Harbour.

The development of the Hong Kong Marathon has been phenomenal. The event was well promoted and successfully conducted the past few years by commercial sponsors. With the full support of the Hong Kong government, the organizers have given the marathon a fun and competetive atmosphere. By 2006, there were almost 40,000 participants from around the world, making the Hong Kong marathon a truly international event: it also formed the final leg of the Greatest Race on Earth (GROE) series, after marathons in Nairobi, Singapore, and Mumbai.

The growth from 1,000 runners in 1997 to more than 50,000 in 2009 was considerably challenging for the organizers, particularly regarding the safety and health of the runners. First aiders, nurses, and doctors from the Auxiliary Medical Service (AMS) are deployed to provide medical care along the course, which is one of the toughest in the world. Runners have to run between skyscrapers and bustling streets along uphill and downhill tracks on the highways.

AMS began its participation in the Hong Kong Marathon in 1998. Since then, it has been associated with the annual international event and has provided first-aid support every year. In the early years, AMS first-aid services were provided mostly at the finish line. Only seasoned and experienced runners participated in the early marathons; hence, there were usually only a handful of injuries. There was a particularly wet, humid, and hot year that affected the event and also required quick evacuation and attention to numerous minor traumas.

With more accumulated experience along with the gradual reinforcement of medical services and recruitment of doctors, AMS decided to establish a committee—the Medical Advisory Board on Major Events (MABOME)—in 2004. This committee's role is to advise AMS's chief staff officer on the medical and logistical needs arising from major events such the marathon and the 2006 Ministers' Conference of the World Trade Organization in 2006. MABOME aims to strengthen the knowledge and skills of AMS members and to upgrade the first-aid equipment and supplies of the supporting team.

Before the marathon, MABOME initiates the preparatory phase. Members discuss pertinent issues regarding equipment, manpower, and training needs for the event. Courses on sports injuries are conducted for members, and preference is given to those who will be on duty for the marathon. An evening is also dedicated to brief all doctors, nurses, and officers taking charge of first-aid and commanding posts. A checklist of personal equipment is issued at this briefing session.

Deployment of duty officers and members is handled by AMS officers in conjunction with other regional and district commanders representing the concerned districts to ensure adequate manpower has been deployed for the event. At the same time, medical staff is actively recruited from various specialties to augment the provision of service.

On the day of the race, every officer and member are in action gear for their specified duties and responsibilities. AMS Headquarters staff, senior officers, and the two marathon medical directors from AMS closely monitor the operations. Data from medical posts are relayed electronically to the control centre next to the finish line in real time. In 2009, a real-time data entry system was used at each first-aid post. These data were collated and compared with previously collected data. Response to problems, such as replenishment of supplies and re-deployment of duty members and ambulances where needed, are made on the spot and based on reports from officers in charge and quarterly statistics collected by the command post at the finish line.

Before and during the marathon, AMS officers and the command post are in close liaison with public hospitals (Hospital Authority) and the ambulance control (Fire Services Department) so that smooth transfer of emergency cases can be carried out. A number of medical and nursing officers on AMS duty during the marathon also work in public hospitals. Hence, communication is generally effective. Marathon organizers and the police are well informed of the medical statistics collected by the AMS command post. In fact, these two groups—the police and the event organizers—are housed under the same marquee to conveniently share these data.

It is always an advantage to learn about how other cities organize marathon races. Representatives have joined the events in Singapore, Beijing, Macau, and Japan's Lake Kawaguchi over the past few years as observers and visiting officials. Discussions with the local organizers added to our understanding of local situations and the preparation needed to support the event. This invaluable knowledge has been very useful to the MABOME.

Within AMS, members learn from each other through sharing of experience. A quarterly meeting has been conducted since 2002 and has been well received by fellow members. Experts are invited to talk on subjects of interest. Emphasis is on the psychological aspect and logistics of the marathon, in addition to the consideration of manpower and data collection.

Scientific and Operational Issues

It is essential to have the right information in order to make the right decisions. A specific form is designed to document information related to medical encounters, including time of admission, runner's number, presented problem, treatment given, and discharge. This information is provided to the command post during the marathon so that contingent decisions can be made, if necessary. After the event, evaluation of the cases is made along with a review of the event's deployment and operations. Suggestions for improvements in equipment, supplies, and manpower planning for the coming year are then proposed and discussed by MABOME.

Statistics are often difficult to evaluate because of the circumstances of the event. The forms may not be appropriately completed, or there may be missing data or wrong information entered by duty members. It is thus difficult to collect good information about injuries. This is further complicated by the term "finishers," i.e., those who crossed the finish line. There are times when injuries are only reported after the event. Runner who reported injuries constitute a biased sample at the emergency department, as a study of only this portion of runners would not have represented those who need medical care after the marathon. In general, doctors or accident and emergency departments see patients several days after the event, with complaints resulting from the long run.

Weather has a significant impact on the marathon, both for runners and for organizers. Everyone has to be prepared for the varying weather of the season (Figures 1 and 2) and the effect on the venue, and contingency measures are of utmost importance during times of unexpected changes. It is essential to keep close track of the weather forecast—particularly the temperature, humidity, rainfall, and pollution—so that emergency measures can be carried out accordingly.

Deployment of medical staff is a special operational issue. Expertise in AMS would enhance the knowledge and experience of duty members, particularly in crowd and disaster management, sports injuries, and prevention of stampedes. In addition, education on psychological support for members is emphasized. Courses on psychological first aid are conducted in preparation for major events.

Logistical support for the marathon involves a supply of medical equipment, electricity and lighting, strategic location of first-aid posts, deployment of staff and duty members, uniforms and special equipment, motorcycle and bicycle first aid, mobile chemical toilets, electrolyte and fluid replacement, and time of stand down.

Current Trends

The racecourse that is currently used in the Hong Kong Marathon was first designated in 2001, when the total number of runners was 10,520 (Table 1). In 2007, the runners totaled well over 40,000 at the starting line on Nathan Road (at Tsimshatsui). This does not include the number of spectators and helpers at the event.

During this time, there have also been increased demands on supporting resources such as transportation facilities, water and food, first-aid equipment, manpower from various bodies such as the police, en-route helpers, bridge and tunnel control, and as well as on deployment of medical support.

Figure 1 Mean temperature in December, January and February in the past 13 years

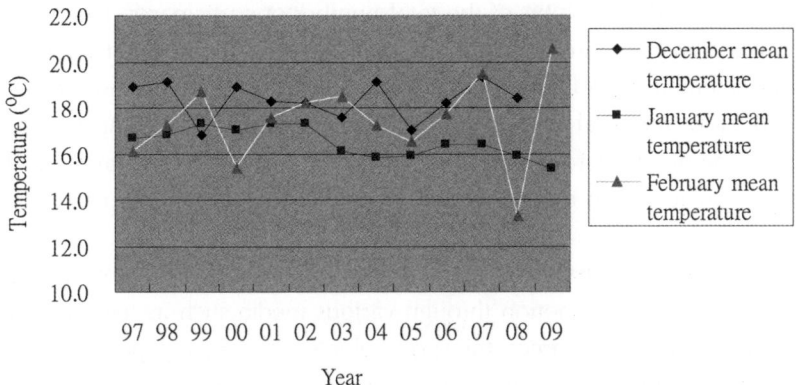

Data from Extract of Meteorological Observations for Hong Kong, Hong Kong Observatory

Figure 2 Mean relative humidity in December, January and February in the past 13 years

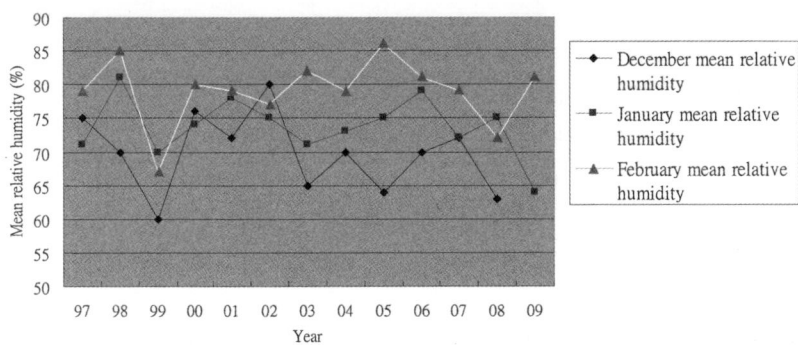

Data from Extract of Meteorological Observations for Hong Kong, Hong Kong Observatory

The increase in runners each year has lead to increased demand of medical assistance for this type of sport event. The number of runners that needed assistance increased yearly from 1,271 in 2002 to 6,249 in 2007, or increase of 9.4% to 14.2% of the total number of participants. The number of runners that required an ambulance transfer to the hospital for further management increased from 8 in 2002 to 35 in 2007, or an increase of 0.05% to 0.07% of the total number of participants (Table 2). During the same period, the number of Auxiliary Medical Service members deployed for this function increased to more than 400 from the original number of less than 200.

The Standard Chartered Hong Kong Marathon has become a social event with lots of promotion through various media such as television and advertisements on the street, transport vehicles, and newspapers. Competitions are also held for poster designs, marathon slogans, and photographs.

Table 1 Number of Participants from 2001 to 2009 (Data provided by the Hong Kong Amateur Athletic Association)

Year	2001	2002	2003	2004	2005	2006	2007	2008	2009
Marathon	1,846	2,345	3,009	3,658	4,983	5,901	6,178	6,237	7,345
Half-marathon	2,734	3,979	4,888	6,982	8,733	10,164	10,714	11,443	13,929
10 km	5,940	7,250	10,489	13,684	17,614	23,752	27,064	32,006	32,908
Total	10,520	13,574	18,386	24,324	31,330	39,817	43,956	49,686	54,272

Table 2 Number of hospital transfers from 2002 to 2009 (Data provided by Auxiliary Medical Service Marathon Working Report)

Year	2002	2003	2004	2005	2006	2007	2008	2009
Number of hospital transfers	— 8	23	13	15	22	35	32	18
Number of medical encounters	1,271	1,766	2,290	2,890	5,094	6,249	6,813	8,170

Moreover, the carnival-like atmosphere at the Marathon Expo further builds up the excitement, which makes this social event the talk of the town. The event starts at dawn when the chief executive of the HKSAR fires the first shot for the tens of thousands of 10 km runners. The carnival atmosphere continues during the 10 km race with fancy clothes, runners carrying small children, and snapshots taken inside the tunnel. The en-route medical support and logistics for the huge crowd are major concerns during the race until the final stand down and resumption of traffic.

The success of this major and significant international event represents the joint efforts of the Hong Kong people and the organizers to enhance its image, but this, in turn, places continuing pressure on the organizers to maintain a high level of quality in future events. Because of this, organizers are forced to make decisions to make the event easier to handle by different parties and the runners. One of the major changes occurred in 2008 when the 10 km route moved to the Eastern Harbour Expressway while the half and full marathon routes continued along the old course. At the same time the finish line was also moved to Victoria Park.

Potential Improvements

Numbers of participants

The number of runners at the starting point has far exceeded the capacity that it can accommodate. Hence, the maximum number of participants will be limited unless there is a change of venue or a change of route so the 10 km race can be conducted separately from the half and full marathon races. The venue for 10km race was later changed in 2008 in view of the above mentioned recommendations. It might even be a good idea to hold that event on a different day. With due consideration by the organizers for available resources, a ceiling on the number of runners was imposed in 2008. There is now potential to have a further increase in the total number of runners.

It is a good idea to have the starting and finish lines situated in a stadium that is large enough to accommodate the expected number of spectators and runners. This also avoids injuries from over-crowding and a stampede at the start. It would also allow more space for the medical team to provide services at the finish, where most of the cases of collapse occur. This will further allow an evacuation route for the ambulances. Moreover, a stadium provides better surroundings for the organizers and runners. The carnival events, or even the 10 km race, can be held inside the stadium while the half and full marathon runners are on the road.

The layout of the route should not aim to build up the number of runners. The image of crowds of runners and spectators only attracts the attention of the media and public. It does not help with the spirit of the event. Furthermore, the running time limit can be lengthened to six or seven hours to ease the tension on the runners and helpers, but this point is arguable because of increased exhaustion during a prolonged event.

Environment

Poor and polluted environmental conditions will adversely affect the performance and health of the runners. Currently, the runners need to run through tunnels, which is undesirable for them if the climate is hot and humid. The ventilation is poor inside the tunnels, and this is only made worse by the huge turnout for the 10 km and half marathon races. Some participants even stop in the tunnel to take pictures, blocking other runners. These conditions have been improved a lot since the shift of the 10 km route to the Eastern Harbour Expressway.

The mean January temperature and relative humidity over the last 13 years were both lower than in February (Figures 1 and 2). We should anticipate mostly hot and humid weather conditions near the end of February and early March, as was the case in 2009 and likely will be in the future, because of global warming.

The 2007 Hong Kong Marathon was held on the 4th of March with the temperature reaching 22.3°C and the relative humidity at 87%.[1] Because of this, we had more cases of collapse due to exhaustion and dehydration that needed to be transferred to the hospital for further management.

a. Timing of the event:

Most other cities, such as Macau, Beijing, or Lake Kawaguchi, hold their marathon races in December or early January when the weather is cooler and less humid.

b. Running inside tunnels:

Many injuries and exhaustion cases occurred inside and right after emerging from the Western Harbour Tunnel. In general, ventilation inside the tunnel must be improved. The number of runners could be spaced out by separating them into more divisions. This would control the number entering the tunnel at once. Since 2008, this problem was alleviated with improvement of ventilation.

c. Redesign of the route:

The goal for runners to have cleaner air during the race can be achieved by shifting the course from city streets to the countryside. This may help avert the issue of air pollution. In addition, the roads from Kwai Chung and Tsuen Wan to Ting Kau have better angles to view the bridges. No one can deny the beautiful scenery along this route.

With the event having been promoted for all these years, the proposed changes are unlikely to create great negative impact on the number of participants, even if the route is re-designed or improved. Certainly, a shift to country roads would not deter genuine runners who are more concerned about safe performance and support. The amateur and fun runners may still be interested to try the new route, and the carnival-like atmosphere will certainly be well maintained by the sponsors. In essence, this great event will continue to attract many sponsors and subscribers.

Most importantly, operational and logistical issues should be the top priority and cater to serious runners, since running the marathon is the main theme of the annual event.

Event promotion

The event has been promoted adequately for the past few years. However, more education and pre-race seminars should be held for participants. It seems that many people are more attracted to or concerned with the social aspects of the marathon, such as taking photographs at certain points, running with dogs, and dressing in less-than-proper sporting gear or fancy clothing during the run. Potential participants should be well informed that this is a sporting event which requires adequate training with appropriate training programs.

Medical fitness

Participants should complete the health assessment form, such as the Physical Activity Readiness Questionnaire (PAR-Q), when they enroll in this event. This will ensure that unfit runners do not place themselves at undue medical risk from the event. The registration form should ask about a history of diabetes, asthma, and coronary artery disease so that specific information with medical advice and safety precautions can be given. A significant past and present medical history, including drugs currently taken, should also be included on the athletes' number bibs.

Monitoring of the event

Water station staff and first-aid helpers should be trained so that they are more alert in spotting runners who appear ill. By doing so, athletes who are unable to finish the race can be identified early and picked up by broom buses. The rule requiring runners to wear number bibs during the race should be strictly observed, and this is even more important due to increased international terrorism. Helicopters hovering over the route can also help to spot adverse events and give prompt support.

To Conclude

Long-distance running, as in the marathon, is a demanding sport that needs physical fitness, endurance, and adequate training to finish. With good support and adequate safety measures from participating organizations, the protection and promotion of good health and in the community can beachieved.

Reference

1. Hong Kong Observatory. 2009. *Extract of Meteorological Observations for Hong Kong, March 2007*. Retireved October 20, 2009, from http://www.weather.gov.hk/wxinfo/pastwx/metob200703.htm

Marathon Media Coverage: Risk or Opportunity?

Professor Anthony FUNG

Media and Publicity Implications

After ten years of marathon coverage in Hong Kong, the dominant image in the mind of the public is related to the spectacle of thousands of people packing Hong Kong's long, winding western highways. This is the media's power to produce a stunning image. However, in addition to this older image, in recent times we have seen a new image: that of increasing casualties, injuries, and even deaths as a result of the marathon. These accidents have gradually begun to supersede the previously festive and celebratory images of the marathon, at least in the eyes of the media. Can the Standard Chartered Marathon maintain its corporate advertisement? Also, what insights can be acquired from examining previous marathon media experiences?

This chapter aims to trace media coverage of the marathon throughout the previous ten years and explicate implications for the general public and society at large. What was the trend? What were the agendas, and were there any changes in orientation in media coverage? If yes, why and how did they occur? What was the impact of marathon media coverage? The significance of this study lies not only in depicting the media image and public perception of the marathon, but also in evaluating the possible consequences of media coverage on Hong Kong society.

A Methodological Note

The illustrations in this chapter are mainly based on a content analysis of the major print media in Hong Kong. The methodology was designed to trace media trends from a historical perspective. Four Hong Kong newspapers were selected for content analysis, namely *Oriental Daily News*, *Apple Daily*, *Ming Pao Daily News*, and *Hong Kong Economic Times*. These papers were selected because they are the most popular and widely-circulated newspapers in Hong Kong. They are representative newspapers from the popular press and intellectual and financial sectors. *The Sun* was not selected, although it is one of the top five newspapers in terms of circulation. This is because *Oriental Daily News* and *The Sun* represent more or less the same kind of newspaper since they belong to the same newspaper group.

Reports from different pages of these newspapers were sampled for analysis. The sample selection relied on a Chinese keyword search— "Chartered Marathon (渣打馬拉松)"—on all coverage between February and April during alternate years. Given the fact that the marathon usually took place in the middle of this period, the selected sample covered all major newspaper reports before and after the event. Because the earliest electronic version of the newspapers was in 1998 (as a limitation), the period analyzed was from 1999 to 2007. Needless to say, in these years, there were other marathons and races which could also be important, but for the purposes of illustration, the "Hong Kong Chartered Marathon" was considered the most important.

Coverage is divided into different categories according to the nature and frequency of the reports. Definitions of the categories are presented in Table 1. It should be noted that, with the keyword search, quite a significant portion of the coverage (25.9%) was found irrelevant to the marathon; such reports were then classified into the "not relevant" category. Other categories reflect the popularity of the marathon, as well as the public and media perception of the marathon.

The Standard Chartered Marathon or The Hong Kong Marathon?

The keyword search for "Chartered Marathon" yielded a comprehensive picture of the public and media concern over the event. In fact, the search not only revealed information about the Hong Kong Standard Chartered event—which is a united front for commercial publicity—but also broadly covered Hong Kong marathons in general, related activities, campaigns, records and figures, anecdotes, public discourse, comments, and the linkage

Table 1 Definition of the categories of coverage in Hong Kong newspapers

Categories	Definition
Details & Preparation	preparation for the marathon, history, related events (e.g., festival), details
Live Reports	day-of-the-race coverage, conditions of the marathon, (e.g., weather), number of people on the spot
Athletes & Competition	coverage featuring individual athletes and their intense competition
Arrangements	arrangements (e.g., transport) made before the marathon
Charity	the charitable nature of the marathon
Sports Promotion	public education and promotion of sports related to the marathon
Health Information	health tips and information
Celebrity	coverage of celebrities (famous stars and officials)
Human Interest	human interest stories (e.g., love affairs, old people) related to the marathon
Sponsorship	coverage featuring the sponsors and sponsorship
Awards	awards given to the champions
Complaints	complaints about the marathon and other environmental factors (e.g., pollution) affecting the marathon
Consumption	marketing products or commercial consumption related to the marathon
Accidents	accidents and casualties
Others	casual coverage of the marathon; comments and other unclassified categories
Not relevant	reports having no direct relevance to the marathon

of marathons to the city. Interestingly enough, although the Hong Kong Standard Chartered Bank is the major sponsor of the event, news reports featuring their sponsorship *per se* were limited (in some years, this report was even absent). In fact, my interpretation is that Hong Kong Standard Chartered Bank's marketing strategy has been very successful: the bank played down its role as primary sponsor and "soft sold" the marathon, which then transformed into a social event for all of Hong Kong.

It is precisely through this transformation that the analysis of marathon coverage and studies in other chapters becomes more meaningful. If the marathon were merely an isolated commercial event, the media portrayal would have only reflected the considerable publicity and resources that the commercial corporation devoted to promotion. In fact, development of the marathon was not just a series of public relations events organized and tightly controlled by the Hong Kong Standard Chartered Bank. Nor was the corporation immune to public criticism and media pressure. By interacting with each other, both the organizers and the media play an important role in steering the direction of marathon coverage.

Increasing Popularity

The coverage of the Standard Chartered Marathon is summarized in Table 2. The figures show that the total coverage was increasing each year. There was a steady upward trend in coverage of the Hong Kong Standard Chartered Marathon from 14 occurrences in 1999 to 83 in 2007. This increase suggests that the media and the public were concerned with and had a growing awareness of the event both directly and indirectly. Among all the categories, the largest deals with the details and preparations prior to marathon day (15 reports in 2007). This means that the marathon is not just a single-day event. It successfully aroused public interest for at least a few months. The general increase in coverage might be due to the fact that the marathon evolved into an event for which news organizations would provide regular coverage by developing a bureaucratic routine with designated manpower. Coverage ten years ago was more ad hoc and not well-planned, and no reports were "bureaucratically organized." (Fishman, 1980: 81)

As for live reports, coverage was initially limited but has also demonstrated a rising trend. In the four newspapers analyzed, the marathon was publicized much more after 2003. Before then, not all newspapers covered the event directly, although other aspects of the marathon might have been mentioned. Live reports emphasized the athletes and competition among the most well-known athletes. Competition, as the marathon gets more and more attention, seems to grow from year to year. As illustrated in Table 2, coverage of the athletes has consistently been high, when compared to many other kinds of reports. Opposition, competition, and even conflict help spur the newsworthiness of the coverage which feeds the main Hong Kong news and sports news pages.

Table 2   Coverage of the Standard Chartered Marathon, 1999–2007 (Feb–Apr) in four selected newspapers (in number of piece of news)

Categories	1999	2001	2003	2005	2007
Details & Preparation	2	0	5	4	15
Live Reports	1	2	3	7	4
Athletes & Competition	5	8	14	11	12
Arrangement	1	5	3	3	1
Charity	2	0	1	3	1
Sport Promotion	0	0	0	4	1
Health Information	0	1	1	3	13
Celebrity	0	1	5	5	5
Human interest	0	0	5	2	6
Sponsorship	2	0	1	0	1
Awards	0	0	0	3	0
Complaints	0	0	0	0	11
Consumption	0	0	0	0	4
Accidents	0	0	0	0	7
Others	1	0	1	3	2
Not relevant	2	5	15	16	14
Total*	14	17	39	48	83

*Note: The total is calculated by adding up occurrences in all categories except "Not relevant"

Changing Concerns

Though the content analysis of the media might not entirely reveal the mentality of the editors and reporters, we can roughly observe their changing agendas and concerns over the past ten years. Besides the routine coverage of marathon events and related activities, public interest was aroused by the involvement of celebrities, including government officials (e.g., the Chief Executive), artists (e.g., artist and former athlete Alex Fong), and famous corporate leaders (e.g., personnel from the Standard

Chartered Bank). Since 2005, there were at least five reports per year covering celebrities' participation in, contributions to, and comments about the marathon. Their involvement attracted public attention and, by extension, promoted participation in the marathon by ordinary people.

"Human interest" stories, with a humanistic, soft, or emotional theme, also became more popular (six stories were printed in 2007). Stories ranged from runners' love stories, the persistence of the elderly in joining the marathon, and the stamina of runners in tackling the training. These reports also indirectly attracted public involvement in the event. As a journalistic practice to cover the marathon for a period of time—before and after—it is necessity for reporters to locate interesting anecdotes and keep the coverage going. The media's quest for stories, particularly ground-breaking ones, explains why, when an "abnormality" in the event occurs, it is amplified for the sake of coverage requirements.

Increased Risks

A banal race every year is not attractive for spectators. Nor is it conducive to sales of newspapers. In contrast, negativity and unexpectedness are of high news value. (Hartley, 1982: 77–79) Thus, when a runner died during the 2006 marathon, the media remembered and looked for death tolls every year thereafter. The media put the blame on organizers and authorities who were not prepared for this outcome. In 2007, among the 11 live reports, four were about the race and seven were about accidents and injuries.

The sudden negative media treatment of the marathon evolved into a crisis for organizers. The public was led to be dubious about the marathon, and an uncontrolled situation could also ruin the overall reputation of the organizers and sponsors. Once a fatality was involved, a previously healthy sporting event suddenly became a public risk, and appropriate measures were needed for organizers to respond to the situation.

It should be noted that the number of complaints has also increased in tandem with the accidents. In 2007, there were 11 reports covering participants' and analysts' complaints about poor arrangements, such as the inadequacy of medical staff to tackle emergencies (which might increase causalities), the unmanageable number of runners (which might include those who are not healthy enough to join the marathon), and the air pollution (which might also increase the risk for runners who rarely exercise). Despite this, I would like to argue that negative news, public criticism, and media challenges in terms of both the perceived risks as well as the various technical problems could eventually be conducive to the development of Hong Kong's marathon and related sports.

More Risks, More Opportunities

It is true that there is ever-increasing negative coverage of the Hong Kong Standard Chartered Marathon, but the growing concern also reflects the fact that the marathon has become a public ritual in Hong Kong. It has become naturalized and normalized as a city event, rather than just a charity event funded by a commercial organization. The ritual is a media event which draws attention to all the people in the city. Through the media, this event has crystallized into a vivid part of history for the Hong Kong people. (Dayan and Katz, 2006) This collective ritual has become more and more important, as evidenced by the increasing concern and wider event coverage from 1999 to 2007. Precisely because the public event has become a part of daily life, it has also drawn public concern and inevitably brings negative coverage as an indirect consequence.

The results of the content analysis have shown that, besides negative coverage such as on air pollution, the lack of athletes' health consciousness, and poor arrangements, there has also been a sudden increase in the amount of health information available in the media. In 1999 and 2001, no coverage focused on health tips and important information for preparing for the race. In 2003, a critical period during which SARS (Severe Acute Respiratory Syndrome) occurred, health discourse started to become prevalent, and it became one of Hong Kong's most prevalent social and media discourses. Since then, coverage of health information has increased and among the four major newspapers in 2007, there were 13 reports primarily featuring marathon-related health information. Reporting on health information is recognized as a palliative measure for stopping further injuries and fatalities.

In a nutshell, the various media events, including marathons and related events, have exposed common health problems and underscored the high health risks faced by most Hong Kong people. However, that higher risk means a greater opportunity for the Hong Kong people. SARS aroused our health consciousness, and the marathons became a means to increase our health awareness in a more subtle and long-term manner.

The perceived risks, in fact, have alerted all affiliated medical and athletic organizations to shoulder greater responsibility and heighten measures over possible casualties during the races. These organizations' efforts, their prescription for the public and the runners, and their further coordination, either among themselves or with the government, are seen as methods to reduce risk.

Conclusion: A Discourse on Health Consciousness

After public panic about bird flu, influenza, and the traumatic experience of SARS, the Hong Kong media in general have developed a discourse on health consciousness. This, to a certain extent, has become an overarching theme in its event coverage and thus is clearly the case in coverage of the Standard Chartered Marathon. In the coverage, it is true that casualties and fatalities are highlighted, but in between these sensational and sometimes horrifying headlines is information about Hong Kong's public health. When a public event such as the marathon becomes a media event, it inevitably draws negative coverage. The latter is not the only by-product, though. The high dosage of health information accompanied by public concern has also produced a public discourse of health awareness in Hong Kong.

While complaints, accidents, and casualties can be considered unfavorable to organizers, sponsors, and the marathon, health information and public education could generate a new image for all parties concerned. The marathon has become an occasion to remind people of their health conditions, and the organizing parties and sponsors have, to some extent, become advocates and forerunners of this movement forward health consciousness. This sort of informal campaign toward health consciousness can be more efficient than any of the formal top-down official health campaigns in increasing public health awareness.

As the famous journalism scholar Herbert Gans (1980: 46) indicated, "responsible capitalism" is one of the enduring values of the local journalism. When corporations deviate from this public norm, they jeopardize their public image, resulting in strong media attacks. By contrast, if they appear to be responsible and enthusiastic in promoting public good, they receive applause from the public. In the long term, if managed carefully as a health campaign, the marathon can build an image of responsible corporation. It is conducive to their reputation as well as that of Hong Kong as an international city.

References

1. Dayan, Daniel, Eilhu Katz. 2006. *Media Events: The Live Broadcasting of History*. Boston, MA: Harvard University Press.
2. Fishman, Mark. 1980. *Manufacturing the News*. Austin, TX: University of Texas Press.
3. Gans, Herbert. 1980. *Deciding what's news: A study of CBS evening news, NBC nightly news, Newsweek, and Time*. New York: Vintage.
4. Hartley, John. 1982. *Understanding News*. London: Routledge.

Marathon Running in Hong Kong
—A Runner's Perspective

Professor Simon YEUNG

Introduction

Of all the Olympic events, the marathon is bestowed with a rich historical heritage that dates back to ancient Greece. The idea of the marathon was inspired by the legend of Phidippides, who died of exhaustion in 490 BC when he carried news of the Greek victory over the Persians in the Battle of Marathon.

Since the marathon's debut in the modern Olympics in 1896, marathon running has remained mainly at a very competitive level. The number of runners grew fairly slowly within the Olympic arena until Frank Shorter's victory in the 1972 Munich Olympics. This captured the hearts of Americans and, thus, the profile of marathon running increased tremendously in the United States. It should be noted that the current marathon distance (26 miles 385 yards, or 42.195 km) was set for the 1908 London Olympics because the course started at Windsor Castle and organizers had to ensure that the Royal Family could watch the finish directly in front of the royal box. This distance was adopted in 1992 as the official marathon distance by the International Amateur Athletic Federations (IAAF).

The popularity of marathons increased when the running route changed from remote to urban areas at the New York marathon in 1976. This route essentially covered a major urban area and attracted a lot of public attention. This was then followed by the Berlin and London marathons in 1980 and 1981 respectively. These events brought the marathon to the attention of the public and attracted massive commercial sponsorships for the promotion of their brands and products. Since then, no major world city has been without its own marathon, and many of these cities make good use of this running event to promote and boost their tourist industries. Today, marathons have become tightly embedded in the distance-running calendar worldwide. There were 285 marathon events organized in 2007. (Marathon guide, 2007) Among these, 24 were in Asia. As of today, the New York marathon still enjoys the largest number of finishers with a record high of 37,866 in 2006. (Association of International Marathon and Distance Races, 2006)

The Hong Kong Marathon

The history of the Hong Kong marathon shares much of the same pattern of development and proliferation of other marathons worldwide. The first international marathon in Hong Kong was held in 1969 to celebrate the opening of Yuen Long Stadium. At that time, only a small number of runners participated in the marathon. The event quieted down in Hong Kong until the late 1970s when the Hong Kong Distance Runners Club (HKDRC) organized its annual marathon. The route at that time looped around Shek Kong and finished at the Shek Kong Army Camp Site. In 1981, the Athletic Veterans of Hong Kong (AVOHK) organized its annual China Coast Marathon, which has a very tough course along the High Island Reservoir of Sai Kung. It was not until the Hong Kong Standard Chartered Bank established its sponsorship for the Hong Kong marathon that the route shifted to a more urban region and stole the limelight of public attention. The event began in 1997 with a group of 1,076 runners crossing the border into Mainland China as part of the hand-over celebrations in Hong Kong. Since then, the participation rate has grown phenomenally from 1,076 runners in 1997 to 43,956 in 2007. Seventy-five thousand runners participated in the full marathon event in 2007, and the Hong Kong marathon is the single largest mass participation sporting event in Hong Kong. With ten years' proliferation of the marathon in our local community, it is indeed timely for us to review the growth of the marathon, both in terms of its depth (our local runners' performance) and width (the marathon as a community sport).

The Flight for International Arena and Elite Status

Before the boom of marathon running in Hong Kong, our runners' performance had already enjoyed a very strong competitive edge in the Asian region. For instance, Yuko Gordon and Winnie Ng represented Hong Kong in the 1984 Los Angeles Olympics. Their personal best times of 2 hr 38 min and 2 hr 42 min were very respectable times in the 1980s. Yuko was the only runner from Hong Kong to represent Asia in the IAAF World Cup in athletics. Her achievement could only be matched by Maggie Chan Man Yee, who represented Hong Kong in the 2000 Sydney Olympics and set a Hong Kong record of 2 hr 35 min 49 sec at the Salt Lake City Marathon, 2004. However, unlike Yuko and Winnie, Maggie's training and competition is essentially based in the United States.

While our male runners did not perform as well as our female runners, our runners were generally very strong in the early to late 1980s. During this time, we had more than five local runners who completed a marathon faster than 2 hr 30 min. These included Ng Fai-yeung (2 hr 24 min 51 sec), Chik Ho-sing (2 hr 25 min 57 sec), Lee Kar-lun (2 hr 27 min 03 sec), Lam Weng-hei (2 hr 28 min 22 sec) and Chung Yan-kwei (2 hr 29 min 07 sec), etc. Furthermore, we had a good base of runners who could complete the marathon faster than 2 hr 35 min. However, we saw a drop in runners' performance since the mid 1990s (Tables 1 and 2). This obviously departs from the continuous improvement of marathon runners' performance in a global perspective. One is left to wonder about the possible causes of this decrease in our runners' performance, despite an increase in the number of marathon runners over the last decade.

I believe that there are two principal reasons that have contributed to our runners' relatively weak performance during the last decade. First, in the 1980s, our distance-running community had a strong base of expatriates that trained and competed in Hong Kong. This provided a competitive training atmosphere for local runners. Just to name a few, we had Adrian Trowell, Ted Turner, Paul Spowage, Keith Crawley, Tim Soutar, Steve Wright, Jean Fasnacht, and John Arnold. The best recorded marathon at that time was made by Ted Turner, a British army officer based in Hong Kong. He achieved a personal best of 2 hr 17 min 27 sec in the 1983 Hong Kong marathon, organized by the HKDRC, at the Hong Kong Sports Institute. The second reason is possibly due to the change in Hong Kong's climate, which has somewhat deterred our runners from training. The general belief is that running performance worsens when the temperature increases. Montain et al. (2007) showed that marathon performance times progressively decrease as weather warms above 5–10°C. Warm and humid weather not only affects performance at the competition, but more importantly, it affects performance during preparation for the marathon.

A typical marathon training regime includes mileage, long runs, speed work, and tapering. Very often, building up mileage is the beginning of one's training, and it is well acknowledged that it normally takes at least six to nine months to properly prepare for a marathon. If we consider that the Hong Kong marathon is scheduled in February, and that many international competitions also take place at a similar time of the year, then our runners need to begin building up their mileage between June and September. This, however, is exactly the hottest season in Hong Kong. As a matter of fact, the weather trend in Hong Kong over the last ten decades has been increasingly warmer. Figure 1 shows a monthly weather comparison between 1960–1990s and 1997–2006. To circumvent this problem and allow our elite distance runners to train properly, their training should be based in cooler regions and at higher altitudes to benefit from lower oxygen concentrations. In this regard, the Hong Kong Amateur Athletic Association should direct the effort to properly groom and train our talented runners so that they can once again shine in the international arena.

Marathon as a Community Sport

Participation in sports and physical activities is increasingly popular in Hong Kong. A telephone survey of 2,652 respondents, conducted by the Social Sciences Research Centre of the University of Hong Kong (Hong Kong Sports Development Board [HKSDB], 1999), indicated that 54% of the Hong Kong adult population participated in at least one sports activity during 1998. This was comparatively higher than 1996 statistics which resulted in only 40% (HKSDB, 1996). Of the top five major sports activities, running (or jogging) is one of the most frequently practiced sports. The number of people who participate in sports has increased tremendously during the last decade. A recent public opinion survey on physical exercise participation in Hong Kong revealed that 80% of Hong Kong people performed physical exercise during the previous three months in 2006. (The government of the Hong Kong Special Administrative Region, 2006) This high participation rate is reflected in the record number of 43,956 runners who took part in the 2007 Standard Chartered Marathon. This trend of increased participation in running as a form of physical activity is a global phenomenon.

Despite the health benefits associated with running, concerns have been raised about injuries associated with running. In a study of the 5,500 participants at the Tsing Ma Bridge International 10 km/marathon run in 1997 (Yeung et al., 1998), the incidence of injured runners seeking physiotherapy because of musculoskeletal complaints was comparable to overseas running competitions. (Crouse and Beattie, 1996; Kretsch et al., 1984) While most of the overuse injuries are minor and might not cause runners to decrease their training levels, repeated and chronic injuries might force runners to give up running permanently. (Koplan et al., 1995) This cannot be taken lightly as this might ultimately negatively affect their interest in the continuation of all sports activities.

In addition to musculoskeletal injuries resulting from overtraining, inadequate or poor training may also have a negative effect. The nature of a marathon run demands an adherence to a persistent and intense load-training program. Under-training will result in an inability to finish the marathon or in injuries sustained during the competition. Indeed, in our study conducted at the Standard Chartered New Airport International Marathon, the findings indicated that the marathon non-finishers were inadequately prepared with an average training distance of only 8.57 km/week (Yeung et al., 2001). The results also reflected that these runners had a poor understanding of proper preparation for a marathon. If time limits had not been set and enforced during this event, this group of runners might have continued to run past their limits to the extent that injuries might have resulted.

The findings of these two studies must be considered in light of the fact that injuries and health problems associated with long-distance running are not uncommon, and few of these may be serious. In order to promote running as a form of physical exercise and to achieve the beneficial health effects while remaining free from injuries, health professionals should seriously emphasize pre-race preparations and the formulation of strategies. This is even more important with the increasing number of novice runners in these competitions. Indeed, the casualty in the 2006 Standard Chartered Marathon has drawn public attention to the issue of safety in marathon running.

The medical and health-care professionals who are committed to provide support to marathon runners should seriously consider possible problems that a marathon runner might sustain during the course of their training and competition, and they should decide what appropriate assistance and advice can be given. For instance, what is the best mode of training progression to successfully complete a marathon? Is the 10% rule of progression an effective mode? Will guided-training programs, education, and practice in injury prevention regimens prevent running injuries and ensure completion of a marathon? What is considered to be proper fluid replacement (Hew-Butler et al., 2006) and how does one prevent hyponatraemia in marathon running? (Chorley, 2007) Advances in the medicine and science of marathon running have been phenomenal, but there is much we have to learn in order to better serve this unique group of athletes.

Table 1 Performance of Hong Kong Male Marathon Runners from 1986–2006

Year	Best time	Name	2nd ranking	Name	3rd ranking	Name
2006	02:33:06	Andrew Naylor	02:33:27	Lai Hok-yan	02:35:44	Ng Kam-tai
2005	02:33:57	Mark William	02:37:24	Andrew Naylor	02:37:26	Lai Hok-yan
2004	02:31:02	Mark William	02:35:42	Lai Hok-yan	02:39:49	Chung Yan-kwei
2003	02:36:45	Ng Hok-ming	02:36:50	Chu Wai-tim	02:37:01	Wu Ki-kai
2002	02:31:54	Kjeld Dissing	02:36:45	Michael Capper	02:37:22	Mo Wai-shing
2001	02:33:40	Mo Wai-shing	02:34:55	Chik Ho-sing	02:36:40	Ho Hoi-to
2000	02:34:21	Kjeld Dissing	02:37:23	Ho Hoi-to	02:39:33	Mo Wai-shing
1999	02:36:34	Chik Ho-sing	02:38:15	Mo Wai-shing	02:39:04	Lee Kar-lun
1998	02:33:55	Chung Yan-kwei	02:34:42	Chik Ho-sing	02:34:59	Lee Kar-lun
1997	02:34:20	Lee Kar-lun	02:34:41	Chik Ho-sing	02:42:12	Ho Kam-fuk
1996	02:27:26	Robereto De Vido	02:34:43	Lee Kar-lun	02:36:08	Fung Wang-tak
1995	02:31:50	Robereto De Vido	02:35:32	Lee Kar-lun	02:38:21	Fung Tze-man
1994	02:25:04	Ng Fai-yeung	02:27:25	Lee Kar-lun	02:28:22	Lam Weng-hei
1993	02:29:19	Lee Kar-lun	02:33:43	Ng Fai-yeung	02:34:19	Cheung Man-ho
1992	02:24:51	Ng Fai-yeung	02:25:57	Chik Ho-sing	02:31:35	Cheung Man-ho
1991	02:27:12	Chik Ho-sing	02:29:26	Ng Fai-yeung	02:29:49	Lee Kar-lun
1990	02:26:53	Ng Fai-yeung	02:27:03	Lee Kar-lun	02:33:28	Wong Chi-sum
1989	02:27:17	Lee Kar-lun	02:27:25	Ng Fai-yeung	02:29:07	Chung Yan-kwei
1988	02:30:24	Lee Kar-lun	02:30:30	Tim Soutar	02:31:37	Chik Ho-sing
1987	02:27:36	Tim Soutar	02:28:39	Chik Ho-sing	02:28:42	Steve Wright
1986	02:25:35	Keith Cawley	02:25:42	Paul Spowage	02:26:12	Tim Soutar

Table 2 Performance of Hong Kong Female Marathon Runners from 1987–2006

Year	Best time	Name	2nd ranking	Name	3rd ranking	Name
2006	02:57:19	Fan Siu-ping	02:58:35	Lai Ka-wai	03:00:34	Leong Yuen-fan
2005	02:57:01	Lai Ka-wai	03:06:53	Lai Yuk-kei	03:07:22	Wong Siu-ping
2004	02:35:49	Chan Man-yee	02:48:43	Christine Double	02:55:07	Lai Ka-wai
2003	02:47:40	Christine Double	02:55:10	Lai Ka-wai	02:58:31	Castka Gillian
2002	02:37:52	Chan Man-yee	02:50:30	Lai Ka-wai	03:08:10	Ng Lai-chu
2001	02:51:48	Christine Double	02:53:43	Lai Ka-wai	02:58:59	Ng Lai-chu
2000	02:53:47	Christine Double	03:00:22	Ng Lai-chu	03:00:23	Lai Ka-wai
1999	02:55:46	Ng Lai-chu	02:59:10	Castka Gillian	03:05:17	Lai Ka-wai
1998	02:54:05	Ng Lai-chu	02:57:23	Lo Man-yi	03:06:04	Altegeld Heidi
1997	02:49:30	Lo Man-yi	02:54:56	Ng Lai-chu	03:41:08	So Suk-fun
1996	02:49:01	Lo Man-yi				
1995	02:55:25	Yuko Gordon	02:56:07	Ng Lai-chu	03:15:42	Cho Yee-wah
1994						
1993						
1992						
1991	02:51:24	Castka Gillian	02:52:54	Lo Man-yi	02:59:00	Wong Fung-fun
1990	02:50:09	Lo Man-yi	02:51:02	Ng Lai-chu	02:58:47	Wong Fung-fun
1989	02:45:36	Ng Lai-chu	03:06:05	Rita Wong	03:07:11	Lau Shuk-yi
1988	02:51:37	Yuko Gordon	03:02:00	Veronica Thresh	03:12:28	Ko Fung-ling
1987	02:38:32	Yuko Gordon	02:52:41	Wong Fung-fun	02:56:03	Alison Robinson

Figure 1 Annual Temperature Pattern between 1960–1990s vs. 1997–2006

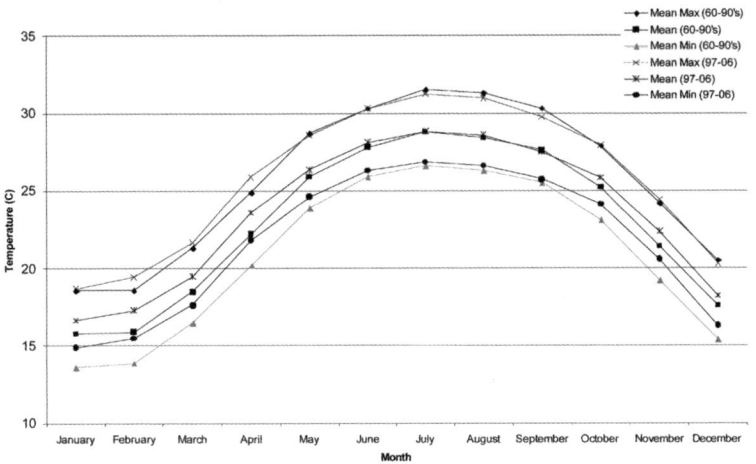

References

1. *The website of the Association of International Marathon and Distance Races.* Retrieved October 20, 2009, from http://www.aims-association.org/

2. Chorley JN. 2007. Hyponatraemia: Identification and evaluation in the marathon medical area. *Sports Med* 37:451–54.

3. Crouse B, Beattie K. 1996. Marathon medical services: strategies to reduce runner morbidity. Med Sci Sports Exerc 28 (9): 1093–96.

4. The government of the Hong Kong Special Administrative Region. *Public opinion survey on physical exercise participation in Hong Kong, 2006.* Retrieved October 20, 2009, from http://www.lcsd.gov.hk/lschemes/cscommittee/form/paper_csc_0806_20061122_annex_e.pdf.

5. Hew-Butler T, Verbalis JG, Noakes TD. 2006. Updated fluid recommendation: position statement from the International Marathon Medical Directors Association (IMMDA). *Clin J Sport Med* 16 (4): 283–92.

6. Hong Kong Sports Development Board. 1999. *Sports participation survey, 1998.* Rerieved October 20, 2009, from http://www.hksi.org.hk/hksdb/html/pdf/research/Report25e.pdf.

7. Hong Kong Sports Development Board. 1996. *Participation in sport—the case of Hong Kong, 1996.* Retrieved October 20, 2009, from http://www.hksi.org.hk/hksdb/html/pdf/research/rl1e.jpg.

8. Koplan JP, Rothenberg RB, Jones EL. 1995. The natural history of exercise: A 10-yr follow up of a cohort of runners. *Med Sci Sports Exerc* 27 (8): 1180–84.

9. Kretsch A, Grogan R, Duras P, Allen F, Sumner J, Gillam I. 1984. 1980 Melbourne marathon study. *Med J Aust* 141 (12–13): 809–14.

10. Marathon Guide. *Marathon directory in 2007.* Retireved October 20, 2009, from http://www.marathonguide.com.

11. Montain SJ, Matthew RE, Cheuvront SN. 2007. Marathon performance in thermally stressing conditions. Sports Med 37 (4–5): 320–23.

12. Yeung SS, Yeung EW, Wong TW. 1998. Provision of physiotherapy at the Tsing Ma Bridge international marathon and 10 km race in Hong Kong. *Br J Sports Med* 32 (4): 336–7.

13. Yeung SS, Yeung EW, Wong TW. 2001. Marathon finishers and non-finishers characteristics: a preamble to success. *J Sports Med Phys Fitness* 41 (2): 170–76.

Elite Female Runners in Hong Kong

Dr. Carina Ll

Most people think that it is not easy to start running in Hong Kong, especially as a female. This is needless to say about long-distance running like marathons; running alone in the streets or country parks can be quite scary for most women when they are young. Women's participation and recognition in sports worldwide have grown dramatically over the past thirty years, and this trend is expected to continue. The situation in Hong Kong is similar. We have more female runners than ever before, and their performance is improving with new records.

A Survey of Elite Female Runners in Hong Kong, 2007

In Hong Kong, there is scant information on running, exercise science, diet, training, and psychology related to females who participate in long-distance running events. Interviewing several elite female runners in Hong Kong has provided us with more ideas about the impact of running on different aspects of their lives. Alternatively, we can look into how our elite female athletes train themselves while also maintaining a busy working life.

This survey was conducted of Hong Kong's elite female runners and sought to gain and compare information related to demographics; athletic and running histories; diet and training; history of injury and health information; and cultural, social, and motivational perspectives.[1] It was conducted after the 2007 Hong Kong racing season. A questionnaire was sent to ten elite female long-distance runners who were ranked, according to the Hong Kong Amateur Athletic Association (HKAAA), among the top ten in different race categories during 2006 and 2007. They were interviewed by telephone. Seven runners responded, and the other three were too busy to respond to the questionnaire.

Results

Demographic data

The mean age was 36.9 years, and the mean height was 161.7 cm. The mean body weight (BW) was 48 kg with a mean body mass index (BMI) of 19.5 kg/cm². (Table 1) All of the runners had a stable body weight over the year (+/– 1.1 kg). Only two runners were not satisfied with their current body weight and wanted to be lighter, although, in both cases, their BMI was less than 22.

Table 1 Demographic Data of Respondents

	Mean	Median	Range
Age	37	35	26–50
Height (cm)	162	161	155–175
BW (kg)	50	48	45–60
Body Mass Index (BMI) (kg/cm²)	19.5	19.5	18.2–21.8

Occupations and social factors

All of the respondents were working full time, and their working hours averaged 47.4 per week. Two were self-employed. They were as busy as most Hong Kong people, yet they could also achieve high mileage during training. As noted in the overseas survey,[1] most of the runners were highly educated, with 71.4% holding university degrees. Only two out of the seven runners were married with children, and this is comparable to another survey[1] in which there were 38.3% married ultramarathon runners. Most of them (57.1%) lived with their families.

Athletic history

All of the respondents had good performance in past races. Some had a short history of marathon running, but they were nevertheless able to attain very good results and personal best times (PB) within one to two years. The median time it took to run a 10 km, half marathon, and full marathon were 4, 7, and 6 years respectively, with a total range of 0–29 years.

The median times for both a first attempt at and a personal best (PB) in a 10 km race was 0:44:30 and 0:39:39, while the overall fastest time was 0:34:17. The median times for both a first and personal best half marathon were 1:50:00 and 1:29:00 respectively, while the overall fastest time was 1:24:28. Lastly, the median times for a first and personal best marathon were 4:11:00 and 3:01:00 respectively, and the best performance time was 2:32:53.

Table 2 Athletic Racing History of Respondents

	Mean	Median	Minimum	Maximum
First 10 km time (hr:min:sec)	0:49:43	0:44:30	0:35:21	1:15:00
Number of years since first 10 km	8	4	0	25
First half marathon time (hr:min:sec)	1:52:22	1:50:00	1:32:00	2:24:00
Number of years since first half marathon	9	7	2	28
First marathon time (hrs:min:sec)	4:09:51	4:11:00	3:36:00	4:49:00
Number of years since first marathon	8	6	1	29
Personal best (PB) 5 km time (hrs:min:sec)	0:18:44	0:18:59	0:16:40	0:20:13
PB 10 km time (hrs:min:sec)	0:39:08	0:39:39	0:34:17	0:42:59
PB 15 km time (hrs:min:sec)	1:04:28	1:03:30	1:01:57	1:08:58
PB half marathon time (hrs:min:sec)	1:30:32	1:29:00	1:24:28	1:39:59
PB full marathon time (hrs:min:sec)	3:04:10	3:01:00	2:32:53	3:23:00

The average age that the women start running consistently was 26 and the median age was 28, with a total range of 17–36. The median number of total years running was 7 with a range of 3–28. This finding showed that these elite performers could have started their running career relatively late in life and could last for more than twenty years. With adequate and consistent training, they could achieve good performance within years. The median longest distance for racing events was 100 km, and this was usually the Hong Kong Trailwalker, an annual fundraising event in Hong Kong. Most (71.4%) of the runners were involved in trail running events, such as the King of the Hill series, the Raleigh Challenge–Wilson Trail, and Trailwalker. Most runners got involved in trail running, but this might be a special finding in Hong Kong, due to the special terrain of the region, where enormous slopes and hills are within a short distance from home and working places. Among these elite runners, the median longest practice distance per week was 36 km. Most of the women surveyed also had good experience in overseas marathons with a median of seven total events, including ones in Macau, Korea, China, Thailand, Japan, Rotterdam-Netherlands, Singapore, and the United States. One of them even joined the ultramarathon in the Sahara Desert with a total distance 243 km.

Table 3 Running and Practice History of Elite Female Runners

	Mean	Median	Minimum	Maximum
Age when consistent running began	26	28	17	36
Number of years running	10	7	3	28
Longest racing distance (km)	100.8	100.0	42.2	243.0
Longest practice distance (km)/week	41	36	25	63
Number of overseas marathons	11	7	1	37
Speed work/week	7	8	4	9
Previous year running distance (km)	2964	3000	2000	4000
Previous week running distance (km)	43	40	6	80

Training program

Four of the respondents were Hong Kong athletics team members and had national team experiences. However, only three had ever had personal trainers or coaches and only two had personal trainers or coaches at the time of the survey. One was a personal trainer herself. Only one knew the maximum oxygen consumption and trained accordingly. None recorded their maximum and resting heart rate, or followed other scientific guidance. Only one had special training experience such as high-altitude and heat/cold training.

All of them were members of a training club and did speed work, such as track, fartlek, and tempo runs as a regular part of their training, with a median of eight runs per month (the range was four to nine). Most of them kept a training log, but the logs were not very systematic. In the previous year, they recorded a median of 3,000 km and the median distance in the week before the survey was 40 km (the range was 6 km to 80 km). This low distance per week was because most of them had rested for eight weeks, during which time they jogged about 23 km per week, but they ran a median distance of 85 km per week when "training hard." This practice might be important for recovery from injuries after racing seasons. If a race were coming up in eight weeks, they would try to accomplish a median number of six (the range was two to nine) long runs of over 20 km each. This is comparable to the overseas survey.[1]

The runners were asked about training in groups or alone, and they were asked to describe their "willingness to train with others" during daily, long-distance, and trail runs.

Table 4 Willingness to Train with Others (frequency)

	Daily runs	Long runs	Trail runs*
Never	0%	14.3 %	0%
Seldom	14.3%	28.6 %	0%
Occasionally	42.9%	14.3%	28.6%
Most of the time	42.9%	14.3%	14.3%
All of the time	0%	28.6%	42.9%

* one runner did not run on trails

It appeared that these women were not afraid to run by themselves during long-distance and trail runs, but they preferred to have company for their daily practice.

The percentage of runners who had cross training was 42.9%. Multiple activities conducted at least once a week were reported as follows: resistance training 42.9%; bicycling 14.3%; aerobics 28.6%; walking 14.3%. Surprisingly, swimming was not chosen as an alternative for cross training. This may be due to inconvenient swimming facilities for training in Hong Kong.

Diet

On average, the respondents ate three meals per day. They had no restriction on their diet, but most preferred to have white meats such as chicken and fish while some preferred high-calorie foods like desserts. Only one runner said she restricted her diet to 2,000–2,500 kcal per day, which is higher than recommended for normal, sedentary people.

Most of the respondents did not consistently take supplements. The majority of them (71.5%) took multi-vitamins, and this was comparable to their overseas counterparts. Other supplements included milk products (42.9%); glucosamine, a cartilage supplement (42.9%); vitamin C (28.6%); soybean milk or products (28.6%); and protein supplements and egg whites (28.6%). One of the runners took a commercial sports supplement with calcium, iron, magnesium, and other contents. Two runners took Chinese herbs and one took fish oil daily.

More than 71% of the respondents said they practiced carbohydrate loading before races. One said that she would taper her running practice to match the carbohydrate loading. None starved themselves to lose weight before a race. Generally, they did not understand the scientific basis for carbohydrate loading. One runner did not practice carbohydrate loading for fear of putting on weight.

During a marathon, they drank a median of 200 ml of water per 5 km (the range was 5 ml to 250 ml). Only one runner, who was more experienced, could point out that the amount of water required is determined by the temperature, rate of evaporation, and humidity. Regarding supplements taken during a marathon, all except one took a carbohydrate supplement with commercial energy gel preparations (usually taken at 20 km and 30 km). None of them ate the food or fruit supplied by the organizers during the run.

Four runners had recovery drinks after the race. Three of them used commercial preparations, but they did not know the contents. They knew they were getting electrolyte supplements. Two knew about the importance of protein supplements for muscle recovery.

Overall, the runners were found to have inadequate knowledge about the importance of carbohydrates, electrolytes, and protein supplements before, during, and after running a marathon. More education on the essential dietary aspects of nutrition is of the utmost importance in order to improve sports performance and, at the same time, decrease injuries related to fatigue, mineral deficiency, heat-related diseases, and hypoglycaemia.

Preparation for races

Apart from dietary supplements, nearly 50% of the respondents said they would have a massage to improve sports performance. Two would have acupuncture if they had injuries. Four said they would rest during the week before the marathon, and two would have a massage during this week. One runner raised the importance of sleep and better hydration. Despite the busy schedule of full-time work and training, they managed to sleep an average seven hours per night during the week of the race. One runner stated that she slept less before the race due to anxiety.

Most of the runners took note of the temperature and humidity of the race day, but only two runners appreciated the importance of wind effects in evaporation and heat loss. Although most of them checked the route before the race, only two completed a mock run before the race.

Health and injuries

All of the runners stopped running for two weeks when they had injuries. None of them had joint injections such as steroids. When they had problems in the joints and muscles, they took advantage of many types of health-care practitioners, including massage therapist 57.4%, physical therapist or physiotherapist 42.9%, acupuncturist and bone setter 14.3%, trainer 14.3%,[1] and homeopathist 14.3%. No one went to chiropractors, orthopedic specialists, sports medicine doctors, podiatrists, family doctors, or nutritionists. Reasons for not consulting these practitioners included "not needed" 57.4%, "expensive" 28.6%, and "not known" 14.3%.

The following is a summary of the major types of injuries reported by the runners: hamstring 71.4%, shin splints 57.1%, compartment syndromes 57.1%, knee 57.1%, plantar fasciitis 28.6%, sciatica 28.6%, back 28.6%, stress fractures of the foot 14.3%, iliotibial band 14.3%, hip 14.3%, sprains 14.3%.

Hard training and racing was also found to have effects on the menstruation pattern. The women presented with either early or delayed onset of menses and pain. One runner had a history of amenorrhea for more than a year and required hormonal therapy. Two experienced rectal or urinary bleeding during their running career, two had a history of anemia, and one had hypothyroidism.

We do not have adequate medical support and education for these elite runners in Hong Kong. Some expressed that most family doctors only asked them to rest but were unable to give a diagnosis or advise them on how to return to racing. This survey revealed a general lack of confidence in physicians.

The Female Athlete Triad

The female athlete triad describes the coexistence of three distinct medical conditions that may occur in female athletes. The triad includes eating disorders/disordered eating behavior, amenorrhea/oligomenorrhea, and decreased bone mineral density (osteoporosis and osteopenia).[14] Coupled with inadequate nutrition, the high caloric expenditure of training results in a sustained negative caloric balance and low energy availability. This situation is exquisitely sensed by the hypothalamus, which initiates a complex neuroendocrine adaptive cascade with changes in the hypothalamic-pituitary-ovarian axis. Estrogen levels decrease, resulting in reproductive dysfunction that may include amenorrhea, oligomenorrhea, or anovulation. Low estrogen levels in otherwise healthy young women is associated with decreased bone mineral density and an increased risk of fractures.[23–26]

Once the triad is detected, multidisciplmary treatment should begin to reduce or prevent long-term adverse sequela to the bone and a recurrence of the triad.[16,17] Physicians caring for such athletes need to keep triad symptoms in mind and recognize their potential severity.[13] Elite training among young girls tends to delay pubertal development, resulting in decreased bone mass accumulation and reduced growth potential.[20] In young athletes, peer support and education are the most important factors for successful detection and treatment.

Gender Differences in Sports Performance

Over the past thirty years, participation by women in marathon running has grown dramatically, and, during the same period, women's marathon performances have improved at a remarkable rate. Societal views of and training practices of female distance runners have changed greatly, especially in Hong Kong. The rate of improvement for women has been extraordinary, and it is larger for longer distance events. The male physiology is more suited to anaerobic strength events while, given increased access and participation, women can be expected to be more on a par with men in some long-distance aerobic events. However, certain performance-related biological differences between men and women are quite unlikely to change. A model predicts that men's world records are nearing asymptotic limits. Many of the established men's and women's endurance running world records are nearing their limits.[39] Will women soon outrun men?

There are physiological and morphological gender differences. These differences become evident in the specific responses or magnitude of response to various training regimens. Men and women experience similar relative strength gains and body composition changes when under the same programs of progressive resistance strength training. While the best marathon times of American men have remained fairly constant in recent decades, the best times of American women have decreased dramatically from 2:47:10 in 1976 to 2:21:25 in 2005, a decrease of 15.6% over thirty years.

A study showed that the physiological characteristics of elite American female marathon runners differ from those of elite male marathon runners (e.g., maximum oxygen uptake = 67.1 +/– 4.2 ml/kg/min against 74.1 +/– 2.6 ml/kg/min).[32] There are no gender differences in central or peripheral cardiovascular adaptations to aerobic training.[33] Sparling and Cureton (1983) have shown that differences in similarly trained male and female distance runners are largely due to body fat percentage, and less to cardiorespiratory fitness and running economy.[34] Pate et al. (1985) determined that men and women who are capable of similar performances (i.e., a 15-mile race), do not differ in body composition, cardiorespiratory response, or metabolic response.[35] There appears to be no difference in the relative increases of maximum VO_2 for men and women when they train under the same mode, intensity, frequency, and duration. However, researchers have suggested that there appears to be less muscle hypertrophy with strength improvement in women when compared to men. On the other hand, women generally have a reduced O_2 carrying capacity.

Endurance performances in a performance-matched event have showed that female subjects performed as well as their male counterparts at 42.2 km, while performances for 90 km were significantly better (P < 0.05) within the female group. The average fraction of maximum VO_2 (F) sustained by each subject indicated that the females achieved their performances by working at a higher F (73.4 +/– 5.5% vs. 66.3 +/– 3.7% for 42.2 km and 59.8 +/– 6.2% vs. 50.2 +/– 3.1% for 90 km). The degree of decline in the fraction of maximum VO_2 sustained as the distance of running increased was significantly less among females. The better performances by females at 90 km was not related to greater maximal aerobic capacity, running economy, training level, or fatty acid metabolism.[34]

It was found that in a study of middle and long-distance runners, when compared in running economy, men used less oxygen (ml/km/kg) at common absolute velocities, but VO2 (ml/km/kg) was not different between men and women at equal relative intensities (%VO2max). Hence, at absolute running velocities, men are more economical than women, but when expressed in ml/km/kg, there are no gender differences at similar relative intensities.[37] When men and women of equal economy or maximum VO_2 are matched, the men show a better aerobic profile. Female ultramarathon runners have greater fatigue resistance than do equally trained men, whose performances are superior up to the marathon distance.[34] In all, men possess a larger aerobic capacity and greater muscular strength, hence the gap in running performances between men and women is unlikely to narrow naturally.

Running is healthy for both men and women

Athletic participation and exercise are healthy for the body, if done appropriately. The benefits of participation in sports and exercise vastly outweigh the risks of permanent injury. It has been shown that women who regularly exercise have a significantly reduced risk of developing hypertension, coronary events, death, and nonfatal stroke.[19] Moreover, exercise has been successfully used as a therapeutic adjunct in a variety of psychiatric disorders.

Ladies and gentlemen, it does not matter who is going to be faster! It is never too late to run and become an elite runner. This athletic goal can be achieved after one has finished raising the family and retired. There are many good psychosocial and physical reasons to run. The following practical tips are especially recommended to those women in Hong Kong who are crazy about dieting and getting slim and fit. **—the author**

Practical tips for carbohydrate loading and hydration during long-distance races

- Consume 7–10 g carbohydrates per kg body mass per day
  (e.g., a person weighing 60 kg should have 420–600 g carbohydrate per day)
  Men generally need more than women, since men burn more calories and have more muscle bulk and less fat. Women burn more fat than men while running, so men need at least four grams of carbohydrates per pound (e.g., 8.8 g/ kg) of body weight daily. Women need three (e.g., 6.6 g/ kg).
- Try to have a de-carbohydrated diet (aiming to deplete the glucogen storage in liver and muscles) before loading for a marathon race, by having fat, protein and fiber but no carbohydrates to maximize the effectiveness of carbohydrate loading in the later phase.
- Do not skip meals, but eat frequent meals and drink water and fluids throughout the day. You can drink sweet drinks and honey water, if desired. If sugar is added as sweetener, add 1 teaspoon sugar per 5 g carbohydrates.
- To prepare for the race, taper your training during carbohydrate loading. Remember not to try unfamiliar foods with adequate hydration. Runner should have a light, high carbohydrate meal two to three hours before the race. Runners need to plan and prepare for the race with appropriate dress, socks and shoes, food and drinks (including maintenance food and post race snacks or recovery drinks.) It would be best to pack up and prepare few days before the race. Good preparation is of utmost importance to alleviate pre-race anxiety. Consider having a trial or mock race in order to record the amount of water, drinks, and food required.

1. Record your sweat rate and salt loss.
2. Practice at the same time of day.
3. Take note of the weather, temperature, humidity, and wind effects.
4. Plan energy/carbohydrate replacement intervals.
5. Route technical points such as hilly slope or turns, narrow route, etc. with strategies.
6. Record your pre-run body weight and calculate the rate of hydration as follows:

Total water required/hour =

$$\frac{\text{weight lost in kg + fluid drunk in the mock run in liters}}{\text{duration in hours}}$$

$$\text{Water required/km} = \frac{\text{Total water required/hour}}{\text{Personal record for km/hour}}$$

Proper preparations for the marathon result in a good performance.

References

1. Rebekah Trittipoe. A Survey of female ultrarunners. Ultrarunning magazine 1997. Retrieved October 20, 2009, from http://www.extremeultrarunning.com/survey.

2. McConnell TR. 1988. Practical considerations in the testing of VO2max in runners. *Sports Med* 5 (1): 57–68.

3. Saunders PU, Pyne DB, Telford RD, Hawley JA. 2004. Factors affecting running economy in trained distance runners. *Sports Med* 34 (7): 465–85.

4. Rehrer NJ. 2001. Fluid and electrolyte balance in ultra-endurance sport. *Sports Med* 31 (10): 701–15.

5. Maughan RJ, Leiper JB, Shirreffs SM. 1997. Factors influencing the restoration of fluid and electrolyte balance after exercise in the heat. *Br J Sports Med* 31 (3): 175–82.

6. Maughan RJ, Noakes TD. 1991. Fluid replacement and exercise stress. A brief review of studies on fluid replacement and some guidelines for the athlete. *Sports Med* 12 (1): 16–31.

7. Cheuvront SN, Haymes EM. 2001. Thermoregulation and marathon running: biological and environmental influences. *Sports Med* 31 (10): 743–62.

8. Johnsen HK, Rognmo A, Nilssen KJ, Blix AS. 1985. Seasonal changes in the relative importance of different avenues of heat loss in resting and running

reindeer. *Acta Physiol Scand* 123 (1): 73–9.

9. Fredericson M, Misra AK. 2007. Epidemiology and aetiology of marathon running injuries. *Sports Med* 37 (4–5): 437–9.

10. Brunet ME, Cook SD, Brinker MR, Dickinson JA. 1990. A survey of running injuries in 1505 competitive and recreational runners. *J Sports Med Phys Fitness* 30 (3): 307–15.

11. Roberts WO. 2000. A 12-yr profile of medical injury and illness for the Twin Cities Marathon. *Med Sci Sports Exerc* 32 (9): 1549–55.

12. Joy EA, Campbell D. 2005. Stress fractures in the female athlete. *Curr Sports Med Rep* 4 (6): 323–8.

13. Zeni AI, Street CC, Dempsey RL, Staton M. 2000. Stress injury to the bone among women athletes. *Phys Med Rehabil Clin N Am* 11 (4): 929–47.

14. Constantini NW, Warren MP. 1994. Special problems of the female athlete. *Baillieres Clin Rheumatol* 8 (1): 199–219.

15. Hirschberg AL, Hagenfeldt K. 1998. Athletic amenorrhea and its consequences. Hard physical training at an early age can cause serious bone damage. *Lakartidningen* 95 (50): 5765–70.

16. Broso R, Subrizi R. 1996. Gynecologic problems in female athletes. *Minerva Ginecol* 48 (3): 99–106.

17. Warren MP. 1992. Clinical review 40: Amenorrhea in endurance runners. *J Clin Endocrinol Metab* 75 (6): 1393–97.

18. Williams M. 1984. Oligomenorrhoea and amenorrhoea associated with exercise. A literature review. *Aust Fam Physician* 13 (9): 659–63.

19. Hale RW. 1983. Exercise, sports, and menstrual dysfunction. *Clin Obstet Gynecol* 26 (3): 728–35.

20. Diddle AW. 1983. Athletic activity and menstruation. *South Med J* 76 (5): 619–24.

21. Shangold MM. 1985. Causes, evaluation, and management of athletic oligo-/amenorrhea. *Med Clin North Am* 69 (1): 83–95.

22. Highet R. 1989. Athletic amenorrhoea. An update on aetiology, complications and management. *Sports Med* 7 (2): 82–108.

23. Anderson JM. 1999. The female athlete triad: disordered eating, amenorrhea, and osteoporosis. *Conn Med* 63 (11): 647–52.

24. Papanek PE. 2003. The female athlete triad: an emerging role for physical therapy. *J Orthop Sports Phys Ther* 33 (10): 594–614.

25. Kleposki RW. 2002. The female athlete triad: a terrible trio implications for

primary care. *J Am Acad Nurse Pract* 14 (1): 26–31.

26. Weight LM, Noakes TD. 1987. Is running an analog of anorexia?: A survey of the incidence of eating disorders in female distance runners. *Med Sci Sports Exerc* 19 (3): 213–17.

27. Hulley AJ, Hill AJ. 2001. Eating disorders and health in elite women distance runners. *Int J Eat Disord* 30 (3): 312–17.

28. Prather H, Hunt D. 2005. Issues unique to the female runner. *Phys Med Rehabil Clin N Am* 16 (3): 691–709.

29. Walther M, Kirschner S. 2004. Is running associated with premature degenerative arthritis of the hip? A systematic review. *Z Orthop Ihre Grenzgeb* 142 (2): 213–20.

30. White KM, Lyle RM, et al. 2006. The acute effects of dairy calcium intake on fat metabolism during exercise and endurance exercise performance. *Int J Sport Nutr Exerc Metab* 16 (6): 565–79.

31. Pate RR, O'Neill JR. 2007. American women in the marathon. *Sports Med* 37 (4–5): 294–98.

32. Sparling PB, Nieman DC, O'Connor PJ. 1993. Selected scientific aspects of marathon racing. An update on fluid replacement, immune function, psychological factors and the gender difference. *Sports Med* 15 (2): 116–32.

33. Lewis DA, Kamon E, Hodgson JL. 1986. Physiological differences between genders. Implications for sports conditioning. *Sports Med* 3 (5): 357–69.

34. Sparling PB, Cureton KJ. 1983. Biological determinants of the sex difference in 12-min run performance. Med Sci Sports Exerc 15 (3): 218-23.

35. Pate RR, Barnes C, Miller W. 1985. A physiological comparison of performance-matched female and male distance runners. Res Q Exerc Sport 56: 245-250.

36. Speechly DP, Taylor SR, Rogers GG.. 1996. Differences in ultra-endurance exercise in performance-matched male and female runners. *Med Sci in Sports Exerc* 28 (3): 359–65.

37. Suter E, Marti B, Tschopp A, Wanner HU. 1991. Effects of jogging on mental well-being and seasonal mood variations: a randomized study with healthy women and men. *Schweiz Med Wochenschr* 121 (35): 1254–63.

38. Chatterjee S, Laudato M. 1995. Gender and performance in athletics. *Soc Biol* 42 (1–2): 124–32.

39. Daniels J, Daniels N. 1992. Running economy of elite male and elite female runners. *Med Sci Sports Exerc* 24 (4): 483–89.

40. Bam J, Noakes TD, Juritz J, Dennis SC. 1997. Could women outrun men in

ultramarathon races? *Med Sci Sports Exerc* 29 (2): 244–47.

41. Nevill AM, Whyte G. 2005. Are there limits to running world records? *Med Sci Sports Exerc* 37 (10): 1785–88.

42. Coast JR, Blevins JS, Wilson BA. 2004. Do gender differences in running performance disappear with distance? *Can J Appl Physiol* 29 (2): 139–45.

43. Marti B. 1991. Health effects of recreational running in women: Some epidemiological and preventive aspects. *Sports Med* 11 (1): 20–51.

44. Van Pelt RE, Jones PP, Davy KP, et al. 1997. Regular exercise and the age-related decline in resting metabolic rate in women. *J Clin Endocrinol Metab* 82 (10): 3208–12.

45. Dishman RK. 1985. Medical psychology in exercise and sport. *Med Clin North Am* 69 (1): 123–43.

46. Masters KS.1992. Hypnotic susceptibility, cognitive dissociation, and runner's high in a sample of marathon runners. *Am J Clin Hypn* 34 (3): 193–201.

47. Chan DW, Lai B. 1990. Psychological aspects of long-distance running among Chinese male runners in Hong Kong. *Int J Psychosom* 37 (1–4): 30–34.

48. Jokl P, Sethi PM, Cooper AJ. 2004. Master's performance in the New York City Marathon 1983–1999. *Br J Sports Med* 38 (4): 408–12.

Addendum: Profiles of Elite Female Runners in Hong Kong

Fan Sui Ping 范瑞萍 (Category 30+)

First Marathon: 2001

Personal best time

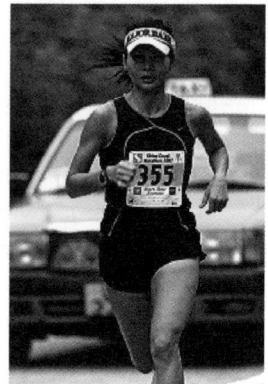

5 km:	00:19:02 (2008)
10 km:	00:39:01 (2009)
Half marathon:	01:24:34 (2008)
Full marathon:	02:49:08 (2008)

Ultra-marathon race: 243 km Sahara Dessert

Trail race: Trailwalker 100km, best time: 14:23:00

The longest running distance for race: 243 km

The longest running distance for practice: 63 km

Experience with overseas marathon race: 25

HK Team Member: Yes

Represent Hong Kong team experience: five

HKSCM 2007 full marathon: Category Senior 2nd position, time 03:03:18, 10 km 00:43:03, 30 km 02:08:56

HKSCM 2009 full marathon: Category Senior Champion, time 02:57:24, 10 km 00:41:03, 30 km 02:04:36

Castka Gillian (Category 45+)

First Marathon: 1978

Personal best time

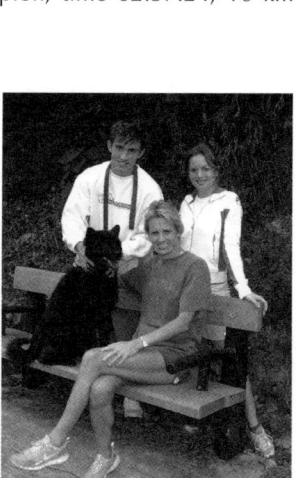

5 km:	00:16:40 (1980)
10 km:	00:34:17 (1987)
Half marathon:	01:13:40 (1984)
Full marathon:	02:32:53 (1984)

Any ultra-marathon race: No

Trail race: Half round the island race 33 km

The longest running distance for race: 42.2 km

The longest running distance for practice: 36 km

Experience with overseas marathon races:

United Kingdom, Japan, North American, Singapore, Bangkok, China, etc. Total 30

HK Team Member: Yes

Represent national team experience: Yes, United Kingdom

HKSCM 2007 Half marathon: Category master two 2nd position, time 01:30:36

HKSCM 2008 Half marathon: Category master two: 2nd position, time 01:30:36

HKSCM 2009 Half marathon: Category master two Champion, time 01:34:30

Leong Yuen Fun 梁婉芬 (Category 30+)

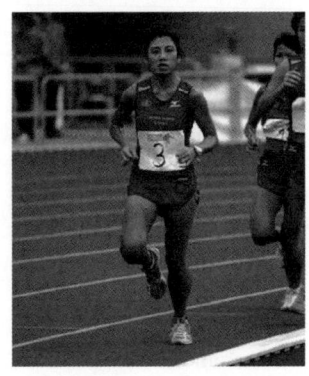

First Marathon: 2003

Personal best time

5 km: 0:18:41(2009)

10 km: 0:39:19 (2006)

15 km: 1:03:12 (2006)

Half Marathon: 1:24:10 (2009)

Full Marathon: 2:56:57 (2008)

Any ultra-marathon race: No

Trail race: Raleigh Challenge-Wilson trail 78 km, 13:20:00

The longest running distance for race: 78 km

The longest running distance for practice: 38 km

Experience with overseas marathon race: Macau, Japan, China- Xiamen, Beijing, India-Mumbai, South Korea-Seoul. Total 8

HK Team Member: yes

Represent Hong Kong experience: 5

HKSCM 2007 full marathon: Category 6th position, time 03:25:09, 10 km 0:45:59, 30 km 2:23:53

HKSCM 2008 full marathon: Category master one 2nd position, time 03:00:49

HKSCM 2009 full marathon: Category 9th position, time 02:59:39,10 km 00:41:30, 30 km 02:04:41

Leung Ying Suet 梁影雪 (Category 25+)
**2005田總全年傑出運動員 (女子成年組) HKAAA Excellent Athlete of the Year 2005
(Women Senior)**
First Marathon: 2006
Personal best time

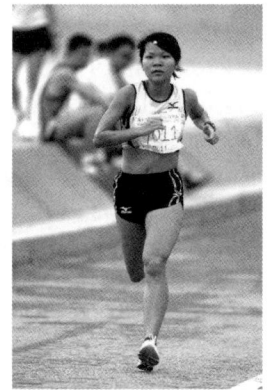

5 km: 00:17:56 (Nov 2007)
10 km: 00:37:20 (2007)
15 km: 1:01:57 (2007)
Half marathon: 01:23:38 (2007)
Full marathon: 03:14:28 (2007)
Any ultra-marathon race: No
Trail race: No
The longest running distance for practice: 42.2 km
The longest running distance for practice: 25 km
Experience with overseas marathon race: 2
HK Team Member: Yes
Represent Hong Kong team experience: Two
HKSCM 2007 full marathon: Female Category Senior 3rd place 03:17:54, 10 km
0:44:05, 30 km 2:16:46
HKSCM 2008 10 km: Senior Champion 00:38:01
HKSCM 2009 half marathon: Senior 5th position 01:31:02

Acknowledgment: The author wishes to thank the elite female runners who contributed their precious time and shared their running secrets for this chapter.

The Making of a Marathon Runner

Dr. HO Chung Ping

My first encounter with the Hong Kong Standard Chartered Marathon was in 2002 at the age of 53. For those who knew me, it was hardly imaginable that I would ever take part in the race. Like many people born soon after World War II, I was brought up in a culture that followed the credo "work hard and play little." Competition in school was intense, and the concept of physical exercise was relatively unknown. There were only one or two weekly physical education (PE) sessions in school, and, during these times, the teachers simply let the students run free in the playground. My school had no changing rooms, and none of us would dream of being able to take a shower after the PE sessions. I was quite happy that, beginning in F.6, PE sessions ceased to exist.

At university, all freshmen were required to take a physical fitness assessment, actively engage in training, and then take another reassessment three months later. We were warned that one of the requirements would be running around the Pokfield Road sports ground three times. I took the threat seriously and practiced a lot. Initially, I was out of breath after running for three minutes, but as I kept running, these symptoms disappeared. The reason for this "second wind" is because organs like the heart and lungs are able to increase their working capacity to cope with increased demand. With practice, I was soon able to comfortably finish three laps.

The reassessment came and after the first year, there were no more compulsory PE sessions. After graduation, life as a young doctor was extremely busy. Sleep was a luxury and exercise remained the privilege of the more senior staff. There was no more jogging during my junior doctor years.

My reunion with jogging was quite accidental. I started my own private practice in a region where there were few car parks. A friend suggested that I join a nearby sports club to use their car park for a monthly fee. After morning rounds, I parked my car at the club and walked the short distance to my office. In the evening, this routine was reversed.

I later noted that there were good sports facilities for tennis, hockey, and lawn bowling in the club. I thought it would be a good idea to get some exercise by jogging on the lawn between the evening clinic and hospital rounds. The idea made sense because it seemed ridiculous to join a club just for its car park facilities. I preferred jogging to ball games because jogging is an independent activity. A doctor's schedule is so hectic and unpredictable that it is often difficult to make and keep appointments with other people. Moreover, jogging made the best use of my available time. Quite a significant portion of ball games is spent passively waiting for the ball.

When I started running, I could only run for 15 minutes at a time. After a short rest, I was able to run for another 15 minutes. After some practice, I could run for 30 minutes non-stop. As extra encouragement, I used to receive cheers from fellow club members, as I was the only regular jogger at the club.

From then on, I became addicted to running. I jogged twice a week. After running, I took a shower at the club and felt relaxed. During clinic hours, the muscles in my body tightened up from mental tension, and jogging was a good way to find relaxation. After a shower, my mood was much improved. The scientific explanation is that exercise causes the brain to secrete a morphine-like substance that makes people feel elated. This substance is thus called endorphin (endogenous morphine). If I stopped running for a couple weeks, I felt an urge to run again, possibly driven by my body's lack of endorphin.

Later, I heard that there was a cross-country race organized by a local athletic association. The word *cross-country* had great appeal to me because my friends who attended schools in the UK talked of their cross-country running experiences at school. I thought it would be a nice way to make up for my "lost" cross-country experience, and I joined the race. I increased the intensity of my practice.

The cross-country race started at the Pineapple Dam in the Shing Mun Reservoir. It was a 10 km race through the area surrounding the reservoir. The uphill portions were quite steep, but I was able to finish in the prescribed time. It was my first experience with "sports competition."

With my growing passion for running, I gave several talks on sports medicine in the Auxiliary Medical Service (AMS) to promote exercise and the proper way to handle sports injuries. The lectures were all well received.

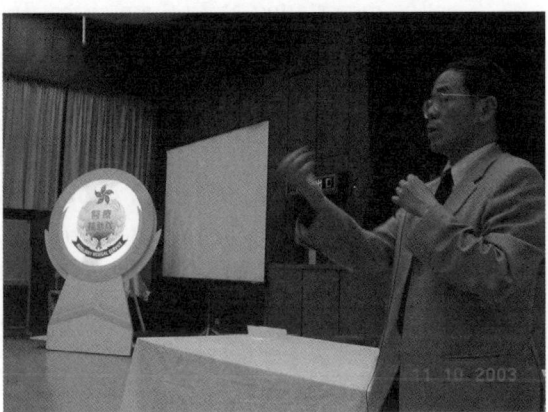

Fig 1 Training AMS members before the Hong Kong Marathon.

In 2001, my friends told me that there was a Standard Chartered Hong Kong Marathon, and I entered for the 10 km race. The race started in Tsim Sha Tsui and, on reaching East Kowloon, we were directed to the Western Harbour Tunnel. My immediate reaction was that, once I crossed the harbor, the Convention Centre would not be far away and the 10 km was too short for me. I decided not go to the tunnel and instead joined the half-marathon group. We ran along Route 3, and it was a pleasant experience to run with many other people. I ran together with my friend Hong until we reached the half-marathon turning point where I turned back and he continued along the full-marathon route.

The island exit of the Western Harbour Tunnel is uphill, but it did not bother me too much. After exiting the tunnel, I noted that many people were walking, due to exhaustion. I prided myself that I was at least still running. When I reached the Convention Centre, I followed the half-marathon entrance but was directed to another lane. I realized that I was treated as a 10 km runner—and a poor one too, since I took so long to reach the finish line. Despite this, it was an excellent experience. Since I did not feel too exhausted after the run, I thought a full marathon was not impossible. For this reason, I increased my practice time until I could run for three hours. The following year, I joined the full race with the thought that, if I could run for three hours, I could finish the full 42 km race with the added help of adrenaline during the race. The adventure was recorded in my e-mail to friends after the event:

> *The race started at 7:00 am sharp. Things were proceeding smoothly like the year before. When I reached Tsing Yi Island, there were occasional calf cramps and I had to stop and do some stretching exercise. When I reached the Tsing Ma Bridge, I was feeling very tired. I used my will power to propel myself along the Ting Kau Bridge and I spent 2 hours 20 minutes at the half-marathon mark. Then I was utterly exhausted and there was pain on the lateral part of my thighs with each step. I thought I could run for a few more km but since I needed to take a rest very frequently, there was no way I could finish the 42 km in time.*

> *When I reached the 26 km mark, I could not continue any longer. Then a bus came along to pick up the wounded and the deserters and I boarded the bus. I felt like a defeated Taliban. But instead of facing beating, extortion and humiliation, I was given water, banana and tin foil blankets. There were even paramedics on board.*

That was the end of my first marathon. At the end of the year, I increased my training with the hope that I could finish the 2004 race. However, I failed to make it and the event was detailed in my e-mail to friends:

> *I did not manage to finish the race. I used 3.5 hours to cover 31 km, and then there was very severe muscle cramps. My cardiovascular system was perfectly OK, I can walk with no problem, but whenever I ran the cramps came back. I calculated that since there was still 12 km to cover and if I walk, I would need 2 hours and I would be overtime. Moreover, it does not look nice to walk in a marathon race. As such I quitted.*

I did not have much time to practice in 2005 because of a family health emergency. I would sometimes practice until 7:30 pm, and then run to the hospital to see my daughter. I also took part in the Marathon Expo to give some advice to the race participants.

On the day of the 2005 race, it was raining at 6:00 am and I was tempted to quit the marathon. Ultimately, I decided to proceed. The full marathon started at 7:45 am, after the half marathon and the 10 km. It was an improvement over past years because marathon runners tended to run more slowly in the initial stages, but the 10 km runners tended to run much faster. Letting the 10 km runners start first avoided the confusion of fast runners overtaking slow runners.

I reached the half-marathon point at 2 hours and 28 minutes, and it was obvious that I could not finish the marathon within the prescribed time of five hours. I struggled to the 28 km point, but my thigh muscles were too sore and I had to walk. Once again, I had to board the bus to carry me to the finish line.

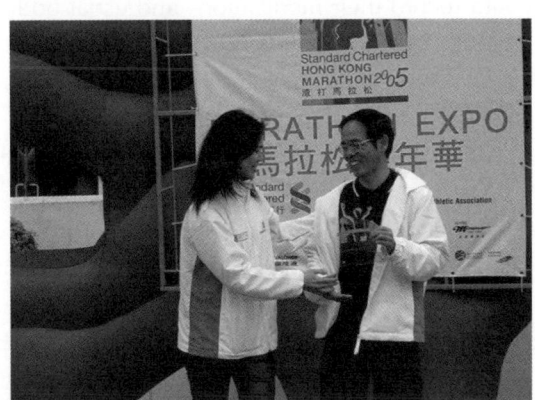

Fig 2 Speaking at the Marathon Expo.

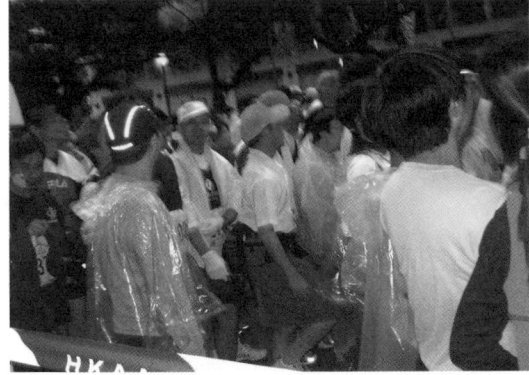

Fig 3 At the starting line of the Marathon.

I did not join the 2006 race because my application was lost in the mail. I was saddened to note that the event ended up with two severely ill patients, one of whom eventually died in the hospital.

This tragedy caused some concern in Hong Kong, and some people blamed the poor air quality. I do not think air pollution was an important factor. Some proposed that all participants should undergo a medical check, but there was no proposal as to what tests should be performed, and the cost of checking all participants would be very high.

To address the public concerns, the Hong Kong Medical Association (HKMA) held a press conference. At the meeting, I proposed that all partici- pants should undertake a self-assessment questionnaire known as the PAR-Q test. Those who showed abnormalities in the test should seek a professional medical opinion. I proposed that it would be much better if the runners could record their medications and usual body weight on the back of their labels to facilitate emergency medical treatment, should it be necessary. Not all of the suggestions were implemented, but the prescribed time for the race was increased to 5.5 hours.

In the summer of 2008, my friend told me that he and his wife followed a training scheme that was suitable for everyone. The scheme was simple: regular practice of 45 minutes three times per week; before the actual race, run 35 km once; then decrease the intensity of training as the race draws near.

I followed this scheme and increased my practice from 30 minutes to 45 minutes. When I had no time for runs three times a week, I compensated with two one-hour practices. By December 2008, the whole city seemed to

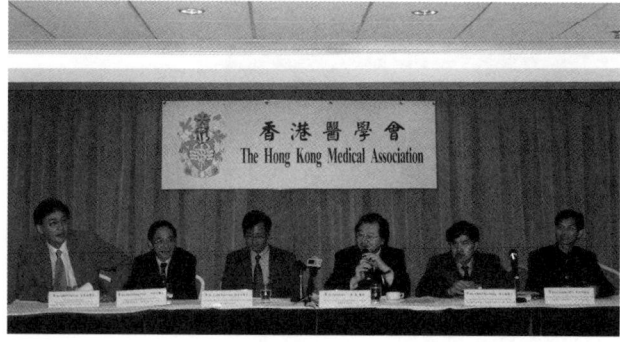

Fig 4 Advising marathon safety in the HKMA press conference.

be preparing for the race. On my way to the hospital, I saw runners jogging along Renfrew Road. I needed to find a more convenient training location, and my friend told me that Kowloon Chai Park, which was very close to my home, had an excellent jogging trail. I went there and found a jogging trail around the main race track that was used by many people. Such a track did not cost much to build but was most useful. There was even a drinking fountain nearby, so there was no need to carry water. I could easily run up to the hospital for medical rounds when needed.

Such practice sessions were good for muscle strengthening, but the 35 km practice was necessary. Practising along the jogging trail would require 70 laps, and this idea was not attractive to me. I decided to do some road practice in Sai Kung.

It was fortunate that the Chinese New Year was in January 2009, well ahead of the race. This gave me time for more practice during the holiday. On New Year's Eve, I drove to Tso Wo Hang Pier, parked my car in the virtually empty car park there, jogged along the Tai Mong Tsai Road to Pak Tam Chung, and entered the country park. Since traffic was restricted in the country park, I did not need to worry about traffic and air pollution. The first part of the MacLehose trail was a long and uphill road but I managed to run all the way up. After this, the road became easy. I ran to the West Dam and had to turn back because of time constraints. The whole trip took 2.5 hours.

Four days later, I ran the route again with an additional mission to test the food I would be carrying during the actual race. Although the organizers provide bananas, many slow runners find that they are all gone when they reach the food stations. My friend Hong told me that he brings chocolate along, but I think chocolate would only provide a short burst of energy. Somebody else suggested energy gel. I tried this in a previous race but did not like the taste and found it to not be readily available. I chose chocolate digestive biscuits, McVitie's®, because the chocolate coating would give instant energy and the wheat flour would provide a sustained energy supply. During my second run, I ran all the way to the East Dam and, on my way back, I tried the biscuits only to find that the chocolate melted away and was quite messy. The whole trip covered 35 km and gave me some confidence in the race. The problem was that there were only about ten days until the race, and my body might not have the time to recover fully. For the remaining days, I stopped all training. I decided to carry lemon puffs in a sports pouch, because the lemon sugar would give quick energy and the biscuits a more sustained supply. I wished to offload as much as possible and would not carry things like a watch, a camera, a mobile phone, or money.

On the day of the race, I went to the starting line by taxi and loaded my luggage into the truck arranged by the organizers. I went to the starting line after warming up only to realize that I forgot to bring the pouch with my cash and ID card. With no food and no cash, I went to an AMS station and asked a member to lend me some money to buy two chocolate bars, knowing that they would melt, so that I would not run hungry.

Due to my improved training, the run was smooth and enjoyable. When I exited the Cheung Tsing Tunnel after the 10 km checkpoint, I experienced some muscle cramps in my calves, but they subsided with some stretching. When I reached the Tsing Ma Bridge, I suddenly fell and landed on my outstretched hands. I sustained two wounds on my palms, but I continued running despite the bleeding. My experience was not unique and a female runner had a similar fall only ten minutes before me.

The Tsing Ma Bridge is a black spot for injuries. It is 18 km from the starting line, and people start to get tired. Some muscle fibers in my calves suddenly gave way, causing the fall. The bridge is open and windy, and those runners who have to take a rest can quickly go into hypothermia.

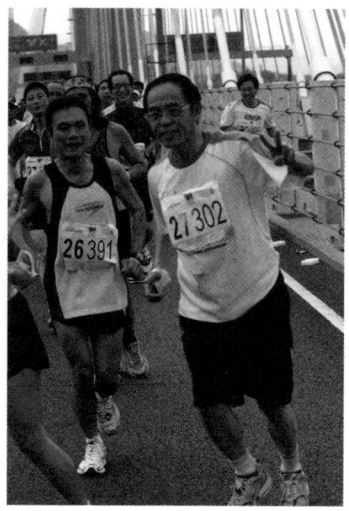

Fig 5 2009 Hong Kong Marathon—turning around at the bridge.

After the Tsing Ma Bridge, we went up the Ting Kau Bridge and back. After exiting the Cheung Tsing Tunnel, I was very happy because, in past races, I dropped out shortly after emerging from the Tunnel. I noted that many people around me were running slowly and that I could easily overtake them. The journey was easier because it was gently sloping downhill. At some of the water stations, there were bananas freely available. When I reached the 30 km mark, the track was less congested, possibly because many runners had left the race. The 30 km point is sometimes called the "30 km barrier," because many people quit before they reach this point. I briefly

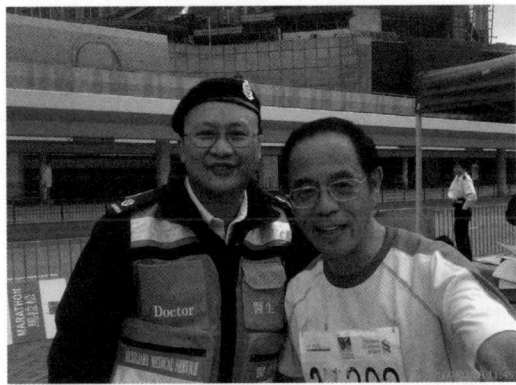

Fig 6 2009 Hong Kong Marathon—reaching the Western Harbour Tunnel.

rested at the entrance of the Western Harbour Tunnel because there was only 10 km to go. After exiting the tunnel, I felt tired and stopped to stretch. For the first time, I had to walk along an uphill section.

After reaching the Convention Centre, I saw a woman lying in a stretcher and surrounded by policeman and first-aid workers. I approached them to see if they needed help. I found our AMS doctor, John, there and he politely sent me away. Days later, John told me that the girl was probably suffering from low blood sugar. The last leg of the race is also a high-risk area because the participants are all exhausted and prone to heat exhaustion and low blood sugar.

The last kilometer was in downtown Wanchai and, since people lined both sides of Jaffe Road to watch and cheer, I had to put up a heroic look despite utter fatigue. The last 100 meters was in the form of a runway in Victoria Park. [figure 7 reaching the finishing point]. I finished the race in 5 hour and 1 minute. It was one of the happiest moments in my life.

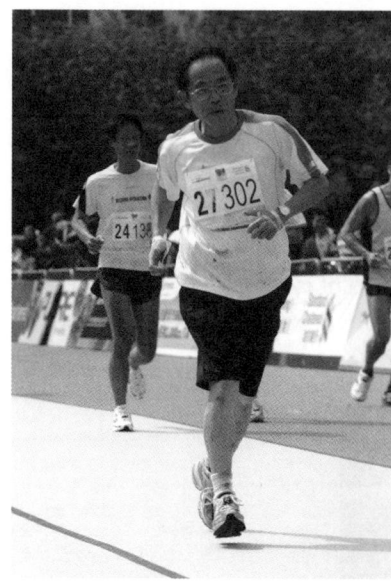

Fig 7 2009 Hong Kong Marathon—
reaching the finishing port.

Fig 8 2009 Hong Kong
Marathon—mission
accomplished.

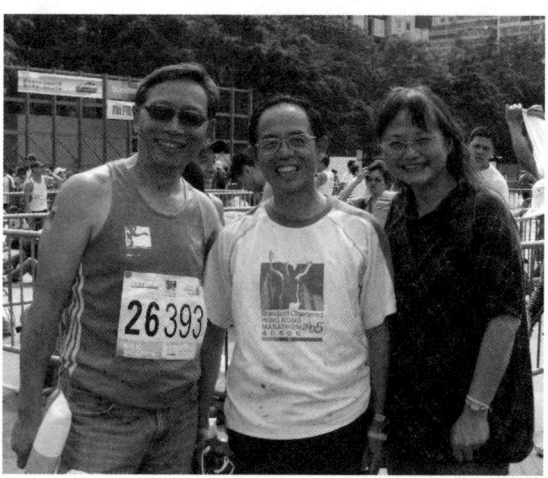

The marathon is the *sine qua non* of all seasoned runners. With a lot of
training and careful planning, anyone can make it.

Review of Medical Encounters in the 2007 Hong Kong Marathon

Dr. Ben FONG

There were 43,956 entrants in the 2007 Hong Kong marathon. Among them, 6,178 (14%) ran the full marathon, 10,714 (24%) ran the half marathon, and 27,064 (62%) ran the 10 km race. These figures have increased 2.5 times in five years, with a larger increase in 10 km runners.

On 4 March 2007, the day of the marathon, 37,438 people began the races and 97.3% of the runners finished. The 10 km race started first in three groups at 5:30, 5:50, and 7:05 am. The half marathon began at 6:10 am and the full marathon began at 7:40 am.

Based on experience from previous years, twenty-three fixed first-aid posts (sixteen in Kowloon and seven on Hong Kong Island) were set up by the Auxiliary Medical Service (AMS) for the marathon. A number of mobile first-aid teams were also deployed at strategic locations, involving nine members in Kowloon and fifty on Hong Kong. In addition, seven AMS ambulances, four motorcycle ambulances, and fifteen first-aid bicycles were on duty during the race. Overall, there were four hundred AMS members and officers, including twenty-eight doctors, on duty for the 2007 marathon.

The command post and responsible AMS staff kept close communication with the six public hospitals and Accident and Emergency Department along the route, in addition to the organizers and police. This ensured a smooth transfer of cases to the hospitals and prompt responses to unexpected incidents. The individual first-aid posts and teams reported to the command post every hour with the number of cases managed in various categories and the details of runners transferred to the hospitals.

Data collection was carried out by duty members and officers at all first-aid posts during the marathon. A simple form was designed by the Medical Advisory Board on Major Events. (Tables 1a and 1b) Essentially, symptoms

Table 1a Auxiliary Medical Service: Record of Cases in Hong Kong Marathon on 4 March 2007

Post :					Time Period							Page No. :	
Order	Arrival Time	Runner's Number	Sex		Treatment							Time Leaving	Remarks
					Massage	Wounds	Blisters	Warming	Ice Pack	Electrolytes	Others		
1			M	F									
2			M	F									
3			M	F									
4			M	F									
5			M	F									
6			M	F									
7			M	F									
8			M	F									
9			M	F									
10			M	F									
11			M	F									
12			M	F									
13			M	F									
14			M	F									
15			M	F									
16			M	F									
17			M	F									
18			M	F									
19			M	F									
20			M	F									
21			M	F									
22			M	F									
23			M	F									
24			M	F									
25			M	F									

Table 1b 醫療輔助隊2007年3月4日香港馬拉松個案處理紀錄

崗位：					時段：							頁數：	
序	接收時間	參賽者號碼	性別		治療							離去時間	備註欄
					拉筋/按摩	傷口/包紮	水泡處理	保暖	冰敷	電解飲料	其他		
1			男	女									
2			男	女									
3			男	女									
4			男	女									
5			男	女									
6			男	女									
7			男	女									
8			男	女									
9			男	女									
10			男	女									
11			男	女									
12			男	女									
13			男	女									
14			男	女									
15			男	女									
16			男	女									
17			男	女									
18			男	女									
19			男	女									
20			男	女									
21			男	女									
22			男	女									
23			男	女									
24			男	女									
25			男	女									

or complaints and treatment given were recorded. Officers in charge of all posts reported the figures to the command post for updating overall hourly statistics. The forms were then collected by AMS Headquarters. Under the circumstances of this major event, we could not expect complete accuracy of the data. Indeed, some of the data on the forms were not completed.

Findings of Medical Encounters

Table 2 Responses to Medical Encounters in the 2007 Hong Kong Marathon

Medical Encounters	Massage	Treatment	Hospital Transfer	Total
Number of Attendances	5,759	455	35	6,249
Percentage of total	92.2%	7.3%	0.6%	100%

Table 3 Actual Affected Cases of Medical Encounters by Type of Race in the 2007 Hong Kong Marathon

Type of Race	Runners (%)	Affected Cases (%)	Medical Encounters (%)
10 km	27,064 (62)	307 (1.1)	369 (1.4)
Half Marathon	10,714 (24)	999 (9.3)	1,387 (12.9)
Full Marathon	6,178 (14)	2,020 (32.7)	4,493 (72.9)
Total	43,956 (100)	3,326 (7.6)	6,249 (14.2)

Table 4 Responses to Medical Encounters by Type of Race in the 2007 Hong Kong Marathon

Medical Encounters	Massage (%)	Treatment (%)	Hospital Transfer (%)	Total (%)
10 km	184 (3.2)	164 (36.0)	20 (57.1)	368 (5.9)
Half Marathon	1,248 (21.7)	132 (29.0)	8 (22.9)	1,388 (22.2)
Full Marathon	4,327 (75.1)	159 (34.9)	7 (20.0)	4,493 (71.9)
Total Number of Attendances	5,759 (100)	455 (100)	35 (100)	6,249 (100)

There were a total of 6,249 medical encounters, 3.5 times more than the total in 2002, but only 3,326 runners (9% of total) were affected. Hence, many runners stopped at the first-aid posts more than once, mostly for massage. Among the affected runners, 307, 999, and 2,020 ran in the 10 km, half marathon, and full marathon races, respectively. In terms of percentage, 1.1%, 10%, and 30% of the runners in these same races were involved.

Most medical encounters occurred in the full marathon runners, who comprised 14% of all runners. Not many 10 km runners required first-aid services, though they accounted for 60% of all participants.

The total number of runners who came for massage for leg cramps was 5,759, or 92.2%. Three-quarters of all attendees to the first-aid centers were full marathon runners. Many were not first-aid services in a strict sense, and hence did not count as clinical cases. On the other hand, 455 runners required genuine first-aid treatment, and this figure doubled from 2006. Of these, 61% had wounds from accidents and 15% had blisters from running.

Thirty-five runners, comprising twenty-eight males and seven females, required hospital transfer to four hospitals. Twenty (57%) were 10 km runners, eight were half marathon runners, and seven were full marathon participants. Twenty-nine were admitted to Ruttonjee Hospital, close to the finish line, three were sent to Kowloon's Kwong Wah Hospital, two were sent to Kowloon's Princess Margaret Hospital, and one was sent to Hong Kong Island's Queen Mary Hospital.

Twenty-one (60%) hospital transfers were cases involving dizziness, three were for wounds, four were for low blood pressure, one was for a fractured finger, one was for chest pain, two were for shock, one was for low body temperature, one was for cramps, and one was for a head injury. Cases transferred to hospitals did not necessarily equate to seriousness of the injuries or bodily complaints. Some were sent to the Accident and Emergency (A&E) Departments because duty officers in charge considered it more appropriate to have the conditions managed in a hospital setting.

During the inspection round on my way to the medical post near the finish line, I advised the transfer of a man who suffered from multiple and fairly deep abrasions to his face, lips and limbs, because he would receive better wound cleansing and care in the A&E Department. This accident occurred very early in the morning before the Sun rose.

Fortunately all patients except six were discharged within the same day, even though the total number of hospital transfers was 1.6 times more than 2006, when there were twenty-two cases. However, a critical case was kept in Ruttonjee Hospital for more than a week, and this case is reported by Dr. Szeto.

Hong Kong was unfortunate to have experienced its first fatality in 2006 with the death of a 53 year-old runner who was a known asthmatic. Despite the fact that a few doctor-runners were there to resuscitate the patient, he subsequently died after hospital admission.

Time Trend

Table 5 Hourly Medical Encounters in the 2007 Hong Kong Marathon

Time (hours)	Massage	Treatment	Hospital Transfer	Hourly Total	Cumulative
0500-0600	2	1	0	3	3
0600-0700	30	39	7	76	79
0700-0800	75	64	9	148	227
0800-0900	639	100	6	745	972
0900-1000	788	75	6	869	1,841
1000-1100	1,201	25	1	1,227	3,068
1100-1200	1,293	28	2	1,323	4,391
1200-1300	1,460	109	2	1,571	5,962
1300-1400	271	14	2	287	6,249
Total	5,759	455	35	6,249	

The number of medical encounters increased progressively with time, most significantly two hours after the first group of 10 km runners began at 5:30 am. (Table 5) This trend was expected because the great majority of cases (92%) came for massage of leg cramps, which was a function and consequence of prolonged running. (Figure 1) The same temporal trend was observed when only the massage cases were examined. (Figure 2)

When treatment cases were examined, a quarter of these encounters occurred in the first two hours and predominantly affected the 10 km runners. (Figure 3) The other three quarters were seen during the hours of 8–9 am, 9–10 am and 12–1 pm. There was an obvious decline during the two hours from 10 am–12 pm. These trends reflect the bulk of the 10 km and half marathon runners, comprising 84% of all runners, before the decline, while the full marathon runners came for treatment during the final hours of the event.

The majority (80%) of hospital transfers took place in the first four

Figure 1 Hourly Medical Encounters in the 2007 Hong Kong Marathon

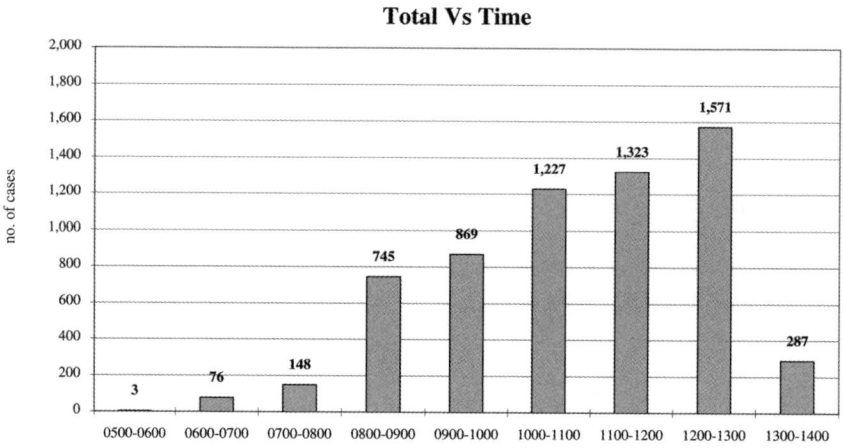

Figure 2 Hourly Medical Encounters requiring Massage in the 2007 Hong Kong Marathon

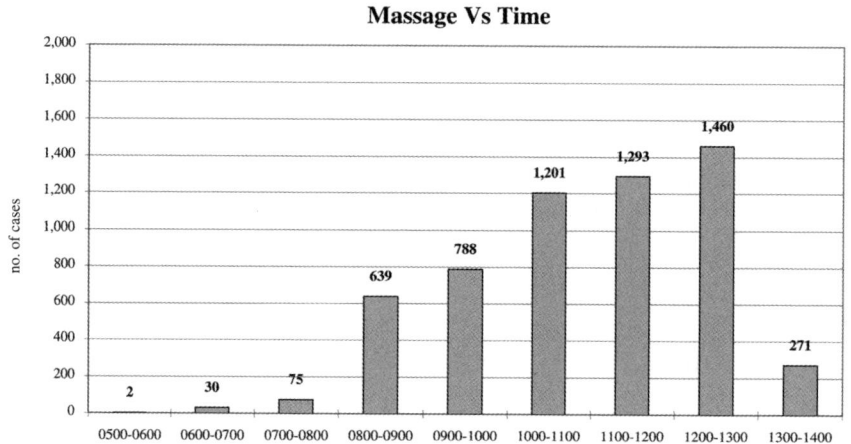

Figure 3 Hourly Medical Encounters requiring Treatment in the 2007 Hong Kong Marathon

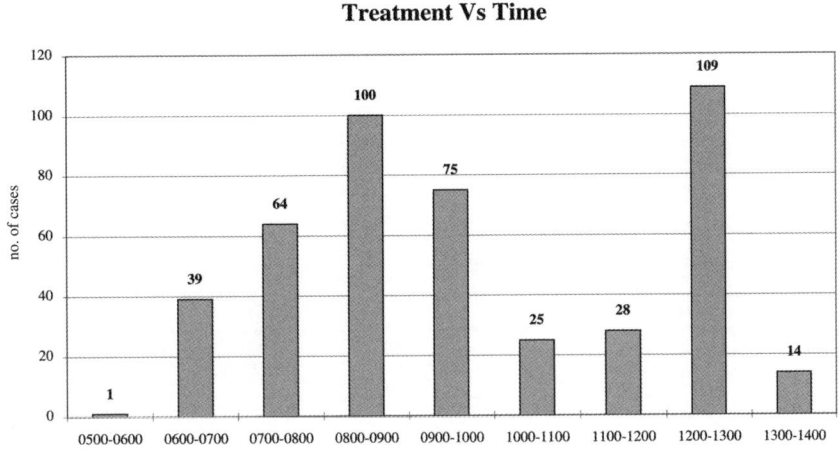

Figure 4 Hourly Hospital Transfers in the 2007 Hong Kong Marathon

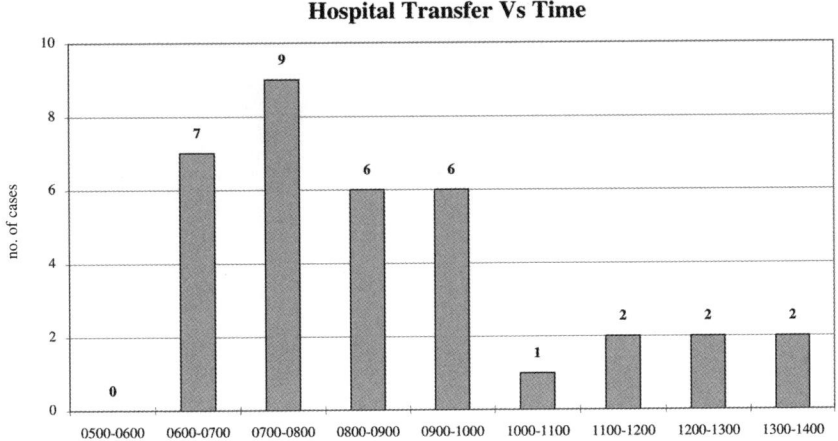

hours. (Figure 4) This trend arose from the fact that 20% (i.e., seven of the thirty-five cases) of the transfers were full marathon runners who were sent to the hospital after 10 am.

Medical Encounters at First-Aid Posts

Table 6 Responses to Medical Encounters at First-Aid Posts during the 2007 Hong Kong Marathon

First-Aid Posts	Massage	Treatment	Hospital Transfer	Total	People on Duty
K1a	0	1	0	1	12
K2a	3	1	0	4	4
K2b	0	1	0	1	5
K3	231	89	0	320	19
K4	476	20	1	497	7
K5	278	7	1	286	4
K6	269	0	0	269	15
K7	377	5	0	382	7
K8	130	8	0	138	7
K9	349	6	0	355	4
K10	118	1	0	119	7
K11	7	2	1	10	14
K12	116	8	2	126	7
K13	422	3	0	425	8
K14	39	3	0	42	41
K1a-1c	840	16	1	857	12
Hla-1c	677	6	1	684	12
H1	400	18	3	421	21
H2a-2b	73	7	0	80	8
H3a-3b	413	3	0	416	8
H4a-4b	74	1	4	79	8
H2	5	4	2	11	7
H5a-5c	131	33	1	165	12
H3	17	15	0	32	18
H4	207	83	15	305	29
H5	40	31	1	72	6
H6	52	65	2	119	15
H7	15	18	0	33	4
Total	5,759	455	35	6,249	321

Medical incidents can never be fully predicted in terms of type, time, and place, particularly during an endurance race like the marathon. Hence, the distribution of medical encounters among the fixed and mobile first-aid posts varied. (Figures 5a and 5b) Similar trends were again observed in the massage and cramp cases, which comprised 92% of encounters. (Figure 6)

Nearly two-thirds, or 62.4%, of medical encounters requiring treatment occurred on Hong Kong Island during the latter legs of the race. (Figure 7) This finding was not unexpected because the finish line was on the island after runners passed through the Western Harbour Tunnel, a rather long and hilly stretch. More treatment cases were found at three particular posts: K3, H4, and H6. K3 was the medical post in Kowloon before the entrance to the Western Harbour Tunnel, and H4 was on Hong Kong Island next to the finish line. H6 was situated inside the Wanchai Sports Ground, where runners picked up their personal belongings after the race. These medical posts, as described in Fung and Shum's chapter on AMS Support and Deployment, were strategically located as a result of past experience and

Figure 5a Total Medical Encounters at First-Aid Posts in the 2007 Hong Kong Marathon

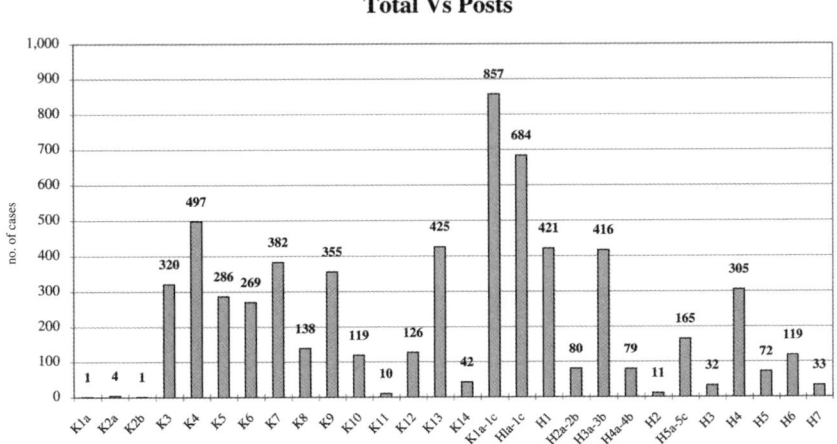

Figure 5b Total Medical Encounters at First-Aid Posts in the 2005 and 2006 Hong Kong Marathon

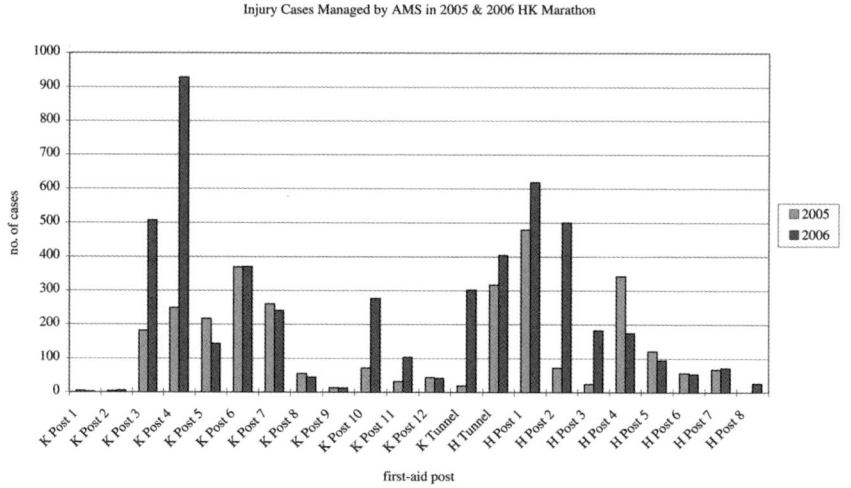

Figure 6 Medical Encounters requiring Massage at First-Aid Posts in the 2007 Hong Kong Marathon

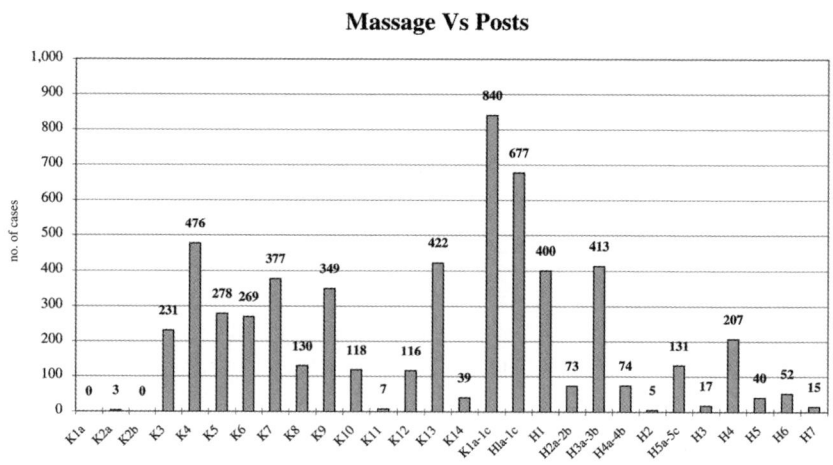

Figure 7 Medical Encounters requiring Treatment at First-Aid Posts in the 2007 Hong Kong Marathon

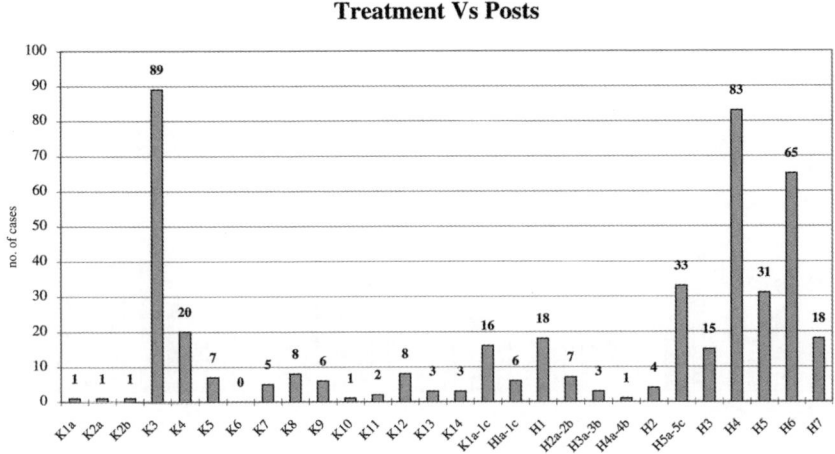

Figure 8 Hospital Transfers from First-Aid Posts in the 2007 Hong Kong Marathon

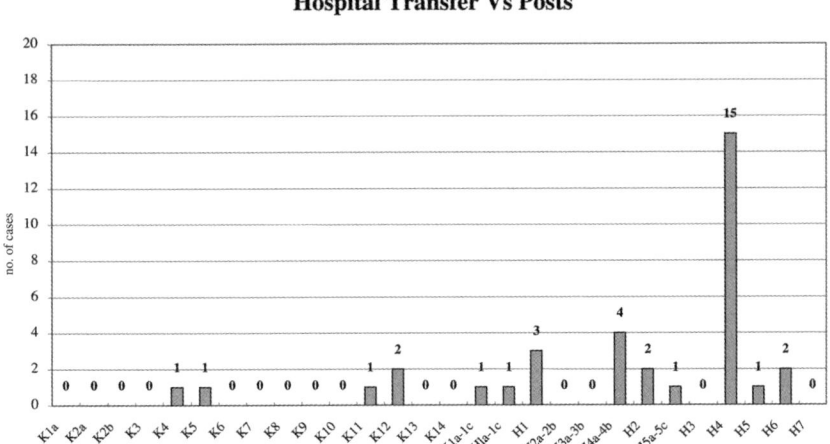

Figure 9 AMS Deployment at First-Aid Posts in the 2007 Hong Kong Marathon

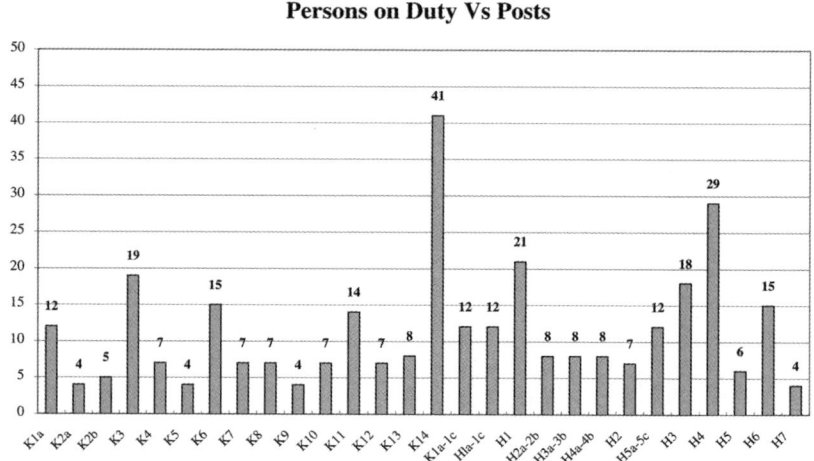

Persons on Duty Vs Posts

statistics. More staffing and related resources were assigned to these three posts.

With respect to encounters that were eventually transferred to hospitals, the vast majority (i.e., thirty out of thirty-five cases) were referred from Hong Kong Island. Among these sick or injured runners, half were encountered at the medical post near the finish line. (Figure 8)

Having considered the statistics of medical encounters for various complaints and conditions, and from past experience and feedback among duty members and officers, deployment of AMS volunteers to the first-aid posts, mobile parties, bicycles, motor bicycles, and ambulances was made in a strategic and practical way, so that the anticipated need could be met with a comfortable safety margin. (Figure 9) Participation by nurses and doctors in recent years further enhanced the professional backup at key posts and, at the same time, boosted the morale among duty members.

Case Report: 28-year-old 10 km Runner Collapses Before the Finish Line

Dr. SZETO King Ho

On 4 March 2007, the accident and emergency department of Ruttonjee and Tang Shiu Kin Hospital received an ambulance with a 28-year-old man who was competing in a 10 km race. He collapsed 500 meters before the finish line, and his wet clothes were removed at the scene. The confused man (Glasgow coma scale E4V2M4) developed respiratory insufficiency and cardiovascular failure with a blood pressure of 70/32 mmHg, a pulse rate of 145 per minute, and respiratory rate of 42 per minute. Core temperature measured by rectal probe was 41.8°C. Oxygen saturation was 96% on room air. Physical examination revealed that his general conditions were critical. His skin was dry, hot, and dehydrated. Both pupils were equal and reactive. There was no focal neurological sign and no scalp wound. Chest and abdominal examinations were unremarkable. Limb muscles were shivering. The combination of hyperpyrexia (elevated core body temperature exceeding 40°C) and predominant central nervous system dysfunction resulting in delirium, convulsion, or coma made exertional heat stroke the top differential diagnosis.

The treatment goals were immediate lowering of the patient's core temperature, intensive-care supportive measures, and workups to exclude other differential diagnoses. A 100% oxygen non-rebreathing mask was applied and two intravenous drips of 2 L 0.9% normal saline were infused at full rate. External cooling measures were ordered by putting ice packs on the groin, axillae, and neck regions. Evaporation heat loss was facilitated by spraying room-temperature water to the whole body. The patient's shivering was controlled by 5 mg intravenous diazepam to prevent further thermogenesis. A paracetamol 500 mg suppository STAT was also prescribed.

Urgent bedside investigation of blood sugar was 6.2 mmol L.

An electrocardiogram showed sinus tachycardia. The chest X-ray was unremarkable. Subsequently, the patient's core temperature was lowered to 38.5°C, and he was transferred to the intensive care unit (ICU).

The patient's identity was finally determined, and we discovered that he underwent a video-assisted bilateral thoracoscopic sympathectomy from T2 to T5 for axillary hyperhydrosis in 2003. According to the information from his family, this was his second attempt to run the 10 km race. He was an amateur long-distance athlete, and had regularly practiced for a month. His body weight was estimated to be 70 kg, and no significant family and drug histories were elicited.

On admission, the biochemical profile was deranged, which suggested multiple organ failure. Impaired liver function and disseminated intravascular coagulopathy (DIC) were manifested as albumin 34 d/L, total bilirubin 5 umol/L, alkaline phosphatase (ALP) 92, alanine aminotransferase (ALT) 20, and a prothrombin time (PT) of 11.3 sec, international normalized ratio (INR) 1.09, and activated partial thromboplastin time (APTT) 32.5 sec. These parameters peaked during day three with albumin 30, bilirubin 149, ALP 128, ALT 7112, PT 30.3, APTT 51.4, and INR 2.42. The complete blood picture showed white cell counts from 8.8 to 13.6×10^9/L, hemoglobin levels from 15.6 g/L to 8.5 g/dL, and thrombocytopenia from 111 to 84 $\times 10^9$/L on day three. Both blood urea and serum creatinine levels were elevated (urea 6.2 to 8.3 mmol/L and creatinine 196 to 389 umol/L), indicating the beginning of acute renal failure.

This situation was further complicated by rhabdomyolysis with creatine kinase (CK) level 399 IU/L and peaked at >20000 IU/L on day three. Urine for myoglobin was later confirmed to be positive. To prevent imminent renal failure, forced alkalinized diuresis was initiated and continued to ensure a urinary excretion rate of more than 100 ml/h. With these aggressive measures, extracorporeal hemofiltration was avoided. The arterial blood gas suggested mixed respiratory alkalosis and metabolic acidosis, presumably from lactate acid overproduction (pH 7.32 pCO_2 3.9 kPa, pO_2 12 kPa, HCO_3 15 mmol/L base excess -9.6mmol/L O_2 saturation 97%). The T troponin was elevated at 0.48 ng/ml. Urine for the toxicology screen and sepsis workup were negative. The brain-computed tomography scan did not reveal any pathology except for ethmoid sinusitis.

At the same time, the hepatobiliary surgical team at Queen Mary

Hospital was consulted to discuss the option of liver transplant. Disseminated intravascular coagulopathy was corrected by fresh frozen precipitate and Vitamin K_1 infusion. Electrolyte imbalance (hypoglycemia, hypokalemia) was corrected as indicated. Supportive measures were given to manage the multi-organ failure. The patient's biochemical profile was stabilized after four days of ICU care. He was discharged after 31 days of hospitalization. The serum CK level finally returned to normal seven weeks after discharge. He was also finally able to resume his work and perform moderate exercise at this time.

Discussion

This case is the first report in the literature that demonstrates bilateral sympathectomy is a risk factor for heat stroke. Diagnosis of heat stroke is, classically, a clinical diagnosis of core temperatures greater than 40°C and central nervous system (CNS) dysfunction. Profuse sweating is a classic sign of exertional heat stroke. Differential diagnoses must exclude drug poisoning (e.g., anticholinergic, serotonin, and amphetamine), CNS injury, hyperthyroid storm, pheochromocytoma, sepsis, neuroleptic malignant syndrome, and malignant hyperthermia.

This case had a provisional diagnosis of heat stroke (at the scene) based on circumstantial evidence and initial vital signs. Past medical, drug, and family histories and extensive investigations ruled out alternative diagnoses. The patient had a clinical course of classic heat stroke with multiple organ failure, including encephalopathy, rhabdomyolysis, myocardial injury, acid-base imbalance, acute renal failure, acute hepatic failure, and DIC. Mortality could be as high as 30%. The prognostic factors include age, past medical health, and time from diagnosis to application of cooling measures to lower the core temperature to 38.5°C. Fortunately, survival in this case was predicted from early recognition, early pre-hospital transfer, early cooling measures, and early ICU care.

Risk factors that increase the likelihood of heat-related illnesses include a preceding viral infection, dehydration, fatigue, obesity, lack of sleep, poor physical fitness, and a lack of acclimatization. This 10 km race, in an ambient temperature of 25°C and a relative humidity 85%, was a moderate heat stress to our patient. The physiological change secondary to sympathectomy may play a significant role in this case. Axillary hyperhydrosis surgically treated by bilateral sympathectomy at the T4 level may later result in compensatory hyperhydrosis in the palms and feet. However, our patient underwent an extensive T2 to T5 sympathectomy in order to provide better satisfaction. It is postulated that the compensatory thermoregulation may be jeopardized in case of a moderate heat stress. So far, no mortality cases due to heat stroke have been reported in any 10 km race in Hong Kong.

In conclusion, heat stroke is a time-sensitive acute medical emergency that carries a high mortality rate unless prompt cooling measures begin during pre-hospital transfer. A physical activity readiness questionnaire may be included for screening. In this particular case, a pre-race medical consultation on his surgical problem should be reviewed. A longer training time for acclimatization and standard medical advice for long-distance running should be employed to prevent possible tragedy.

Auxiliary Medical Service
—Support and Deployment

Dr. Marcus FUNG & Mr. James SHUM

Introduction

Since 1997, first-aid coverage for the Hong Kong Marathon has been provided by the Auxiliary Medical Service (AMS), which is a government department under the Security Bureau. AMS comprises more than 4,000 trained volunteer members from all walks of life, including doctors and nurses.

The AMS Medical Advisory Board on Major Events (MABOME), on which most members are doctors and senior officers, provides medical advice for major events. Technique and Experience Sharing Meetings are also held before and after each major event. Since 2006, a medical director and a deputy medical director were appointed annually to oversee the marathon's medical-related matters. Both directors were invited as observers of marathons organized by neighboring countries. After that, they gave presentations about first-aid and medical support to AMS members involved in marathon duties.

Allocation of Posts, Manpower, and Equipment

The strategic allocation of first-aid posts, manpower, and equipment for the marathon is a great challenge. Careful design with close monitoring and prompt response are necessary to optimize first-aid support during the marathon.

The 2007 Hong Kong Marathon was held on 4 March 2007. The running route covered the West Kowloon Highway, Cheung Tsing Tunnel, Tsing Ma Bridge, Kap Shui Mun Bridge, Ting Kau Bridge, West Harbour Tunnel, and main roads along the Western District, Central District, and

Wanchai. According to the operation order, AMS members were requested to provide first-aid and ambulance services along the running route. Details of manpower allocation in each of the first-aid posts are summarized in Table 1. Ambulance standby locations are listed in Table 2.

Table 1 Post Details and Manpower Allocation

Post number	Duty location	Manpower			
		Officer	Member	Doctor	Nurse
K1a	Starting line—Junction of Kimberley Road outside Hotel Miramar	1	8	2	1
K1b	Junction of Nathan Road & Austin Road	-	6	-	-
K2a	Junction of Nathan Road & Peking Road	-	4	-	-
K2b	Junction of Nathan Road & Haiphong Road (near the mosque)	1	4	-	-
K3	Entrance of West Harbour Tunnel (southbound) (**W3**) (Sick Bay)	3	10	2	1
K4	Flyover between Tonkin Street & Hing Wah Street (southbound) (**W4**)	1	6	-	-
K5	Flyover between HK International Container Terminal (**W5**)	-	-	-	-
K6	Return point for half marathon (**between W5 & W6**)	1	6	2	1
K7	Flyover facing the container terminal & Godown, near Terminal 4 (**W6**)	1	6	-	-
K8	Exit of Cheung Tsing Tunnel (westbound) (**W7**)	1	6	-	-
K9	Return point for full marathon (**between W7 & W8**)		4	-	-
K10	First main pole of Tsing Ma Bridge (westbound) (**W8**)	1	6	-	-

K11	Passing Tsing Ma Bridge about 500 m (full marathon turning point) **(W9)**	1	6	1	1
K12	First main pole of Ting Kau Bridge near Tsing Yi **(W10)**	1	6	-	-
K13	Junction of Tuen Mun Road & Tsing Long Highway **(W11)**	6	1	-	1
K14	Mobile first-aid parties (en-route bus services)	1	40	-	-
K15	Mobile parties inside West Harbour Tunnel	-	12	-	-
K16	First-aid bicycles—return point for half marathon **(between W5 & W6)**	-	3	-	-
K17	First-aid bicycles—return point for full marathon **(W9)**	-	6	-	-
H1	Exit of West Harbour Tunnel (southbound) **(W2)**	4	12	2	2
H2	Lung Wui Road **(W1)**	1	6	-	-
H3	Finish line (next to monument)	1	10	2	2
H4	Expo Drive next to physiotherapy area (Sick Bay)	5	16	4	4
H5	Convention Avenue, bus terminus (next to Harbour Road Indoor Games Hall)	-	6	-	-
H6	Wanchai Sports Ground	1	12	-	1
H7	Central Plaza, Harbour Road	1	12	-	1
H8	Mobile parties (inside the West Harbour Tunnel)	-	12	-	-
H9	Mobile parties (from H1 to Flyover o/s Rumsey Street)	-	8	-	-
H10	Mobile parties (from Flyover o/s Rumsey Street to the entrance of the Pedder Street underpass)	-	8	-	-
H11	Mobile parties (from the entrance of Pedder Street underpass to H2)	-	8	-	-

H12	Mobile parties (to and from H2 & H4)	-	12	-	-
H13	First-aid bicycles (station next to H1)	-	6	-	-
Kowloon Control Room	AMS Headquarters	1	22	-	-
Hong Kong Control Room	Inside Hong Kong Convention and Exhibition Centre	4	1	-	-
Store & Logistics	Hong Kong Store	-	20	-	-

Table 2 Ambulance Standby Locations

Ambulance	Duty location (standby)	Manpower		
		Officer	Nurse	Member
Amb 1	Entrance of West Harbour Tunnel (southbound)	-	1	3
Amb 2	Turning point for half marathon **(between W5 & W6)**	-	1	3
Amb 3	Passing Tsing Ma Bridge about 500 m (turning point for full marathon)	1	1	3
Amb 4 (motorcycle)	Entrance of West Harbour Tunnel (southbound) **(W3)**	-	-	1
Amb 5 (motorcycle)	Flyover facing Hong Kong International Container Terminal **(W5)**	-	-	1
Amb 6 (motorcycle)	Second turning point for full marathon **(between W7 & W8)**	-	-	1
Amb 7 (motorcycle)	Passing Tsing Ma Bridge about 500 m (turning point for full marathon) **(W9)**	-	-	1
Amb 8	Mobile Command Post—along the route from Kowloon to Hong Kong	2	-	3
Amb 9	Inside Expo Drive next to physiotherapy area	-	1	3
Amb 10	Inside Expo Drive next to physiotherapy area	-	1	3

Amb 11	Inside Expo Drive next to physiotherapy area	-	1	3
Amb 12	Exit of West Harbour Tunnel (southbound)	-	1	3

Allocation of first-aid posts and manpower

In the 2007 Hong Kong Marathon, there were 19 first-aid posts set up in Kowloon and 13 first-aid posts on Hong Kong Island. More than 400 members were deployed, including 15 doctors and 22 nurses. Among these posts, K3 (outside the Kowloon side of the Western Harbour Tunnel) and H4 (near the finish line) were purposely set up as sick bays. These posts were set up with medical tents, additional medical equipment, and extra manpower.

Ambulances were assigned to standby near the sick bays. Patients with unstable conditions could be transferred to the Accident and Emergency Departments of the closest hospital within the shortest time. Generally, all sick bays were established under the same principle in Diagram 1.

During the race, AMS command post officers kept close communication with the Accident and Emergency Departments of six Hospital Authority hospitals along the route.

The selection criteria of the locations and the scale of first-aid posts were based upon the recommendation by the event's organization committee, expected number of casualties, and members' feedback during the previous years. Visibility and accessibility to the runners were also very important. The posts were situated very close to water stations set up by the organizers, and these corresponded to W1–W9 in Table 1. Prominent and clear signage for the first-aid posts was installed. In case of an emergency, real-time communication with the organizers could easily identify the exact location. In regions where vehicles could not access, mobile first-aid teams (K14–K15 and H8–H12) and bicycle first-aid teams (K16–K17 and H13) were deployed to provide the service. Such mobile services were particularly important inside the Western Harbour Tunnel.

Moreover, emergency evacuation routes were taken into consideration. Since the police denied vehicle access for practical reasons, evacuation of patients and the supply of additional emergency equipment could be very difficult; therefore, the location of such posts and evacuation routes had

Diagram 1 General Layout of Sick Bays

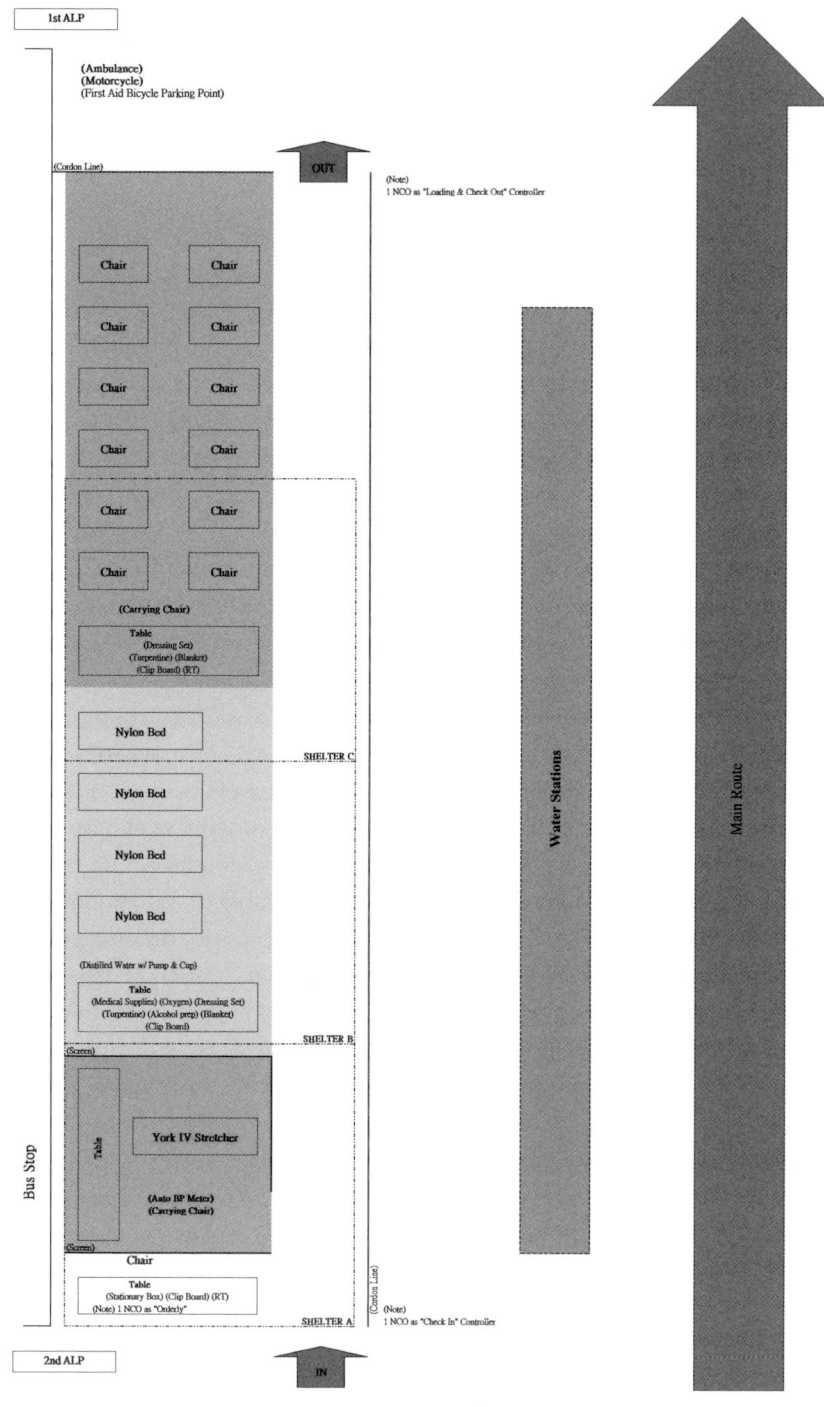

been carefully planned to allow patient removal over the shortest possible distance. All duty members were briefed about the emergency evacuation routes close to their first-aid posts.

Allocation of equipment

The allocation of equipment is in accordance with the type and nature of first-aid posts. The equipment items listed in Table 3 are available to all first-aid posts, which are managed by first responders. Each first responder carries a first-aid kit which includes the equipment items listed in Table 4.

Sick bays are managed by doctors and nurses, in addition to first responders. Table 5 lists the additional equipment items that are available in the sick bays. Also, spare first-aid kits and medical supplies are stored in the sick bays. In case of a supply shortage, members can request replacements from the nearest sick bay.

Apart from the usual set-up, modifications of first-aid supplies are made according to the weather forecast provided by the Hong Kong Observatory. The temperature, relative humidity, and wind speed are of particular importance. If the weather is cold and windy, additional blankets are shipped to prepare for hypothermic cases. For hot and dry weather, additional sponges, water, and ice will be prepared for heat stroke. Additional electrolyte fluids will also be prepared. Twenty members stand ready in the AMS Hong Kong Store to provide logistic support, additional equipment, and medical supplies, when necessary.

Other Considerations

Privacy

As most of the first-aid posts are located in open areas, maintaining patient privacy is a challenge. Members have been trained to use blankets to provide a partition for patients during treatment. Mobile partitions are available in the sick bays to ensure privacy, particularly during medical examinations and resuscitation. Moreover, general consensus has been made between the organizer and media that reporters will not take photographs of patients inside the first-aid posts.

Signage

Clear signs are displayed to show the location of the first-aid posts. All AMS members wear reflective vests with the first-aid logo—a green background with a white cross—in the front and on the back for easy identification. Signboards are set up to clearly indicate the entrance, zones of treatment, and exit in the sick bays. Patients are requested only to leave at the exit of the sick bay to make sure that the officer-in-charge can accurately record the designation of patients after treatment. Outside each sick bay, a signboard reading "AMBULANCE LOADING POINT" is set up to facilitate easy identification of the point where ambulance crews pick up patients.

Communication

During the marathon, at least one radio telephone (RT) machine is allocated to each first-aid post. However, only emergency cases are reported to the command posts via the radio system. This is to avoid jamming lines when multiple people are using the same channel. Telephone numbers for the medical director and deputy medical director are available at all posts. In case of emergency, members can request medical advice and receive a response in real time. For other inquires, and for reporting patient information, members are requested to use mobile phones to communicate with the command posts. The officer-in-charge of each first-aid post reports regularly to the command post about the number of cases treated and detailed information about the casualties who were transferred to the hospital.

The Hong Kong Control Post is located next to the command posts of other government departments and the organizing committee. Information about the number of casualties and the condition and designation of individual patients can be shared with other parties in real time. The organizing committee can then provide real-time information about the number and designation of casualties to the media upon request.

Table 3 First-Aid Post Equipment

Automatic external defibrillator (AED)
Oxygen regulating system with D-size oxygen cylinders
Bag valve mask and face masks
Bottled distilled water
Portable stretchers
Chairs
Tables
Towels
Blankets
RT machine
Signage for first-aid post
Pens and patient record forms

Table 4 First-Aid Kit Contents

Pocket mask
Elastic bandages
Tape scissors
Dressing pads
Disposable dressing kits
Turpentine
Pens and papers for record collection
Latex gloves
Bandages
Skin disinfectants
Adhesive bandages
Triangular bandages
Gauze pads
Cold pack
Disposable gloves
Surgical masks

Table 5 Sick Bay Medical Equipment

Automatic external defibrillator (AED)
Pocket mask + filter
Portable sphygmomanometer
Electrical automatic sphygmomanometer (Dinamap)
Stethoscopes
Pen torch
Glucometer and strips
Electrical thermometer and disposable caps
Tourniquet
Scissors
Dressing kits
Oxygen tanks (D-size and K-size)
Oxygen regulation system
Nasal cannula
Oxygen extension tubing
Oxygen masks and non-rebreather masks
Laryngeal mask airways
Laryngoscope and disposable blades
Endotracheal tubes, stylette, elastic gum bougie, disposable tube holders
Adult Magill forceps
Artery forceps
KY jelly
Portable suction
Bacterial filters
Bag valve mask and face masks
Oro- and naso-pharyngeal airways
Pulse oximeter
Syringes (3 mL, 5 mL, 10 mL)
Angiocaths (16 G, 18 G, and 20 G)
Intravenous fluid pump sets
Intravenous fluid infusion sets
Normal saline for intravenous use, 500 mL and 1 L
5% dextrose for intravenous use, 500 mL
50% dextrose for intravenous use
Water for injection
Syringes (3 mL, 5 mL, 10 mL)
3-way connector
Kidney dish and gallipots

Foley catheter
Glucose-electrolyte drink
Super York IV stretcher
Long spinal board
Sharp boxes
Alcohol swabs
Disposable & sterile gloves
Surgical masks
Micropore tape
Duoderm
Primapore dressing
Adhesive bandages
Triangular bandages
Elastoplasts
Tegaderm
Cotton wool & gauze swab
Cold pack
Wooden applicator & tongue depressor
Medications: paracetamol tablets, TNG tab, Ventolin puff
CPR resuscitation drugs: adrenaline, atropine sulphate, dextrose D50, chlorpheniramine maleate BP (Piriton), Voltaren injection, Lignocaine

Medical Case Studies from the Hong Kong Marathon

Dr. LAM Kin Kwan & Dr. Marcus FUNG

Preparation

Over the past ten years, the number of marathon participants has been increasing, as has the number of injuries. The pre-hospital environment is a challenge to medical staff because of unfamiliar working environments and limited medical supplies. Literature on the epidemiology of common injuries related to marathon running is limited. Equipment provisions are based on limited reports provided by first responders over the years. Overseas lessons always provide valuable information for the optimal planning of medical support.

First-aid Posts

Two kinds of first-aid posts are set up by the Auxiliary Medical Service (AMS) during the marathon. Most are essentially first-aid posts managed by first responders. Two selected first-aid posts are designated as medical tents to accommodate more serious cases and the expected large number of encounters. They are located at the Kowloon end of the Western Harbour Tunnel and near the finish line. Extra medical and nursing staff and first responders are deployed to these medical tents.

Medical Tents at the Finish Line

A triage system and zoning approach are used in the medical tents to manage multiple injuries and conditions. This approach is modified from the Advanced Trauma Life Support (ATLS) proposed by the American College of Surgeons. The cases are triaged to receive service in either the red, yellow, or green zones. Patients who need urgent resuscitation are treated in the red zone. Those who have unstable conditions are treated in the yellow zone. Minor injuries and mild conditions are managed in the green zone.

In the yellow and red zones, patients are treated on portable beds with medical equipment close to the beds for easy access. Super York IV ambulance stretchers are used in the red zone so that patients can be elevated to receive treatment in appropriate positions. Moreover, the stretchers also have the advantage of rapid transfer and loading directly to ambulances without the need of changing beds.

Typical Cases Encountered during the Marathon

The following are typical cases encountered during the marathon.

Case 1: *Hypothermia*
A 28-year-old lean woman complained of dizziness after running for two hours on a cool day.
The initial vital signs were: blood pressure 105/70 mmHg; pulse 65 beats/min; Glasgow Coma Scale 15/15; temperature 34.6°C.
She was shivering and had cold extremities.
She was insulated with a blanket and then took a warm sports drink. She was continuously monitored and was discharged 30 minutes later. Her temperature returned to 36.2°C before discharge.

Marathons require prolonged running activity. Runners usually wear insufficient clothing but are exposed to increased wind chill factors.[1,2] They are also dehydrated and exhausted near the end of a long race. Patients with mild hypothermia (33–35°C) should be removed from the cold. They can be safely re-warmed with appropriate insulation, such as blankets, in the non-hospital setting. They feel comfortable after drinking warm sports drinks and can be safely discharged soon thereafter.

Moderate hypothermia (31–32°C) or severe hypothermia (<31°C) are less often encountered in the Hong Kong Marathon. These patients should be continuously monitored for arrhythmia and hypotension. Intravenous rehydration and treatment of arrhythmia should be done as indicated. Patients should be transferred to a hospital for re-warming.

Case 2: *Hypoglycemia*

A 54-year-old man was confused after he crossed the finish line. He was disoriented and aggressive to the medical personnel.

The vital signs were: blood pressure 145/90 mmHg; pulse 110 beats/min; Glasgow Coma Scale 13/15; temperature 35.8°C.

The hemoglucostix was 3 mmol/L (Reference range: 3.9–6.1 mmol/L).

Intravenous glucose (40mL of 50% dextrose solution) was infused.

He gradually returned to full consciousness and his vitals became normal. He then drank sweet sports drinks and was discharged one hour later.

Hypoglycemia should be considered for patients with altered mental status.[3] When marathon runners present with dizziness or confusion, a glucometer should rapidly be used to detect the glucose status. For mild hypoglycemia, the patients are conscious but may present with sweating, headaches, and tremors. They recover after drinking a glucose-electrolyte solution. However, semiconscious or unconscious patients need urgent intravenous glucose administration. Hospital admission is indicated if the patient does not regain consciousness after correction of hypoglycemia.

Case 3: *Heat exhaustion*

A 35-year-old man complained of dizziness, weakness, and leg cramps after running for two hours on a warm and humid day.

The vital signs were: blood pressure 130/89 mmHg; pulse 105 beats/min; Glasgow Coma Scale 15/15; temperature 39.0°C.

The hemoglucostix was normal.

He was irrational and shouted at nurses. He took off his T-shirt and sat on a stretcher, but he refused to lie down.

After resting for a moment in a cool place, he drank a sports drink. His temperature lowered to 37.8°C after 45 minutes. In the end, he apologized for his initial behavior and was accompanied home by a friend.

Marathon runners have high metabolic rates, which may cause high body temperatures.[4,5] After cessation of exercise and appropriate cooling, the temperature usually returns to normal. These heat exhaustion patients usually do not require hospital admission. However, in case of heat stroke with a temperature above 41°C and neurological symptoms, rapid cooling and intravenous fluid replacement are important. The patient usually needs urgent hospital admission.

Case 4: *Exercise-associated collapse*

A 60-year-old man was escorted by two runners to a medical tent after completing the marathon. All of them were overseas medical doctors. The patient collapsed a moment after he crossed the finish line. He complained of dizziness, nausea, and weakness.

The vital signs were: blood pressure 90/60 mmHg; pulse 60 beats/min; Glasgow Coma Scale 14/15; temperature 38.2°C.

The hemoglucostix was 7.3 mmol/L. He also had leg cramps.

He was lying supine on a stretcher with legs elevated. Two doctors were stretching his limbs. After five minutes, his blood pressure returned to 115/85 mmHg. He felt better and drank a cup of warm sports drink. He recovered well, walked unaided 30 minutes after arrival and left the tent with his friends. His vitals were normal at discharge.

Exercise-associated collapse is a common medical condition presented to the medical tent after the finish line. This could be caused by post-exercise hypotension in marathon runners.[8] This postural hypotension is due to pooling of blood in the lower limbs. Patients are treated by lying in the Trendelenburg position with pelvis and legs elevated above the level of heart.[9] This restores the right atrial filling pressure and reverses vasodilatation caused by the Barcroft-Edholm reflex.[10] In this way, most athletes with this problem will recover within 30 minutes and do not require hospitalization.

Case 5: *Runner's diarrhea*

A 26-year-old woman complained of abdominal colicky pain. The pain started during running and persisted after she completed the race.

The initial vital signs were: blood pressure 110/85 mmHg; pulse 95 beats/min; Glasgow Coma Scale 15/15; temperature 37.2°C.

An abdominal examination showed increased bowel sound.

She felt better after passing stool later.

Diarrhea and abdominal colic are frequent in long-distance runners.[11] Relative intestinal ischemia, increased intestinal mobility, and anxiety associated with competition may be contributing factors.[12] These athletes often do not seek further medical attention, so it is important to rule out other serious causes of abdominal pain. The simple "runner's diarrhea" can be treated with dietary advice and anti-spasmodics.

Case 6: *Cardiac arrest*
A middle-aged man collapsed just before the finish line. He had no pulse, but he exhibited shallow breathing.
Cardiopulmonary resuscitation (CPR) was started immediately. Bag-valve-mask ventilation with high-flow oxygen and chest compressions were provided by an AMS medical team. The automated external defibrillator (AED) was attached which showed "No Shock Indicated."
The patient had a spontaneous return of circulation three minutes later and was escorted by doctors to the closest hospital. He made good recovery in the cardiac care unit and was neurologically intact at discharge.

Sudden cardiac arrest is uncommon but a serious cause of collapse.[13] Coronary artery disease is the most common cause of exercise-related deaths in athletes over 35 years of age.[14] Hypertrophic cardiomyopathy is a common cause of cardiac death in young athletes.[15] High-quality CPR should be delivered immediately. An AED will defibrillate ventricular fibrillations and pulseless ventricular tachycardia. CPR, AED, and prompt initiation of advanced cardiac life support improve the chance of survival of cardiac arrest victims.[16] Further discussion can be found in Chapter 15 of this book.

Observations

Most medical cases treated during the marathon are minor conditions and are treated on site. However, some runners need urgent attention and resuscitation, and a number of the more severe cases are transferred to the nearest Accident and Emergency Department, which has been on alert for the event. Close communication with the command post and headquarters of the Auxiliary Medical Service, the organizers, and the receiving public hospitals has been shown to enhance smooth operations of the marathon's medical and first-aid services over the years.

References

1. Armstrong LE, Epstein Y, Greenleaf JE, Haymes EM, Hubbard RW, Roberts WO, et al. 1996. American College of Sports Medicine position stand. Heat and cold illnesses during distance running. *Med Sci Sports Exerc* 28 (12): i–x.

2. Castellani JW, Young AJ, Ducharme MB, Giesbrecht GG, Glickman E, Sallis RE, et al. 2006. American College of Sports Medicine position stand: prevention of cold injuries during exercise. *Med Sci Sports Exerc* 38 (11): 2012–29.

3. Malouf R, Brust JCM. 1985. Hypoglycemia: causes, neurological manifestations, and outcome. *Ann Neurol* 17 (5): 421–30.

4. American College of Sports Medicine, Armstrong LE, Casa DJ, Millard-Stafford M, Moran DS, Pyne SW. 2007. American College of Sports Medicine position stand. Exertional heat illness during training and competition. *Med Sci Sports Exerc* 39 (3): 556–72.

5. Noakes TD, Myburgh KH, du Plessis J, Lang L, Lambert M, van der Riet C, et al. 1991. Metabolic rate, not percent dehydration, predicts rectal temperature in marathon runners. *Med Sci Sports Exerc* 23 (4): 443–49.

6. Armstrong LE, Crago AE, Adams R, Roberts WO, Maresh CM. 1996. Whole-body cooling of hyperthermic runners: comparison of two field therapies. *Am J Emerg Med* 14 (4): 355–58.

7. Roberts WO. 2007. Heat and cold: What does the environment do to marathon injury? *Sports Med* 37 (4–5): 400–403.

8. Holtzhausen LM, Noakes TD. 1995. The prevalence and significance of post-exercise (postural) hypotension in ultramarathon runners. *Med Sci Sports Exerc* 27 (12): 1595–1601.

9. Holtzhausen LM, Noakes TD. 1997. Collapsed ultraendurance athlete: proposed mechanisms and an approach to management. *Clin J Sport Med* 7 (4): 292–301.

10. Noakes TD. 2003. The forgotten Barcroft/Edholm reflex: potential role in exercise-associated collapse. *Br J Sports Med* 37 (3): 277–78.

11. Rao SS, Beaty J, Chamberlain M, Lambert PG, Gisolfi C. 1999. Effects of acute graded exercise on human colonic motility. *Am J Physiol* 276 (5 Pt 1): G1221–6.

12. Rao SS, Hatfield RA, Suls JM, Chamberlain MJ. 1998. Psychological and physical stress induce differential effects on human colonic motility. *Am J Gastroenterol* 93 (6): 985–90.

13. Garson A Jr. 1998. Arrhythmias and sudden cardiac death in elite athletes. American College of Cardiology, 16th Bethesda Conference. *Pediatr Med Chir* 20 (2): 101–103.

14. Wike J, Kernan M. 2005. Sudden cardiac death in the active adult: causes, screening, and preventive strategies. *Curr Sports Med Rep* 4 (2): 76–82.

15. Link MS, Homoud MK, Wang PJ, Estes NA. 2001. Cardiac arrhythmias in the athlete. *Cardiol Rev* 9 (1): 21–30.

16. International Liaison Committee on Resuscitation. 2005. *2005 International consensus on Cardiopulmonary Resuscitation and Emergency Cardiovascular Care science with treatment recommendations.* 112:IV–57–IV–66.

Evaluation of the 2007 AMS Sports Injuries Course

Dr. Marcus FUNG, Dr. WAI Heung On & Dr. Ben FONG

The AMS Sports Injuries Course: An Introduction

The Sports Injuries Certificate Course has been conducted for Auxiliary Medical Service (AMS) members annually since 2004. The purpose of this course is to provide additional training for front-line members involved in sports-related first-aid duties, like the Hong Kong Marathon and Trailwalker. The certificate course lasts three evenings and the 2007 course outline is tabulated in Table 1. Lectures are given by AMS doctors and physiotherapists. So far, more than 300 members have passed this certificate course.

Table 1 Course Outline of the 2007 Sports Injuries Course

Day 1	Introduction of common causes of sports injuries
	Sports medicine—an introduction
Day 2	Physiotherapy management of sports injuries
	Hyperthermia and hypothermia
	Metabolism and electrolyte imbalance
	Management of blisters
Day 3	First-aid management of common sports injuries
	Examination

Evaluation of the 2007 AMS Sports Injuries Course

Introduction

The aim of this study was to investigate the change in self-perceived understanding and ability in managing common sports injuries before and after the 2007 AMS Sports Injuries Course.

Methods

This was a self-reported questionnaire study that included two parts. Part 1 was completed at the beginning of the course and Part 2 was completed at the end of the course. The purpose and the design of this study were explained to participants at the beginning of the course. All members who took the 2007 Sports Injuries Certificate Course were invited to participate in this study. The study was conducted anonymously. If the members did not want to participate, they just needed to return the blank questionnaire.

Each questionnaire (Appendix 1) of Part 1 was numbered (1–150) and randomly distributed to members. Members were requested to record the questionnaire number because they needed to collect and complete Part 2 of the same questionnaire at the end of the course.

The information collected in Part 1 included the experience of managing common sports injuries over the previous twelve months, participants' self-perceived ability and competence in managing common sports injuries, participants' background, and two main purposes for taking the course.

Part 2 of the questionnaire (Appendix 2) mainly focused on self-perceived ability and competence in managing common sports injuries after the completion of the course.

The data were collected and entered into an Excel file and then analyzed with the statistical software SPSS version 13.0 (SPSS Inc. Chicago, Illinois, USA). The descriptive data were tabulated and a paired *t*-test was used to test for statistically significant differences in self-perceived ability and competence in managing common sports injuries before and after the course.

Results

Among the 133 questionnaires distributed, 130 were completed and returned. The response rate was 97.7%. Among the participants, 58.5% were male and 41.5% were female. Most of them (93.1%) were rank-and-file members. During the previous twelve months before the study, the mean number of sports-related duties taken by the participants was 4.4, and only 20 participants did not have experience in sports-related duties.

The participants' mean years of service in AMS was 7.32, and the range was 1–33 years. Figures 1 and 2 summarize the years of service in AMS and the highest education attained by the participants, respectively. The participants' main purposes for taking the course were preparation of AMS duties and increased personal knowledge.

The participants' experience in managing common sports injuries during the twelve months before the course is summarized in Figure 3. Participants' self-perceived ability and competence in managing common sports injuries before and after the course are summarized in Figures 4 and 5, respectively. There were statistically significant changes in participants' self-perceived ability and competence in managing strain ($p=0.002$), hypoglycemia ($p=0.010$), electrolyte imbalance ($p<0.001$), and coma ($p=0.016$) after the course.

Discussion

The response rate of this study was high, despite the fact that this was the first time a self-reported questionnaire was used to study the change of self-perceived ability and competence in managing common sports injuries before and after the sports injuries course. This might be due to the participants' understanding that the information collected could be useful for planning future courses. Also, as the study was conducted anonymously, participants could express themselves without much concern. As the questions were simple and direct, most members could answer them without much difficulty.

By the end of this course, participants had significantly higher self-perceived ability and competence in managing strain, hypoglycemia, electrolyte imbalance, and coma. In their usual first aid training, management of these types of conditions was less emphasized compared to CPR and the management of wounds and fractures. However, these sports injuries conditions were more common or critical in the Hong Kong Marathon or Trailwalker. The Sports Injuries Course will enhance participants' knowledge; however, some might not have the chance to take up duties in these major events, despite the mean number of sports-related duties taken by participants. Furthermore, doctors and physiotherapists using clinical cases and pictures could enhance understanding of how to manage these sports injuries.

Conclusion

After the 2007 AMS Sports Injuries Course, participants improved their ability and competency to manage common sports injuries, especially the management of strain, hypoglycemia, electrolyte imbalance, and coma.

Figure 1 Participants' Years of Service in AMS

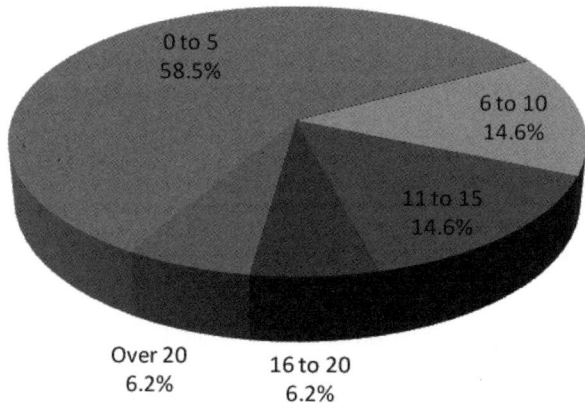

Figure 2 Participants' Highest Education Level Attained

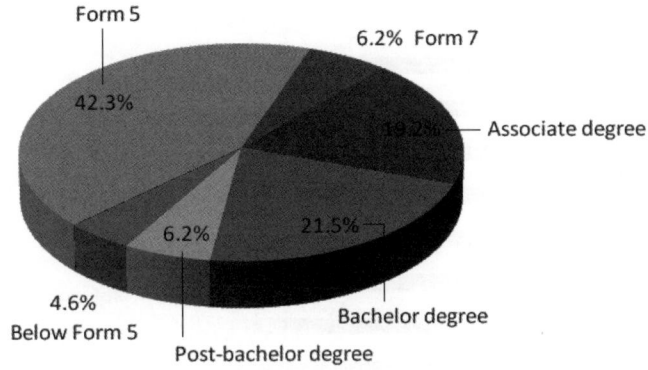

Figure 3 Participants' Experience Managing Common Sports Injuries

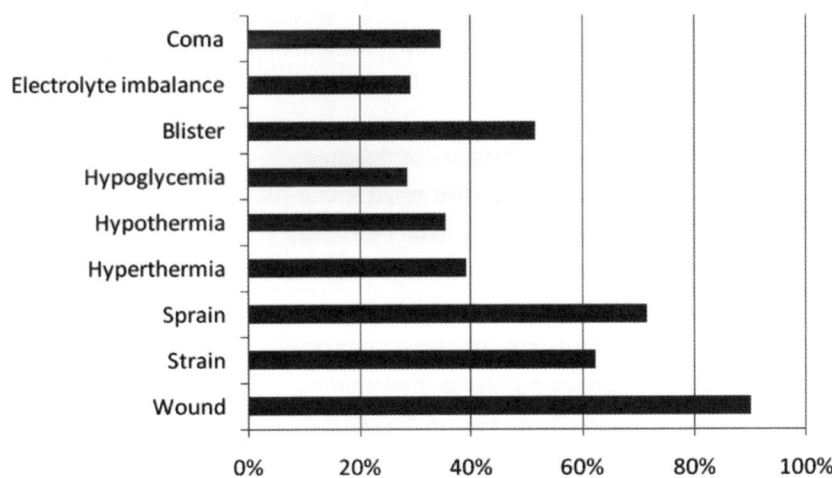

Figure 4 Participants' Self-Reported Ability and Competence Managing Common Sports Injuries Before the Course

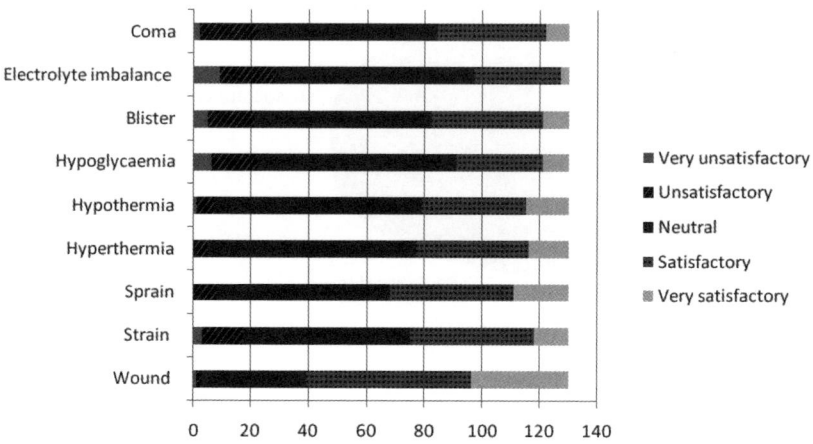

Figure 5 Participants' Self-Reported Ability and Competence Managing Common Sports Injuries After the Course

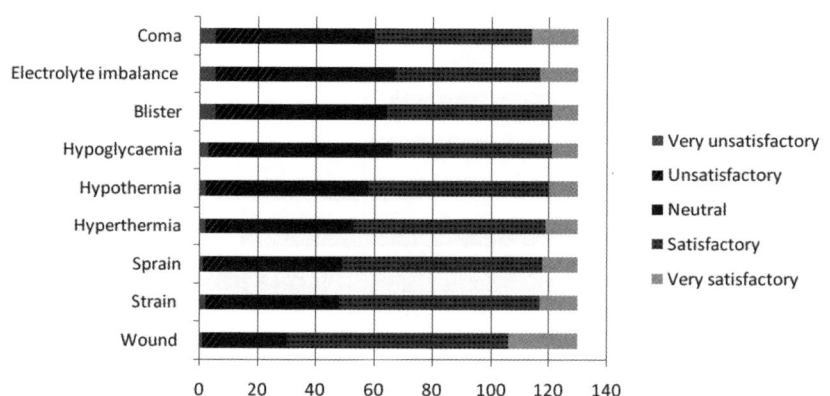

Appendix 1

Part 1 Questionnaire (to be completed at the beginning of the course)

醫療輔助隊運動創傷證書課程問卷調查

<u>第1部份</u>

1. 你有否在過往的12個月參與跟運動有關的當值？ 有／沒有

2. 如過往的12個月你曾參與跟運動有關的當值，你的總當值次數為_____次

3. 在你跟運動有關的當值時，你有否遇見過以下的情況？請同時列出你覺得你對以下各種情況的理解及處理能力。

情況	經驗	理解及處理能力				
傷口處理	有／ 沒有	1	/ 2	/ 3	/ 4	/ 5
拉傷	有／ 沒有	1	/ 2	/ 3	/ 4	/ 5
扭傷	有／ 沒有	1	/ 2	/ 3	/ 4	/ 5
體溫過高	有／ 沒有	1	/ 2	/ 3	/ 4	/ 5
體溫過低	有／ 沒有	1	/ 2	/ 3	/ 4	/ 5
血糖過低	有／ 沒有	1	/ 2	/ 3	/ 4	/ 5
水泡處理	有／ 沒有	1	/ 2	/ 3	/ 4	/ 5
電解質不平衡	有／ 沒有	1	/ 2	/ 3	/ 4	/ 5
失去知覺／昏迷	有／ 沒有	1	/ 2	/ 3	/ 4	/ 5

（1）十分不理想／ （2）不理想／ （3）一般／ （4）理想／ （5）十分理想

4. 你參加本課程的主要目的是（最多2個）

1	消閒
2	為有關當值作準備
3	為個人／朋友比賽作準備
4	增進知識
5	與正職相關
6	個人興趣
7	隊長推薦參加
8	其他原因：_____

5. 你在AMS服務的總年份為_____年

6. 你的性別是　男／女

7. 你在AMS服務的職級是

1	一級長官
2	二級長官
3	三級長官
4	三級以上長官

8. 你的最高學歷為

1	中五以下
2	中五
3	中七
4	大專
5	大學學士
6	大學學士以上

*** 問卷完，多謝你的積極參與 ***

Appendix 2

Part 2 Questionnaire (to be completed at the end of the course)

醫療輔助隊運動創傷證書課程問卷調查

第2部份

請列出你覺得你對以下各種情況的理解及處理能力。

情況	經驗	理解及處理能力
傷口處理	有／沒有	1 ／ 2 ／ 3 ／ 4 ／ 5
拉傷	有／沒有	1 ／ 2 ／ 3 ／ 4 ／ 5
扭傷	有／沒有	1 ／ 2 ／ 3 ／ 4 ／ 5
體溫過高	有／沒有	1 ／ 2 ／ 3 ／ 4 ／ 5
體溫過低	有／沒有	1 ／ 2 ／ 3 ／ 4 ／ 5
血糖過低	有／沒有	1 ／ 2 ／ 3 ／ 4 ／ 5
水泡處理	有／沒有	1 ／ 2 ／ 3 ／ 4 ／ 5
電解質不平衡	有／沒有	1 ／ 2 ／ 3 ／ 4 ／ 5
失去知覺／昏迷	有／沒有	1 ／ 2 ／ 3 ／ 4 ／ 5

（1）十分不理想／ （2）不理想／ （3）一般／ （4）理想／ （5）十分理想

*** 問卷完，多謝你的積極參與 ***

SECTION III

Advice to Serious Runners

Potential Medical Problems in Marathon Runners

Dr. SIA Yin-Shan Jacky

Introduction

Running is regarded as one of the easiest ways to exercise and marathon is considered to be the most challenging and exciting. It is the holistic achievement of endurance, courage, balance, running strategy, and nutritional tactics. Despite the fact that most problems are musculoskeletally-related, medical problems related to marathons should not be ignored.

Medical Problems

1. Exercise-associated collapse

Exercise-associated collapse (EAC) is the result of interactions between the runner and the environmental conditions, and can include dehydration, exhaustion, hyperthermia, and hypothermia. Clinical features include dizziness, nausea, blurred vision, chest discomfort, blackout, and syncope. EAC is very common during marathons.[1] Some authors have proposed that the definition of EAC should be reserved for those runners with no other identifiable cause for their collapse and who recover within 30 minutes.[2] A diagnostic classification matrix was developed by W. O. Roberts (Table 1).[3] It allows the on-site physician or paramedics to make a prompt assessment based on the mental status and the vital signs of the athlete. One study has found that EAC occurs most commonly about 3.5 hours after the start, i.e., the time that most runners finish the event.[1] The sudden cessation of running is proposed to be one of the precipitating factors for EAC due to activation of the vagal tone. This is especially true when runners compete in hot and humid weather. Immediate management includes rest, leg elevation, and oral or intravenous rehydration. If the condition does not improve after 30 minutes, or if it deteriorates, the runner has to be transferred to the hospital for further evaluation and treatment. Those who collapse before the finish line are more likely to have other medical problems.[3,4]

Table 1 Exercise-Associated Collapse Classification Matrix

	Mild	Moderate	Severe
Clinical features	Conscious	No oral intake	Mental changes including confusion and syncope
	Able to walk with or without assistance	Excessive fluid loss, e.g., sweating, vomiting	
		Muscle cramp and spasm	
		Not able to walk	
Hypothermia	T°C ≤ 36°C	T°C ≤ 35°C	T°C ≤ 32°C
Normothermia	36°C ≤ T°C ≤ 39.5°C		
Hyperthermia	T°C ≥ 39.5°C	T°C ≥ 40.5°C	T°C ≥ 41°C

2. Headache

Headache is another common medical problem related to marathons. Most runners may experience headaches of different severities during training or competition. The pathophysiology of running-related headaches is complex and multi-factorial, including the interaction of neurotransmitters, vascular dilatation, and perivascular inflammation.

There are different types of headaches, including migraines, cluster headaches, tension headaches, and exertional headaches. Most marathon-related headaches are exertional. According to the International Headache Society Classification, an exertional headache is defined as a headache that occurs when the runner starts. The onset is gradual, and it increases in severity as running continues. Nevertheless, there are many risk factors that precipitate or increase the severity of the headache, including:

- diet: dehydration, alcohol, caffeine, nicotine
- medical issues: cardiac problems, hypoglycemia, hypertension

- drugs: nitrates, hydralazine, thermogenic agents, steroids (e.g., oral contraceptive pills)

Pain is usually resolved four to six hours after cessation of running. Hence, most cases are self-limiting, but it has been estimated that 10% of cases have intracranial pathologies such as a tumor or aneurysm. Medical attention should be sought if one notices that the headache is getting worse, sudden blasting in nature, or associated with neurological symptoms.[5]

3. Heat-related illness

Heat-related illness represents a collection of medical conditions including heat cramp, heat syncope, heat exhaustion, and heat stroke. The first three are relatively benign, whereas the last could be fatal. A study has shown that the temperature of post-marathon runners is consistently high.[6] One study found that runners suffer from hyperthermia (rectal temperature above 40°C) even when the ambient temperature is around 4°C–11°C.[1] This implies that prolonged running increases body temperature substantially. However, it is unclear whether these athletes took medication, such as aspirin, that raises metabolic rate. Most heat-related illnesses can be treated with rest or oral or intravenous rehydration. A heat stroke case was found in the 2007 Hong Kong Marathon, and is reported by Dr K. H. Szeto in Chapter 10.

4. Cardiac problems

Cardiac problems—such as rhythm disturbances, cardiogenic syncope, or even cardiac arrest—do occur in runners, despite relatively few incidences. Further details are elaborated in Chapter 15, by Dr. John Wong.

5. Respiratory problems

There are two main respiratory problems that are important and life-threatening. One is called exercise-induced asthma (EIA) and the other is known as non-cardiogenic pulmonary edema (NCPE).

Exercise-induced asthma is defined as a bronchospasm that occurs soon after the runner starts. Patients with asthma or allergic rhinitis are more prone to have EIA.[5] Two theories have been proposed as triggering factors. One is the hyperosmolarity theory and the other is the thermal expenditure theory. The pathophysiological mechanism is shown in Figure 1.[6,7] The former theory is the most widely accepted one and claims that EIA occurs typically after 5 to 20 minutes of running and can last for 20 to 60 minutes. The runner inhales cooled air that induces histamine released from mast cells and subsequently causes bronchospasms. In addition, ventilation-perfusion mismatch, alveolo-arterial oxygen tension discrepancy, and physiological dead space are all increased in asthmatics during exercise without medication. Other high-intensity physical exertion, such as cross-country skiing, ice skating, and ice hockey, are particularly dangerous. The thermal expenditure theory explains why runners present with persistent shortness of breath even after the event has stopped. Despite these theories, studies have not shown any difference in cardio-pulmonary response in asthmatics compared to non-asthmatic subjects.[8,9]

Clinical features of EIA include dry cough, irritated cough, chest tightness, fatigue, breathing difficulty, and wheezing. The administration of inhaled or oral beta 2 agonist 30 to 60 minutes before the marathon could prevent EIA from occurring.[5,7,10,11]

Non-cardiogenic pulmonary edema (NCPE) is another important respiratory problem. Clinical presentations include nausea, vomiting, headache, pinkish frothy sputum, severe respiratory distress, or even respiratory arrest. Death has been reported due to brain herniation.[12] This life-threatening edema is directly related to hyponatremia, which in turn is associated with other risk factors.[13] One proposed mechanism is the preferential distribution of blood into the working muscle when one starts to run. When one stops, a large volume of blood will be returned to the gut causing hyponatremia. Clinical severity depends on the serum sodium level and is categorized as mild (130–135 mmol/L), moderate (120–130 mmol/L), and severe (below 120 mmol/L) hyponatremia.[13] Symptoms vary from asymptomatic in mild cases to cerebral edema and NCPE in severe cases. Latter cases should be sent to the hospital and treated promptly by intravenous hypertonic saline.[12]

Figure 1 The patho-physiological mechanism for exercise induced asthma

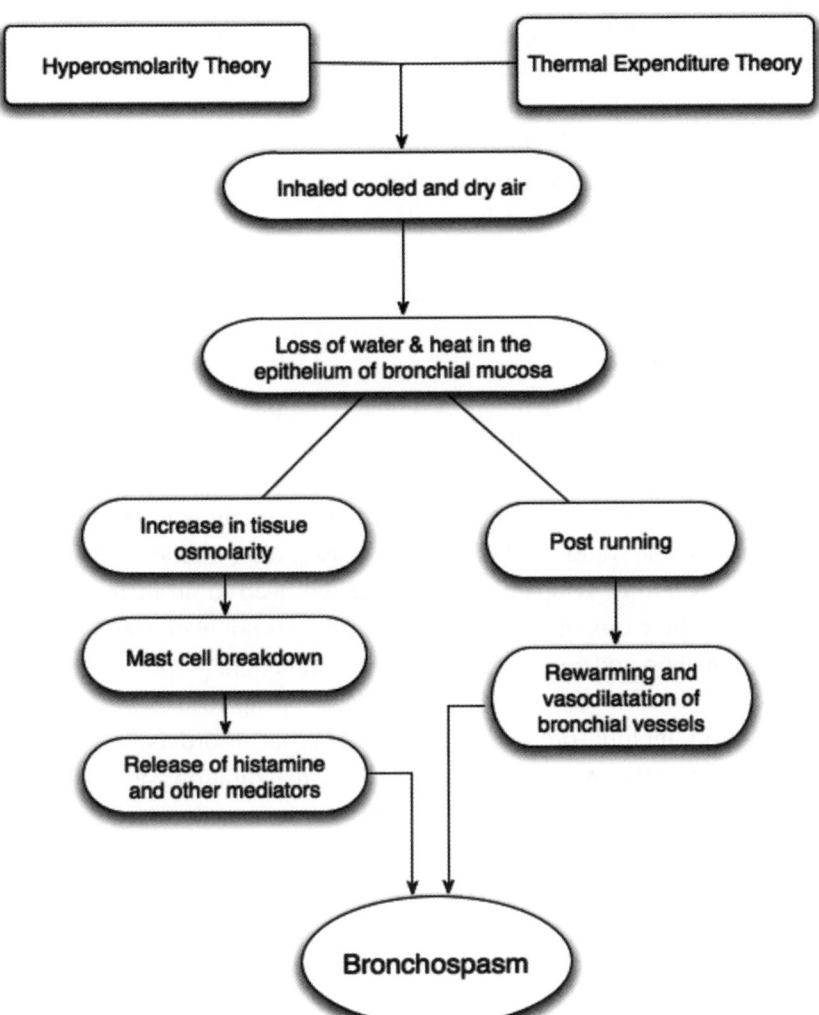

6. Gastrointestinal problems

Gastrointestinal disturbance is common (30% to 80%) in runners. Presentation is variable, including belching, nausea, abdominal pain, diarrhea, colitis, and even gastrointestinal bleeding.[2,14]

Abdominal pain is commonly reported in young and inexperienced runners.[15] Reasons for the pain are multi-factorial. First, it has been postulated that anxiety and stress could be precipitating factors. The second reason is hypoperfusion and ischemia of the gut, due to the shunting of blood to the working muscle.[16,17] The third precipitating factor is the release of hormones such as vasoactive intestinal peptide and prostaglandins (PG).[18] Finally, mechanical strain to the gut, causing mild shearing force, is also proposed.[15]

Diarrhea is frequently noted in runners. The pathophysiology is due to the increase in colonic motility after exercise and is directly related to the intensity of the exercise. During running, blood is shunted to the muscle, resulting in a slowdown of gut motility. The contraction is further inhibited by sympathetic activation. When running ceases, redistribution of the blood and the cessation of sympathetic discharge will lead to an increase in gut activity and, therefore, diarrhea develops.[19] There is no relationship between this phenomenon and age or fiber or milk consumption.[16]

Occult blood in the stool has been reported up to 87%.[20,21] Precipitating factors include pre-existing gastrointestinal disorders, use of non-steroidal anti-inflammatory drugs (NSAIDs), dehydration, non-occlusive mesenteric ischemia, and repetitive mechanical strain to the viscera.

Bloody diarrhea is usually self-limiting within 24 to 48 hours, and the patient recovers after conservative treatment.[22] It is not contraindicated for runners to continue training. However, if the symptoms persist after two days, medical consultation should be sought so as to discover any underlying pathology.

7. Hepatic problem

There is no contraindication for a chronic hepatitis patient or mild acute viral hepatitis patient to participate in a marathon. However, liver enzymes, including serum glutamate oxaloacetate transaminase, alanine aminotransferase, aspartate aminotransferase, alkaline phosphatase, and bilirubin, may be elevated due to hepatic hypoperfusion. These runners should consult their doctors or appropriate specialists to monitor their enzyme levels. Fortunately, these enzymes will be restored to normal levels after seven days.[5]

8. Renal problems

Hematuria and proteinuria are two main marathon-related renal problems. Renal functions, including renal blood flow, glomerular filtration rate, sodium excretion, and urine flow rate, will be reduced during exercise, due to the shunting of blood. The blood could be glomerular or come from the lower urinary tract. Running will increase the body temperature, which in turn redistributes blood from the kidneys to the working muscle. Prolonged muscular activities induce lactic acidosis and hypoxic and ischemic damage to the kidneys. If the runner takes NSAIDs, such as ibuprofen, then this will further compromise the renal perfusion significantly. However, marathon-related hematuria and proteinuria are usually resolved spontaneously after cessation of running and with adequate rehydration. Acute renal failure and rhabdomyolysis have been reported.[23] The proposed pathophysiological mechanism is summarized in Figure 2.[24]

9. Electrolyte disturbance

Hyponatremia is a well-documented and widely studied aspect of the marathon.[25,26] Retrospective analysis and a literature search have shown that this condition is associated with multiple factors (Table 2).

Table 2 Risk Factors for Hyponatremia

Strong evidence	Equivocal evidence
Excessive fluid intake	Female
Weight gain after the race	Use of NSAIDs before or during the race
Long racing time	Amateur runner
High ambient temperature	Low body-mass index (< 20)
	Short distance between water stations

Figure 2 The patho-physiological mechanism for running induced hematuria. (Courtesy of Sia et al. HKJEM)

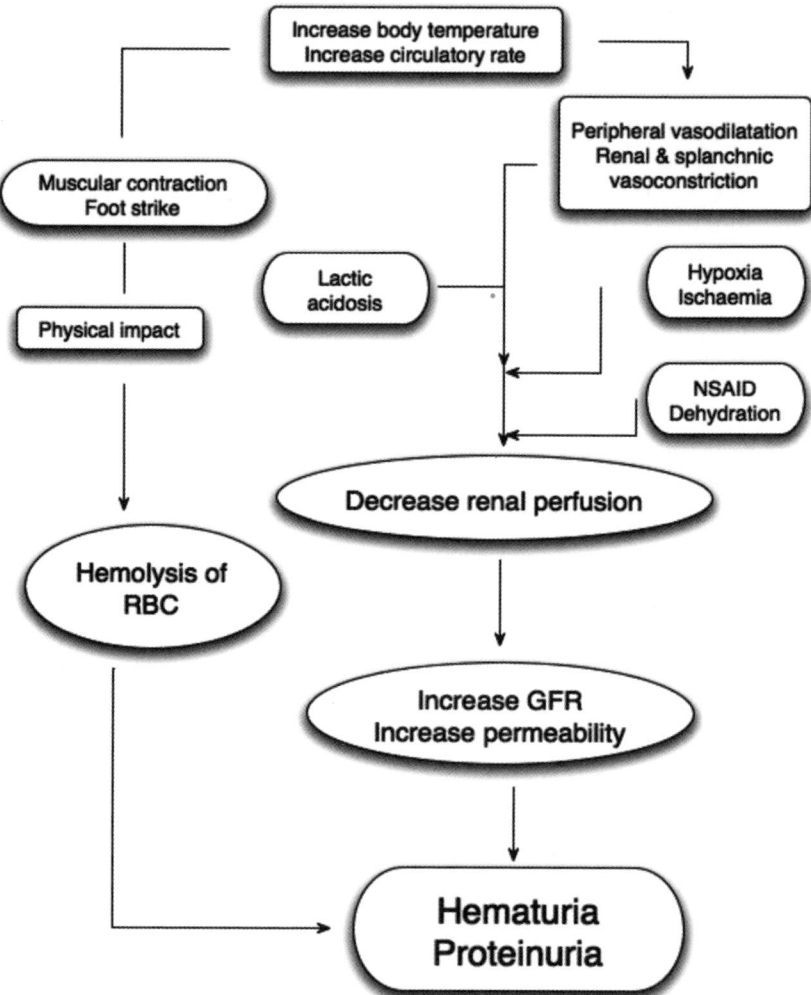

Figure 3 The relationship between numbers of cups of water consumed and hyponatremia

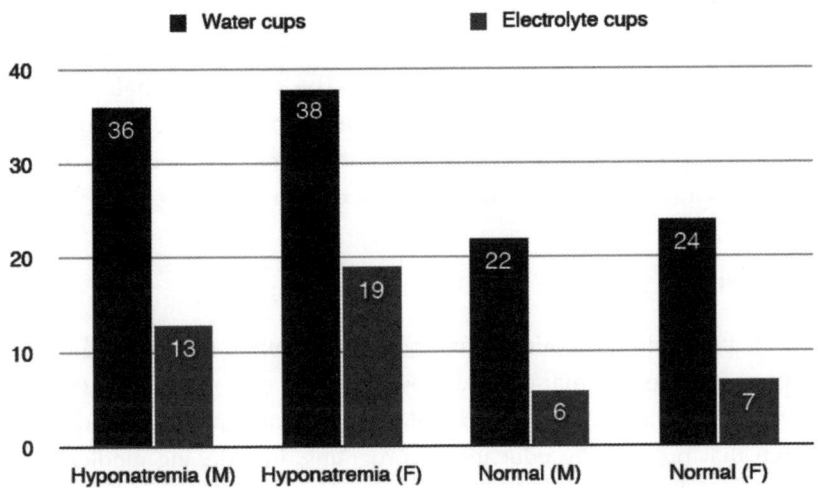

M: male

F: female

Over-consumption of water is undoubtedly one of the reasons. It has been found in the hyponatremic group more than the normal subjects (Figure 3). Similarly, weight gain after the marathon indicates excess water intake leading to hyponatremia.[13,27]

A long finishing time is considered to be another important factor. Runners who require more than four hours to finish the event are found to have the highest incidence of hyponatremia. Slow runners tend to drink water more than faster runners. This is especially true when runners compete in high ambient temperatures.[13] The longer that slower runners take to finish the marathon, the more likely they will be to drink excessively; the corollary is hyponatremia.[12,13,27,28] The ideal distance between water stations has been reported to be five kilometers, rather than 1.6 kilometers, to prevent iatrogenic hyponatremia.[2]

Non-steroidal anti-inflammatory drugs (NSAIDs) are believed to be a cause of hyponatremia. Runners use NSAIDs to blunt their pain response during marathons. It has been reported that as many as 30% of runners use NSAIDs for pain relief.[13,29] NSAIDs inhibit the release of PG, a natriuretic peptide responsible for vasodilatation, and depresses glomerular filtration rate. As a result, they impair water excretion and cause hyponatremia. In severe cases, acute renal failure results.[32] The shorter the half life of the NSAID, the more significantly negative effect it has on renal perfusion.[30,31] In addition, pre-existing renal disease, gender, lack of experience, and low body-mass index are also important risk factors for hyponatremia.[12,13,27-29]

Conclusion

This chapter delivers a brief summary of some important potential medical problems related to marathons. Most illnesses and mortalities could be prevented if both organizers and athletes adequately prepare. Studies have shown that preparatory educational programs, introducing medical problems before the marathon, decrease the incidence of adverse emergencies.[33] Detailed knowledge and anticipation of medical problems supported by scientific evidence are of paramount importance in reducing the morbidity and mortality of the event.

References

1. Roberts WO. 2000. A 12-yr profile of medical injury and illness for the Twin Cities marathon. *Med Sci Sports Exerc* 32 (9): 1549–55.

2. Sanchez LD, Corwell B, Berkoff D. 2006. Medical problems of marathon runners. *Am J Emerg Med* 24 (5): 608–15.

3. Roberts WO. 1989. Exercise-associated collapse in endurance events: a classification system. *Phys Sportsmed* 17 (5): 49–55.

4. Holtzhausen LM, Noakes TD, Kroning B, de Klerk M, Roberts M, Emsley R. 1994. Clinical and biochemical characteristics of collapsed ultra-marathon runners. *Med Sci Sports Exerc* 26 (9): 1095–1101.

5. Francis GOC, Roberts PW. 2001. *Textbook of running medicine.* New York: McGraw-Hill, Medical Publishing Division.

6. Cheuvront SN, Haymes EM. 2001. Thermoregulation and marathon running: biological and environmental influences. *Sports Med* 31 (10): 743–62.

7. Satta A. 2000. Exercise training in asthma. *J Sports Med Phys Fitness* 40 (4): 277–83.

8. Wilber RL, Rundell KW, Szmedra L, Jenkinson DM, Im I, Drake SD. 2000. Incidence of exercise-induced bronchospasm in Olympic winter sport athletes. *Med Sci Sports Exerc* 32 (4): 732–37.

9. Clark CJ. 1993. The role of physical training in asthma. *Principles and practice of pulmonary rehabilitation.* Ed. Casaburi R, Petty TL. Philadelphia: WB Saunders Co., 1993:424–38.

10. McFadden ER. 1984. Exercise performance in the asthmatic. *Am Rev Respir Dis* 129 (Supp): S84–7.

11. Tan RA, Spector SL. 1998. Exercise-induced asthma. *Sports Med* 25 (1): 1–6.

12. Ayus JC, Varon J, Arieff AI. 2000. Hyponatremia, cerebral edema, and noncardiogenic pulmonary edema in marathon runners. *Ann Intern Med* 132 (9): 711–14.

13. Hew TD, Chorley JN, Cianca JC, Divine JG. 2003. The incidence, risk factors, and clinical manifestations of hyponatremia in marathon runners. *Clin J Sport Med* 13 (1): 41–47.

14. Riddoch C, Trinick T. 1988. Gastrointestinal disturbances in marathon runners. *Br J Sports Med* 22 (2): 71–74.

15. Dimeo FC, Peter J, Guderian H. 2004. Abdominal pain in long distance runners: case report and analysis of the literature. *Br J Sports Med* 38 (5): e24.

16. Sullivan SN, Wong C. 1992. Runners' diarrhea. Different patterns and associated factors. *J Clin Gastroenterol* 14 (2): 101–104.

17. Gil SM, Yazaki E, Evans DF. 1998. Aetiology of running-related gastrointestinal dysfunction. How far is the finishing line? *Sports Med* 26 (6): 365–78.

18. MacLaren DP, Raine NM, O'Connor AM. 1995. Human gastrin and vasoactive intestinal polypeptide responses to endurance running in relation to training status and fluid ingested. *Clin Sci (Lond)* 89 (2): 137–43.

19. Rao SSC, Beaty J, Chamberlain M, Lambert PG, Gisolfi C. 1999. Effects of acute graded exercise on human colonic motility. *Am J Physiol* 276 (5 Pt 1): 1221–26.

20. Rudzki SJ, Hazard H, Collinson D. 1995. Gastrointestinal blood loss in triathletes: it's etiology and relationship to sports anaemia. *Aust J Sci Med Sport* 27 (1): 3–8.

21. Choi SC, Choi SJ, Kim JA, Kim TH, Nah YH, Yazaki E, et al. 2001. The role of gastrointestinal endoscopy in long-distance runners with gastrointestinal

symptoms. *Eur J Gastroenterol Hepatol* 13 (3): 1089–94.

22. Lucas W, Schroy PC 3rd. 1998. Reversible ischemic colitis in a high endurance athlete. *Am J Gastroenterol* 93 (11): 2231–34.

23. van Zyl-Smit R, Mills P, Vogelpoel L. 2000. Case report: unrecognized acute renal failure following the Comrades Marathon. *S Afr Med J* 90 (1): 39–40.

24. Sia JYS, Wong YT. 2005. Sweat and blood—runner's haematuria: discharge or further evaluate? *Hong Kong J Emerg Med* 12:32–35.

25. Speedy DB, Rogers IR, Noakes TD, Thompson JM, Guirey J, Safih S, et al. 2000. Diagnosis and prevention of hyponatremia at an ultradistance triathlon. *Clin J Sport Med* 10 (1): 52–58.

26. Speedy DB, Noakes TD, Rogers IR, Thompson JM, Campbell RG, Kuttner JA, et al. 1999. Hyponatremia in ultradistance triathletes. *Med Sci Sports Exerc* 31 (6): 809–15.

27. Almond CSD, Shin AY, Fortescue EB, Mannix RC, Wypij D, Binstadt BA, et al. 2005. Hyponatremia among runners in the Boston Marathon. *N Engl J Med* 352 (15): 1550–56.

28. Davis DP, Videen JS, Marino A, Vilke GM, Dunford JV, Van Camp SP, et al. 2001. Exercise-associated hyponatremia in marathon runners: a two-year experience. *J Emerg Med* 21 (1): 47–57.

29. Reid SA, Speedy DB, Thompson JM, Noakes TD, Mulligan G, Page T, et al. 2004. Study of hematological and biochemical parameters in runners completing a standard marathon. *Clin J Sport Med* 14 (6): 344–53.

30. Murray MD, Brater DC. 1990. Adverse effects of nonsteroidal anti-inflammatory drugs on renal function. *Ann Intern Med* 112 (8): 559–60.

31. Stürmer T, Erb A Keller F, Günther KP, Brenner H. 2001. Determinants of impaired renal function with use of non-steroidal anti-inflammatory drugs: the importance of half life and other medications. *Am J Med* 111 (7): 521–27.

32. MacSearraigh ETM, Kallmeyer JC, Schiff HB. 1979. Acute renal failure in marathon runners. *Nephron* 24 (5): 236–40.

33. Speedy DB, Thompson JM, Rodgers I, Collins M, Sharwood K, Noakes TD. 2002. Oral salt supplementation during ultradistance exercise. *Clin J Sport Med* 12 (5): 279–84.

Sudden Cardiovascular Death in Marathons

Dr. John T. WONG

Introduction

In Hong Kong, the number of both amateur and professional participants in certain commercially sponsored marathon events has soared during recent years. Although there has only been one marathon-associated sudden death over the past ten years, high participation levels have raised questions and concerns about the causes and frequency of such death during these sporting events. Sudden deaths in athletes are mostly caused by previously undiagnosed cardiovascular disease.[2-10]

The Benefits and Risks of Exercise

Regular aerobic exercise, particularly in the form of distance running, has become increasingly common and gained much interest as a public health initiative during the past decade.[11] Based on more than 40 observational epidemiological studies, physical inactivity and a sedentary lifestyle are recognized as major risk factors for the development of coronary artery disease (CAD), adverse cardiovascular events, and mortality.[12-24] Regular aerobic exercise, either during occupational or leisure time, confers many health benefits. It may reduce the risk for fatal and nonfatal myocardial infarction and other coronary events,[12-32] and it has been promoted as a national health agenda in several countries, including Hong Kong, for both primary and secondary prevention of cardiovascular disease.[19,21,27-31,33-34]

On the other hand, acute and vigorous physical exertion may trigger sudden death or myocardial infarction (MI)[3-4,7-10,35-43] in the presence of underlying heart disease,[3] especially in individuals not accustomed to such activity or regular exercise.[35-38,41-45] When sedentary individuals begin or restart an exercise program, there is a certain period of elevated risk during which exertion can provoke a cardiac event; such risk associated with habitual exercise in active individuals is relatively low.[35] Furthermore, it is generally assumed that particularly strenuous exertion or sports competition may predispose athletes to greater cardiac risk than non-strenuous physical activity. Nevertheless, there is abundant evidence that the overall benefits of exercise usually outweigh the associated risks.[12–34,38] Mechanisms by which exercise may protect patients from coronary events have also been proposed.[44–45]

The Risk of Sudden Cardiac Death in Athletes

The frequency with which sudden cardiac death (SCD) occurs in both young (under 35 years of age) and master athletes (over 35 years of age) is not precisely known. A few U.S. studies have reported the risk of sudden death due to undiagnosed cardiovascular disease in young high school and college-aged athletes as between 1 in 200,000 and 1 in 300,000 per academic year.[48–49] However, these studies have been criticized for underestimating such risk since they relied on reports from individual schools and institutions or on media accounts. A prospective population-based study in the Veneto region of Italy reported an incidence of sudden death of 2.3 (2.62 in males and 1.07 in females) per 100,000 athletes per year from all causes, and of 2.1 per 100,000 athletes per year from cardiovascular disease.[50]

The overall prevalence of sudden cardiac death associated with the U.S. marathon population was 0.002%,[40] much lower than other risk variables for premature death calculated in the general American population, namely CAD, automobile accidents, violence-related deaths, etc. The risk of sudden death from a single marathon race was estimated at about 1/100 of the annual overall risk associated with the activity of daily living, regardless of cardiac status. The only activity associated with a lower risk than marathon running was commercial airline travel, with a risk of death of about 0.0001%.

Therefore, although highly trained athletes such as marathon runners may harbor underlying and potential lethal disease, commonly of cardiovascular origin, the risk for SCD is extremely small. This low risk implies that routine preparticipation screening for cardiovascular disease may not be justified.

Causes of Sudden Cardiac Death in Athletes

Unlike athletes over 35 years of age, in whom atherosclerotic CAD is by far the most common cause of fatal events,[7-10] a variety of largely congenital but clinically unsuspecting cardiovascular diseases have been casually linked to sudden death in young trained athletes[2-6,52-59,85] (Figure 1). Essentially, any disease capable of causing sudden death in young people may potentially do so in young competitive athletes. However, it should be stressed that these cardiovascular disorders may be relatively common among young athletes dying suddenly. They are unusual in the general population. Moreover, disorders responsible for sudden death occur with different frequency.

Hypertrophic cardiomyopathy (HCM) and congenital coronary artery anomalies account for more than half of all sudden deaths, and most of the other conditions are responsible for less than 5% (Figure 1). Cardiovascular diseases causing SCD among young athletes include myocarditis (~7%); arrhythmogenic right ventricular dysplasia (~4%); atherosclerotic coronary artery disease (~3%); valvular heart disease, particularly aortic stenosis (~3%); tunneled coronary artery (~3%); and dilated cardiomyopathy (~2%).[2-59,85] A brief review of the more common and important ones is presented in the following section.

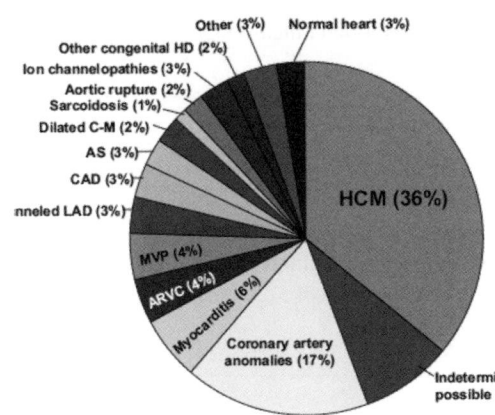

Figure 1[85] Distribution of cardiovascular causes of sudden death in 1435 young competitive athletes. From the Minneapolis Heart Institute Foundation Registry, 1980 to 2005. ARVC indicates arrhythmogenic right ventricular cardiomyopathy; AS, aortic stenosis; CAD, coronary artery diseases; C-M, cardiomyopathy; HD, heart disease; LAD, left anterior descending; LVH, left ventricular hypertrophy; and MVP, mitral valve prolapse.

Hypertrophic cardiomyopathy (HCM)

HCM has been implicated as the principal cause of sport-related cardiac arrest, accounting for more than 1/3 of sudden deaths in the U.S.[2-3,14,49,51,59,85] HCM is an inherited cardiac muscle disorder disease that affects sarcomeric proteins, resulting in small vessel disease, disorganized myocytes and myofibrillar configuration, and fibrosis with or without myocardial hypertrophy.

The expression of disease is age related, and usually occurs during or soon after periods of rapid somatic growth. Its clinical course in adults is usually benign in the majority of cases. Most affected individuals go unrecognized and are either asymptomatic or experience only paroxysmal manifestations.[67] Chronic symptoms such as exertional chest pain and dyspnea can be secondary to myocardial ischemia, diastolic dysfunction, congestive cardiac failure, or any combinations thereof. Symptoms tend to become worse gradually with age.

In general, it is standard practice to treat those patients who have survived cardiac arrest and/or experienced sustained or symptomatic ventricular arrhythmias (secondary prevention) using ICDs, because of the high risk of recurrence of these events.[68,71] Recognized markers for increased risk of sudden death is presented in Table 1.

Table 1 Recognized markers of increased risk of sudden death in HCM

Risk factors

For secondary prevention
- Previous episodes of cardiac arrest or haemodynamically significant ventricular arrhythmias[68,71]

For primary prevention
- Unexplained syncope[72]
- Family history of premature sudden death (< 45 years old)[64,72]
- Severe left ventricular hypertrophy > 3 cm[73-74]
- Non-sustained VT on Holter or exercise[75-76]
- Abnormal exertional blood pressure response (defined as a failure to either augment and/or sustain a systolic blood pressure of > 25 mm Hg above the resting systolic blood pressure during exercise)[77]

Congenital anomalies of coronary arteries

The second most common cardiovascular cause of SCD in young athletics is congenital anomalies of coronary arteries.[2-4,51,53,58,78-79,85] Most of these anomalies are of little clinical impact and are only detected during cardiac catheterization for other reasons. Clinical events occur only when the anomalously connecting artery passes between the aorta and the pulmonary trunk.[80] Cheitlin at el. (1974) pointed out the pathologic significance of such anomalies so that the coronary artery can be compressed between the aorta and the pulmonary artery during exercise.[81] This pathological process could be predisposed to fatal ventricular tachyarrhythmias by providing an electrically unstable myocardial substrate and has shown a striking incidence of exertion-related sudden unexplained death in the affected adolescents and young adults.

The possibility of a coronary anomaly should always be considered in any young athletes with exertional chest pain or cardiac syncope.[83] Since myocardial ischemia is episodic, patients often do not have abnormalities on resting 12-lead or exercise electrocardiograms (ECGs).[58,78,84] Transthoracic or transesophageal echocardiography and magnetic resonance imaging can be used to diagnose the anomaly, and can be confirmed by diagnostic coronary angiography.[58,84]

Myocarditis

Myocarditis can be rather challenging to diagnose clinically because of its insidious nature, and most affected individuals have no symptoms at all.[86] This diagnosis may be suggested in the absence of symptoms on the basis of ECG abnormalities alone, which include heart block and ventricular arrhythmias.[11,87] The inflammatory process of myocarditis is usually triggered by several viral agents, most commonly enterovirus (e.g., coxsackie virus) and adenovirus.[88] The use of a reverse-transcriptase-polymerase-chain-reaction assay to identify a viral genome in endomyocardial-biopsy specimens has enhanced the yield and helped to verify the diagnosis of myocarditis.[88]

Myocarditis is usually a transient illness, and the affected athletes should be allowed to return to competition if they satisfy the following criteria:

- a convalescent period of six months after the onset of symptoms
- normalization of ventricular dimension and function
- absence of clinically significant arrhythmias during ambulatory monitoring and stress tests[11]

Arrhythmogenic right ventricular cardiomyopathy

Arrhythmogenic right ventricular cardiomyopathy (ARVC) is a familial condition that may be associated with important ventricular arrhythmias.[4,89-90] ARVC is characterized histologically by midmural or external myocardial replacement with a fibrolipomatous infiltrate.[91] The degree of right ventricular involvement varies from diffuse to localized infiltrations, which can give a picture of focal akinesia or dyskinesia.[91]

Coronary artery disease

Atherosclerotic coronary artery disease deserves specific attention, as it is the predominant cause of SCD in master athletes (over 35 years of age),[7-10] but it only accounts for few SCD, about 2%–3%, in young athletes under 35 years of age.[2,4,6,51,85,93-94] Especially in older men with underlying CAD, exertion-related SCD is usually associated with the acute rupture of unstable coronary plaque.[93,94] The disease is usually confined to the left anterior descending artery and is due to obstructive fibrous and smooth muscle cell plaques in the absence of acute thrombus.

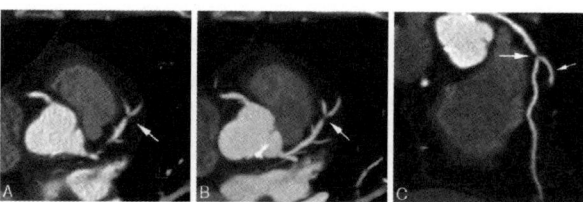

Fig A,B,C: Computed Tomographic coronary angiography (CTCA) showing critical stenosis at mid left anterior descending artery (LAD) (white arrow).

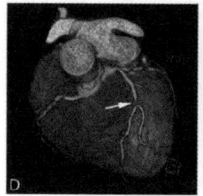 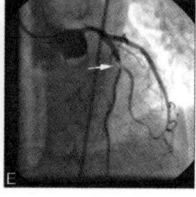

Fig D: 3D reconstruction of above images again showing critical LAD lesion (white arrow). Fig E: coronary angiography showing the same lesion, confirming CTCA findings.

The Role of Preparticipation Screening

Considerable interest has been raised regarding the role of preparticipation screening for early identification of those cardiovascular disorders responsible for athletic field deaths, with the expectation that disqualification of those high-risk athletes may eventually prevent sudden death.[51,52,95] Although some critics have queried the effectiveness of cardiovascular screening,[51,96] overwhelming support for the principle of this public health initiative exists in both the medical and lay communities.[97–100]

Recommendations from the European Society of Cardiology (ESC)[99] and the American College of Cardiology/American Heart Association (ACC/AHA)[85] have generated a debate regarding the most appropriate strategy for screening trained athletes and other sports participants.

Screening protocol in the United States and Europe (Italy)

The 2007 AHA recommendations,[85] which are virtually identical to those proposed in the 1996 AHA Scientific Statement,[51] promote personal and family history and physical examinations as a potential effective strategy to raise the suspicion of cardiovascular disease in both large and small screening populations of high school and college student athletes. The 2007 AHA recommendations consist of 12 items (eight for personal and family history and four for physical examinations) (Table 2). At the discretion of the examiner, a positive response in any one or more of the 12 items may be judged sufficient to trigger a referral for cardiovascular evaluation. The recommendations advocated by ESC (Table 3) are very similar to those of AHA, which also emphasize medical history (personal and family) and physical examinations.[99] The most essential difference between the two is the inclusion of a resting 12-lead ECG in the former.

The AHA guidelines[51,85] assume that a 12-lead ECG is not a cost-effective instrument for screening a large population of young athletes, due to its low specificity. Such a screening strategy has limited power to detect potential lethal cardiovascular abnormalities in young athletes mainly because of the high frequency of ECG alterations associated with normal physiological adaptations of the trained athlete's heart.

In contrast, the ESC guidelines support a 12-lead ECG as an effective

Table 2 The 12-Item AHA Recommendations for Preparticipation Cardiovascular Screening of Competitive Athletes[51,85]

Medical History

(*Parental verification is recommended for high school and middle school athletes*)

Personal

- Exertional chest pain/discomfort
- Unexplained syncope/near syncope, especially exertional (excluding vasovagal)
- Excessive exertional and unexplained fatigue, associated with exercise
- Prior recognition of a heart murmur
- Elevated systemic blood pressure

Family

- Premature death (sudden and unexpected or otherwise) before 50 years of age due to heart disease, in one or more relative
- Disability from heart disease in a close relative <50 years of age
- Specific knowledge of certain cardiac conditions in family members: hypertrophy or dilated cardiomyopathy, long QT syndrome or other ion channelopathies, Marfan syndrome, or clinically important arrhythmias

Physical examination

- Heart murmur*
- Femoral pulses to exclude aortic coarctation
- Physical stigmata of Marfan syndrome
- Brachial artery blood pressure (sitting position and preferably in both arms)

* Auscultation should be performed in both supine and standing positions (or with the Valsalva maneuver), specifically to identify murmurs of dynamic left ventricular outflow tract obstruction

screening tool, with the potential to enhance sensitivity of detecting cardiovascular diseases with the risk of sudden death.[99] In fact, ECG is abnormal in up to 95% of patients with HCM,[101] which is the leading cause of sudden death in athletes.

The European guidelines base their recommendations on nearly 30 years of experience in a systemic preparticipation screening program in Italy.[52,92,102] Italian law requires that everyone from 12 to 35 years of age participate on an organized team or in individual sports to obtain an annual

Table 3 The ESC Recommendations for Preparticipation Cardiovascular Screening of Competitive Athletes[99]

Medical history

Personal

- Exertional chest pain or discomfort
- Syncope or near syncope
- Irregular heart beat or palpitations
- The presence of shortness of breath or fatigue out of proportion to the degree of exertion

Family

- Close relatives have experienced a premature heart attack or sudden death (<55 years of age in males and <65 years in females)
- The presence of a family history of cardiomyopathy, Marfan syndrome, long QT syndrome, Brugada syndrome, severe arrhythmias, coronary artery disease, or other disabling cardiovascular diseases.

Physical Examination

- Physical stigmata of Marfan syndrome
- Diminished or delayed femoral artery pulses
- The presence of mid or end-systolic clicks
- The presence of a second heart sound single or widely split and fixed with respiration
- Marked heart murmurs (any diastolic and systolic grade >or =2/6)
- Brachial blood pressure >140/90mmHg (on >1 reading)

Investigation

- Resting 12-lead ECG

---

medical clearance by accredited sports medicine physicians. Recent data suggest that this screening strategy may indeed be life-saving by reducing cardiovascular events in athletes. A substantial decline (almost 90%) in the annual incidence of sudden cardiovascular death in competitive athletes, largely attributable to reduced deaths from cardiomyopathies, in the Vento region of northeastern Italy has been reported.[103]

AHA supports any public health initiative (i.e., the inclusion of a resting 12-lead ECG in the preparticipation screening program) with the potential to identify adverse cardiac abnormalities on humanitarian medical grounds. Nevertheless, it has been admitted that there are multiple major issues to overcome before such changes can be implemented in the U.S.[85] The AHA has concluded that this is probably impractical and would require considerable resources that do not currently exist; however, such an initiative would have benefits in term of detecting greater numbers of athletes at risk of SCD.[85]

At the moment, there is insufficient data to recommend which protocol to adopt for Hong Kong, as the factors regarding participating athletics—such as demographics, genetics, prevalence of undiagnosed cardiovascular disorders, and other social factors (e.g., economic resources, manpower resources, and logistics involved in such a screening program)—differ significantly from those in the U.S. and Europe.

Conclusion

Although acute vigorous physical exertion may trigger sudden death or MIs in the presence of underlying heart disease, such risk associated with habitual exercise in active individuals is relatively low. As such, it is generally agreed that the overall benefits of exercise usually outweigh associated risks.

The role of preparticipation screenings for early identification of cardiovascular disorders responsible for athletic field deaths has always attracted considerable interest in the medical community. Recently, recommendations by ESC and ACC/AHA have generated a new debate regarding the most appropriate strategy for screening trained athletes and other sports participants. Recent data have suggested that this screening strategy may reduce cardiovascular events in athletes by as much as 90%.

It is difficult to recommend which protocol to adopt for Hong Kong, as the risk factors differ significantly from those in the U.S. and Europe. Hopefully, more local studies will be conducted in the future, and they will guide us in formulating the most appropriate screening strategy for Hong Kong.

References

1. Maron BJ. 1993. Sudden death in young athletes: lessons from the Hank Gaithers affair. *N Engl J Med* 329:55–57.

2. Burke AP, Farb A, Virmani R, Goodin J, Smialek JE. 1991. Sports-related and non-sports-related sudden cardiac death in young adults. *Am Heart J* 121: 568–75.

3. Maron BJ, Shirani J, Poliac LC, Mathenge R, Roberts WC, Mueller FO. 1996. Sudden death in young competitive athletes: clinical, demographic and pathological profiles. *JAMA* 276 (3): 199–204.

4. Corrado D, Thiene G, Nava A, Rossi L, Pennelli N. 1990. Sudden death in young competitive athletes: clinicopathologic correlations in 22 cases. *Am J Med* 89 (5): 588–96.

5. Drory Y, Turetz Y, Hiss Y, Lev B, Fisman EZ, Pines A, et al. 1991. Sudden unexpected death in persons less than 40 years of age. *Am J Cardiol* 68 (13): 1388–92.

6. Liberthson RR. 1996. Sudden death from cardiac causes in children and young adults. *N Eng J Med* 334: 1039–44.

7. Thompson PD, Stern MP, Williams P, Duncan K, Haskell WL, Wood PD. 1979. Death during jogging or running: a study of 18 cases. *JAMA* 242 (12): 1265–67.

8. Thompson PD, Funk EJ, Carleton RA, Sturner WQ. 1982. Incidence of death during jogging in Rhode Island from 1975 through 1980. *JAMA* 247 (18): 2535–38.

9. Waller BF, Roberts WC. 1980. Sudden death while running in conditioned runners aged 40 years or over. *Am J Cardiol* 45 (6): 1292–1300.

10. Virmani R, Robinowitz M, McAllister HA Jr. 1982. Nontraumatic death in joggers: a series of 30 patients at autopsy. *Am J Med* 72 (6): 874–82.

11. Maron BJ, Mitchell JH. 1994. 26th Bethesda Conference: Recommendations for determining eligibility for competition in athletes with cardiovascular abnormalities. *J Am Coll Cardiol* 24:845–99.

12. Paffenbarger RS Jr, Hyde RT, Wing AL, Hsieh CC. 1986. Physical activity, all-cause mortality, and longevity of college alumni. *N Engl J Med* 314 (10): 605–13.

13. Paffenbarger RS Jr, Hyde RT, Wing AL, Lee IM, Jung DL, Kampert JB. 1993. The association of changes in physical activity level and other lifestyle

characteristics with mortality among men. *N Engl J Med* 328 (8): 539–45.

14. Lee IM, Hsieh CC, Paffenbarger RS Jr. 1995. Exercise intensity and longevity in men: the Harvard Alumni Health Study. *JAMA* 273 (15): 1179–84.

15. Kushi LH, Fee RM, Folsom AR, Mink PJ, Anderson KE, Sellers TA. 1997. Physical activity and mortality in postmenopausal women. *JAMA* 277 (16): 1287–92.

16. Bijnen FC, Caspersen CJ, Feskens EJ, Saris WH, Mosterd WL, Kromhout D. 1998. Physical activity and 10-year mortality from cardiovascular diseases and all causes: the Zutphen Elderly Study. *Arch Intern Med* 158 (14): 1499–1505.

17. Erikssen G, Liestøl K, Bjørnholt J, Thaulow E, Sandvik L, Erikssen J. 1998. Changes in physical fitness and changes in mortality. *Lancet* 352 (9130): 759–62.

18. Kujala UM, Kaprio J, Sarna S, Koskenvuo M. 1998. Relationship of leisure-time physical activity and mortality: the Finnish twin cohort. *JAMA* 279 (6): 440–44.

19. Morris JN, Everitt MG, Pollard R, Chave SP, Semmence AM. 1980. Vigorous exercise in leisure-time: protection against coronary heart disease. *Lancet* 2 (8206): 1207–10.

20. Gibbons RJ, Balady GJ, Beasley JW, Bricker JT, Duvernoy WF, Froelicher VF, et al. 1997. ACC/AHA guidelines for exercise testing: a report of the American College of Cardiology/American Heart Association Task Force on Practice Guidelines (Committee on Exercise Testing). *J Am Coll Cardiol* 30 (1): 260–311.

21. Leon AS, Connett J. 1991. Physical activity and 10.5-year mortality in the Multiple Risk Factor Intervention Trial (MRFIT). *Int J Epidemiol* 20 (3): 690–97.

22. Wannamethee SG, Shaper AG, Walker M. 1998. Changes in physical activity, mortality, and incidence of coronary heart disease in older men. *Lancet* 351 (9116): 1603–08.

23. Villeneuve PJ, Morrison HI, Craig CL, Schaubel DE. 1998. Physical activity, physical fitness, and risk of dying. *Epidemiology* 9 (6): 626–31.

24. Blair SN, Kohl HW III, Barlow CE, Paffenbarger RS Jr, Gibbons LW, Macera CA. 1995. Changes in physical fitness and all-cause mortality: a prospective study of healthy and unhealthy men. *JAMA* 273 (14): 1093–98.

25. Fletcher GF, Balady GJ, Blair SN, Blumenthal J, Caspersen C, Chaitman B, et al. 1996. Statement on exercise: benefits and recommendations for physical activity programs for all Americans: a statement for health professionals by the Committee on Exercise and Cardiac Rehabilitation of the Council on Clinical Cardiology, American Heart Association. *Circulation* 94 (4): 857–62.

26. Pate RR, Pratt M, Blair SN, Haskell WL, Macera CA, Bouchard C, et al. 1995.

Physical activity and public health: a recommendation from the Centers for Disease Control and Prevention and the American College of Sports Medicine. *JAMA* 273 (5): 402–407.

27. U.S. Department of Health and Human Services, Centers for Disease Control and Prevention, National Center for Chronic Disease Prevention and Health Promotion, The President's Council on Physical Fitness and Sports. 1996. *Physical Activity and Health: A Report of the Surgeon General.* Atlanta, GA.

28. Fletcher GF, Balady G, Blair SN, Blumenthal J, Caspersen C, Chaitman B, et al. 1992. Statement on exercise: benefits and recommendations for physical activity programs for all Americans: a statement for health professionals by the Committee on Exercise and Cardiac Rehabilitation of the Council on Clinical Cardiology, American Heart Association. *Circulation* 86 (1): 340–44.

29. Physical activity and cardiovascular health. NIH Consensus Development Panel on Physical Activity and Cardiovascular Health. 1996. *JAMA* 1996 276 (3): 241–46.

30. Williams C (Ed.). 1999. *Physical Activity and Cardiovascular Disease Prevention in the European Union.* Brussels, Belgium: European Heart Network.

31. Bijnen FC, Caspersen CJ, Mosterd WL. 1994. Physical inactivity as a risk factor for coronary heart disease: a WHO and International Society and Federation of Cardiology position statement. *Bull World Health Organization* 72 (1): 1–4.

32. Fletcher GF, Balady G, Froelicher VF, Hartley LH, Haskell WL, Pollock ML. 1995. Exercise standards: a statement for healthcare professionals from the American Heart Association. *Circulation* 91 (2): 580–615.

33. Snell PG, Mitchell JH. 1999. Physical inactivity: an easily modified risk factor? *Circulation* 100 (1): 2–4.

34. Fletcher GF. 1997. How to implement physical activity in primary and secondary prevention: a statement for healthcare professionals from the Task Force on Risk-reduction, American Heart Association. *Circulation* 96 (1): 355–57.

35. Siscovick DS, Weiss NS, Fletcher RH, Lasky T. 1984. The incidence of primary cardiac arrest during vigorous exercise. *N Engl J Med* 311 (14): 874–77.

36. Mittleman MA, Maclure M, Tofler GH, Sherwood JB, Goldberg RJ, Muller JE. 1993. Triggering of acute myocardial infarction by heavy physical exertion. Protection against triggering by regular exertion. Determinants of Myocardial Infarction Onset Study Investigators. *N Engl J Med* 329 (23): 1677–83.

37. Willich SN, Lewis M, Löwel H, Arntz HR, Schubert F, Schröder R. 1993. Physical exertion as a trigger of acute myocardial infarction: Triggers and

Mechanisms of Myocardial Infarction Study Group. *N Engl J Med* 329 (23): 1684–90.

38. Vuori I. 1986. The cardiovascular risks of physical activity. *Acta Med Scand Suppl* 711:205–14.

39. Gibbons LW, Cooper KH, Meyer BM, Ellison RC. 1980. The acute cardiac risk of strenuous exercise. *JAMA* 244 (16): 1799–1801.

40. Maron BJ, Poliac LC, Roberts WO. 1996. Risk for sudden cardiac death associated with marathon running. *J Am Coll Cardiol* 28 (2): 428–31.

41. Thompson PD. 1996. The cardiovascular complications of vigorous physical activity. *Arch Intern Med* 156 (20): 2297–2302.

42. Balady GJ, Chaitman B, Driscoll D, Foster C, Froelicher E, Gordon N, et al. 1998. Recommendations for cardiovascular screening, staffing, and emergency policies at health/fitness facilities. *Circulation* 97 (22): 2283–93.

43. Kujala UM, Sarna S, Kaprio J, Koskenvuo M, Karjalainen J. 1999. Heart attacks and lower-limb function in master endurance athletes. *Med Sci Sports Exerc* 31 (7): 1041–46.

44. Albert CM, Mittleman MA, Chae CU, Lee IM, Hennekens CH, Manson JE. 2000. Triggering of sudden death from cardiac causes by vigorous exertion. *N Engl J Med* 343 (19): 1355–61.

45. Maron BJ. 2000. The paradox of exercise. *N Engl J Med* 343 (19):1409–11.

46. Hambrecht R, Wolf A, Gielen S, Linke A, Hofer J, Erbs S, et al. 2000. Effect of exercise on coronary endothelial function in patients with coronary artery disease. *N Engl J Med* 342 (7): 454–60.

47. Roberts WC. 1984. An agent with lipid-lowering, antihypertensive, positive inotropic, negative chronotropic, vasodilating, diuretic, anorexigenic, weight reducing, cathartic, hypoglycemic, tranquilizing, hypnotic and antidepressive qualities. *Am J Cardiol* 53 (1): 261–62. Editorial.

48. Van Camp SP, Bloor CM, Mueller FO, Cantu RC, Olson HG. 1995. Nontraumatic sports death in high school and college athletes. *Med Sci Sports Exerc* 27 (5): 641–47.

49. Maron BJ, Gohman TE, Aeppli D. 1998. Prevalence of sudden cardiac death during competitive sports activities in Minnesota high school athletes. *J Am Coll Cardiol* 32 (7): 1881–84.

50. Corrado D, Basso C, Rizzoli G, Schiavon M, Thiene G. 2003. Does sports activity enhance the risk of sudden death in adolescents and young adults? *J Am Coll Cardiol* 42: 1959–63.

51. Maron BJ, Thompson PD, Puffer JC, McGrew CA, Strong WB, Douglas PS, et al. 1996. Cardiovascular preparticipation screening of competitive athletes: a statement for health professionals from the Sudden Death Committee (clinical cardiology) and Congenital Cardiac Defects Committee (cardiovascular disease in the young), American Heart Association. *Circulation* 94 (4): 850–56.

52. Corrado D, Basso C, Schiavon M, Thiene G. 1998. Screening for hypertrophic cardiomyopathy in young athletes. *New Engl J Med* 339 (6): 364–69.

53. Maron BJ. 1998. Cardiovascular risks to young persons on the athletic field. *Ann Intern Med* 129 (5): 379–86.

54. Van Camp SP, Bloor CM, Mueller FO, Cantu RC, Olson HG. 1995. Nontraumatic sports death in high school and college athletes. *Med Sci Sports Exerc* 27 (5): 641–47.

55. Thiene G, Nava A, Corrado D, Rossi L, Pennelli N. 1988. Right ventricular cardiomyopathy and sudden death in young people. *N Engl J Med* 318 (3): 129–33.

56. Furlanello F, Bettini R, Cozzi F, Del Favero A, Disertori M, Vergara G, et al. 1984. Ventricular arrhythmias and sudden death in athletes. *Ann N Y Acad Sci* 427:253–79.

57. Thiene G, Pennelli N, Rossi L. 1983. Cardiac conduction system abnormalities as a possible cause of sudden death in young athletes. *Hum Pathol* 14 (8): 704–709.

58. Basso C, Maron BJ, Corrado D, Corrado D, Thiene G. 2000. Clinical profile of congenital coronary artery anomalies with origin from the wrong aortic sinus leading to sudden death in young competitive athletes. *J Am Coll Cardiol* 35:1493–1501.

59. Maron BJ, Carney KP, Lever HM, Lewis JF, Barac I, Casey SA, et al. 2003. Relationship of race to sudden cardiac death in competitive athletes with hypertrophic cardiomyopathy. *J Am Coll Cardiol* 41:974–80.

60. Richardson P, McKenna W, Bristow M, Maisch B, Mautner B, O'Connell J, et al. 1996. Report of the 1995 World Health Organization/International Society and Federation of Cardiology Task Force on the Definition and Classification of cardiomyopathies. *Circulation* 93 (5): 841–42.

61. Maron BJ, Gardin JM, Flack JM, Gidding SS, Kurosaki TT, Bild DE. 1995. Prevalence of hypertrophic cardiomyopathy in a general population of young adults. Echocardiographic analysis of 4111 subjects in the CARDIA study. Coronary Artery Risk Development in (Young) Adults. *Circulation* 92 (4): 785–89.

62. Nistri S, Thiene G, Basso C, Corrado D, Scognamglio R, Maron BJ. 1999. Preparticipation Military Screening and Echocardiographic (phenotypic) Prevalence of Hypertrophic Cardiomyopathy. *Eur Heart J* 20:16–16.(Abstract)

63. McKenna WJ, Spirito P, Desnos M, Dubourg O, Komajda M. 1997. Experience from clinical genetics in hypertrophic cardiomyopathy: proposal for new diagnostic criteria in adult members of affected families. *Heart* 77 (2): 130–32.

64. Elliott PM, Poloniecki J, Dickie S, Sharma S, Monserrat L, Varnava A, et al. 2000. Sudden death in hypertrophic cardiomyopathy: identification of high risk patients. *J Am Coll Cardiol* 36:2212–18.

65. Maron BJ, Casey SA, Poliac LC, Gohman TE, Almquist AK, Aeppli DM. 1999. Clinical course of hypertrophic cardiomyopathy in a regional United States cohort [published erratum appears in *JAMA* 1999 Jun 23–30; 281 (24): 2288]. *JAMA* 281:650–55.

66. Maron BJ, Spirito P, Wesley Y, Arce J. 1986. Development and progression of left ventricular hypertrophy in children with hypertrophic cardiomyopathy. *N Engl J Med* 315 (10): 610–14.

67. McKenna W, Elliott PM. 1998. Hypertrophic Cardiomyopathy. In E. J. Topol (Ed.), *Comprehensive Cardiovascular Medicine* (pp. 775–98). Philadelphia, New York: Lippincott Williams & Wilkins.

68. Maron BJ, Shen WK, Link MS, Epstein AE, Almquist AK, Daubert JP, et al. 2000. Efficacy of implantable cardioverter-defibrillators for the prevention of sudden death in patients with hypertrophic cardiomyopathy. *N Engl J Med* 342 (6): 365–73.

69. Nicod P, Polikar R, Peterson KL. 1988. Hypertrophic cardiomyopathy and sudden death. *N Engl J Med* 318:1255–57.

70. Stafford WJ, Trohman RG, Bilsker M, Zaman L, Castellanos A, Myerburg RJ. 1986. Cardiac arrest in an adolescent with atrial fibrillation and hypertrophic cardiomyopathy. *J Am Coll Cardiol* 7:701–704.

71. Elliott PM, Sharma S, Varnava A, Poloniecki J, Rowland E, McKenna WJ. 1999. Survival after cardiac arrest or sustained ventricular tachycardia in patients with hypertrophy cardiomyopathy. *J Am Coll Cardiol* 33 (6): 1596–1601.

72. McKenna W, Deanfield J, Faruqui A, England D, Oakley C, Goodwin J. 1981. Prognosis in hypertrophic cardiomyopathy: role of age and clinical, electrocardiographic and hemodynamic features. *Am J Cardiol* 47 (3): 532–38.

73. Spirito P, Bellone P, Harris KM, Bernabo P, Bruzzi P, Maron BJ. 2000. Magnitude of left ventricular hypertrophy and risk of sudden death in hypertrophic

cardiomyopathy. *N Engl J Med* 342 (24): 1778–85.

74. Elliott PM, Gimeno BJ, Mahon NG, et al. 2001. Relation between severity of left-ventricular hypertrophy and prognosis in patients with hypertrophic cardio-myopathy. *Lancet* 357:420–24.

75. Maron BJ, Savage DD, Wolfson JK, Epstein SE. 1981. Prognostic significance of 24 hour ambulatory electrocardiographic monitoring in patients with hypertro-phic cardiomyopathy: a prospective study. *Am J Cardiol* 48 (2): 252–57.

76. McKenna WJ, Franklin RC, Nihoyannopoulos P, Robinson KC, Deanfield JE. 1988. Arrhythmia and prognosis in infants, children and adolescents with hy-pertrophic cardiomyopathy. *J Am Coll Cardiol* 11 (1): 147–53.

77. Sadoul N, Prasad K, Elliott PM, Bannerjee S, Frenneaux MP, McKenna WJ. 1997. Prospective prognostic assessment of blood pressure response during exercise in patients with hypertrophic cardiomyopathy. *Circulation* 96 (9): 2987–91.

78. Davis JA, Cecchin F, Jones TK, Portman MA. 2001. Major coronary artery anomalies in a pediatric population: incidence and clinical importance. *J Am Coll Cardiol* 37 (2): 593–97.

79. Roberts WC, Kragel AH. 1988. Anomalous origin of either the right or left main coronary artery from the aorta without coursing of the anomalistically arising artery between aorta and pulmonary trunk. *Am J Cardiol* 62 (17): 1263–67.

80. Kragel AH, Roberts WC. 1988. Anomalous origin of either the right or left main coronary artery from the aorta with subsequent coursing between aorta and pulmonary trunk: analysis of 32 necropsy cases. *Am J Cardiol* 62 (10 Pt 1): 771–77.

81. Cheitlin MD, DeCastro CM, McAllister HA. 1974. Sudden death as a compli-cation of anomalous left coronary origin from the anterior sinus of Valsalva: A not-so-minor congenital anomaly. *Circulation* 50:780–87.

82. Cohen AJ, Grishkin BA, Helsel RA, Head HD. 1989. Surgical therapy in the management of coronary anomalies: emphasis on utility of internal mammary artery grafts. *Ann Thorac Surg* 47 (4): 630–37.

83. Goldschlager N, Epstein AE, Grubb BP, Olshansky B, Prystowsky E, Roberts WC, et al. 2003. Etiologic considerations in the patient with syncope and an apparently normal heart. *Arch Intern Med* 163 (2): 151–62.

84. Post JC, van Rossum AC, Bronzwaer JGF, de Cock CC, Hofman MB, Valk J, et al. 1995. Magnetic resonance angiography of anomalous coronary arteries: a new gold standard for delineating the proximal course? *Circulation* 92 (11): 3163–71.

85. Maron BJ, Thompson PD, Ackerman MJ, Balady G, Berger S, Cohen D, et al. Recommendations and Considerations Related to Preparticipation Screening for Cardiovascular Abnormalities in Competitive Athletes: 2007 Update. A Scientific Statement From the American Heart Association Council on Nutrition, Physical Activity, and Metabolism: endorsed by the American College of Cardiology Foundation. *Circulation* 2007; 115 (12): 1643–55.

86. McCaffrey FM, Braden DS, Strong WB. 1991. Sudden cardiac death in young athletes: a review. *Am J Dis Child* 145 (2): 177–83.

87. Feldman AM, McNamara D. 2000. Myocarditis. *N Engl J Med* 343 (19): 1388–98.

88. Pauschinger M, Bowles NE, Fuentes-Garcia FJ, Pham V, Kühl U, Schwimmbeck PL, et al. 1999. Detection of adenoviral genome in the myocardium of adult patients with idiopathic left ventricular dysfunction. *Circulation* 99: 1348–54.

89. Corrado D, Basso C, Thiene G, et al. 1997. Spectrum of clinicopathological manifestations of arrhythmogenic right ventricular cardiomyopathy/dysplasia: a multicenter study. *J Am Coll Cardiol* 30: 1512–20.

90. McKenna WJ, Thiene G, Nava A, Fontaliran F, Blomstrom-Lundqvist C, Fontaine G, et al. 1994. Diagnosis of arrhythmogenic right ventricular dysplasia/cardiomyoapthy. *Br Heart J* 71 (3): 215–18.

91. Marcus FI, Fontaine G. 1995. Arrhythmogenic right ventricular dysplasia/cardiomyopathy: a review. *Pacing Clin Electrophysiol* 18:1298–1314.

92. Pelliccia A, Maron BJ. 1995. Preparticipation cardiovascular evaluation of the competitive athlete: perspectives from the 30-year Italian experience. *Am J Cardiol* 75: 827–28.

93. Corrado D, Basso C, Poletti, A, Angelini A, Valente M, Thiene G. 1994. Sudden death in the young. Is acute coronary thrombosis the major precipitating factor? *Circulation* 90 (5): 2315–23.

94. Burke AP, Farb A, Malcom GT, Liang YH, Smialek JE, Virmani R. 1999. Plaque Rupture and Sudden Death Related to Exertion in Men With Coronary Artery Disease. *JAMA* 281:921–26.

95. Maron BJ, Bodison SA, Wesley YE, Tucker E, Green KJ. 1987. Results of screening a large group of intercollegiate competitive athletes for cardiovascular disease. *J Am Coll Cardiol* 10 (6): 1214–21.

96. Best TM. 2004. The preparticipation evaluation: an opportunity for change and consensus. *Clin J Sport Med* 14 (3): 107–108.

97. Estes NAM III, Link MS, Cannom D, Naccarelli GV, Prystowsky EN, Maron BJ,

et al. 2001. Report of the NASPE policy conference on arrhythmias and the athlete. *J Cardiovasc Electrophysiol* 12 (10): 1208–19.

98. Maron BJ, Zipes DP. 2005. 36th Bethesda Conference: eligibility recommendations for competitive athletes with cardiovascular abnormalities. *J Am Coll Cardiol* 45:1312–75.

99. Corrado D, Pelliccia A, Bjørnstad HH, Vanhees L, Biffi A, Borjesson M, et al. 2005. Cardiovascular pre-participation screening of young competitive athletes for prevention of sudden death: proposal for a common European protocol. Consensus Statement of the Study Group of Sport Cardiology of the Working Group of Cardiac Rehabilitation and Exercise Physiology and the Working Group of Myocardial and Pericardial Diseases of the European Society of Cardiology. *Eur Heart J* 26 (5): 516–24.

100. Preparticipation Physical Evaluation Task Force. 2005. *Preparticipation Physical Evaluation. 3rd ed.* Minneapolis: McGraw-Hill/The Physician and Sportsmedicine.

101. Maron BJ. 2002. Hypertrophic cardiomyopathy: a systemic review. *JAMA* 287 (10): 1308–20.

102. Decree of the Italian Ministry of Health, February 18, 1982. Norme per la tutela sanitaria dell'attività sportive agonistica (Rules concerning the medical protection of althletic activity). *Gazzetta Ufficiale* March 5, 1982:63.

103. Corrado D, Basso C, Pavei A, Michieli P, Schiavon M, Thiene G. 2006. Trends in sudden cardiovascular death in young competitive athletes after implementation of a preparticipation screening program. *JAMA* 296:1593–1601.

Nutrition for Marathon Runners

Ms. Daphne WU

Nutrition Overview

Optimal nutrition plays an important role in helping marathon runners to enhance their running performance.

Marathon running is a typical form of endurance exercise. Many marathon runners believe that their nutrient needs are different from other athletes and community-based participants. Male marathon runners have body fat percentages below 6%, while for female marathon runners the fat percentage ranges from 6% to 15% (Lohman, 1992; Houtkooper and Going, 1994; Sinning, 1996; ACSM, ADA, and Dietitians of Canada, 2000). They expect themselves to have lower or even super low body weights and body fat levels to achieve a high power-to-mass ratio, save energy costs, and improve their heat dissipation and aerobic capacity. They tend to seek the right nutritional strategies to drop unnecessary weight with the same goal: to enhance their performance and success in races.

Marathon runners are encouraged to eat healthily to achieve this goal and to follow proper training regimens. A good diet that provides adequate energy and nutrients definitely helps to normalise the immune system (Table 1), minimise the occurrence of injury, and optimise performance and recovery. Likewise, a poor diet has detrimental effects on performance and health. In this chapter, the dietary strategies applied to daily training, before, during, and after a marathon run will be discussed.

Nutrition for Daily Use

A healthy eating pattern, including the major nutrients that an active body requires, can be classified into the following:

- Carbohydrate
- Protein
- Fat
- Vitamins and Minerals
- Fluid

Table 1 Potential Nutrients for Immune Enhancement

Category	Immune promoting nutrients
Energy	carbohydrate, fat and protein
Protein	arginine, glycine, cysteine; branched chain amino acids (leucine, isoleucine, and valine)
Fats	essential fatty acids, such as arachidonic acid (AA), docosahexaenoic acid (DHA), and eicosapentaenoic acid (EPA)
Vitamin	Vitamins A, C, E, B_6 (pyridoxine) and B_{12} (cobalamin)
Mineral	copper, iron, selenium, zinc

Carbohydrate

Marathon runners have great reliance on carbohydrate metabolism for energy.

The general healthy eating guideline recommends 50%–60% of an adult's total energy come from carbohydrates. Marathon runners are expected to consume more carbohydrates as carbohydrates are the major energy source for endurance exercise. Glucose, the end product after digestion of carbohydrates, is absorbed, transported to muscle cells, and eventually stored as muscle glycogen. Carbohydrate ingestion generally sustains carbohydrate availability, delays the onset of fatigue (particularly at the later stage of prolonged exercise), and thus optimises exercise performance. Insufficient intake of carbohydrates increases the rate of perceived exertion (RPE) during prolonged exercise (Burgess et al., 1991; Timmons and Bar-Or, 2003) and level of cortisol, which is a stress hormone associated with protein catabolism in breaking down muscle membranes and mobilising amino acids from muscle to liver for gluconeogenesis (Anderson et al., 1991; Deuster et al., 1992; Kirwan et al., 1990; Mitchell et al., 1990).

Different types of carbohydrates have different rates of digestion and absorption that subsequently affect the rates of muscle glycogen storage, availability, and recovery. Some runners look for the right carbohydrates to maximise the beneficial effects on performance. There exist several ways to categorise the rates of carbohydrate availability.

Glycaemic index

The glycaemic index was established in the early 1980s as a measure of the rate that certain complex carbohydrates produce sugar. Jenkins et al. (1981) developed a ranking system called the glycaemic index (GI) to classify carbohydrates according to the rate of digestion and absorption inside the human body. The GI is defined as "the incremental area under the blood glucose response curve expressed as a percentage of the response to the same amount of carbohydrates from a standard food taken by the same subject" (FAO/WHO, 1998). The standard food is usually either white bread or glucose containing 50 g of carbohydrates.

$$\text{Glycaemic Index (GI)} = \frac{\text{Blood glucose area of a test food}}{\text{Blood glucose area of a standard food}} \times 100$$

The GI is considered to be a glucogenic indicator of the biological value of carbohydrates (Foster-Powell and Miller, 1995). The conventional concept that complex carbohydrates require more time to be broken and produce a slower rise in blood glucose and insulin levels than simple sugars is no longer valid. Certain complex carbohydrates with a high GI have a greater impact on blood glucose and insulin levels than simple sugars with a low GI. The GI of foods is categorised as:

Low = GI less than or equal to 55
Medium = GI between 56 and 69
High= GI greater than or equal to 70

Although the GI seems to be useful to estimate the rate of carbohydrate availability in the body, the use of GI seems to be limited at the academic level. The GI of a food can be affected by several factors, such as cooking time and method, amount of food, and the combination with other nutrients such as fat and protein. Table 2 shows the GI value of common foods containing 50 g of carbohydrates. However, a wide variety of GI values

Table 2 Carbohydrate Content and GI of Selected Foods (each item contains 50 g carbohydrate)

Food Group	Food Item	Weight	Serving Size	GI*
Cereals and grains	Cornflakes	60 g	2 cups	81
	Soda cracker	72 g	12 crackers	74
	White bread	110 g	2 large slices	70
	White rice, boiled	180 g	1.5 cups	64
	Udon, cooked	200 g	1 pc	62
	Rice vermicelli, cooked	230 g	1.25 cups	58
	Spaghetti, white; boiled	220 g	1.5 cups	44
Starchy Vegetables	Baked potato	250 g	1 large	76
	Sweet potato	240 g	1 large	48
	Baked beans	250 g	1 cup	40
	Lentils, boiled	250 g	1.25 cups	29
Fruits	Raisin	70 g	0.5 cup	64
	Banana, 7.5 inch long	210 g	2 pcs	51
	Orange	430 g	3 large	42
	Apple juice	500 ml	2 cups	41
	Pear/Apple	330 g	2 medium	38
Dairy Products	Fruit yogurt, low-fat, sweetened	270 g	1 cup	33
	Non-fat milk	1,000 ml	4 cups	32
Others	Sports drink	750 ml	3 cups	78
	Jelly beans	54 g	19 pcs	78
	White sugar	50 g	10 tsps	68
	Soft drink	500ml	2 cups	53
	Chocolate	80 g	4/5 bar	45

*Glucose is used as the reference (GI=100).

Source: www.glycemicindex.com; USDA National Nutrient Database for Standard Reference

Table 3 Common Food Sources of Carbohydrates

Food Groups	Examples
Cereals and grains	Breads, granola bar, muesli, noodles, oats, pastas, rice
Starchy vegetables	Carrots, chestnuts, corn, potatoes, sweet potatoes
Fruits	Apples, grapefruit, orange juice, raisin
Beans and bean products	Baked beans, chick peas, hummus, red kidney beans, soy milk
Dairy products	Milk and yogurt
Sugary foods and beverages	Candy, lollipops, sodas, sorbets

exists for the same type of foods produced at different areas or by different manufacturers (Foster-Powell et al., 2002).

Since many natural and processed foods contain carbohydrates (Table 3), marathon runners should bear in mind that a sufficient intake of carbohydrates supports routine training and can be obtained from natural sources without the use of supplements which may be more expensive, have a lower nutrient content, and be monotonous in taste.

Protein

Adequate protein intake, together with appropriate exercise, promotes muscle gain.

Proteins are absolutely essential to life. They have a wide range of functions to the body such as supporting growth, repairing body tissues, and maintaining the immune system. From ancient Greece to modern societies, a majority of athletes believe that their protein requirements should be higher than those of other people. The general recommendations for adult protein intake are between 0.8–1.0 g protein per kilogram of body weight or 10%–15% of total energy. Currently, the protein intake of many athletes is much higher than these guidelines for muscle growth. In fact, consuming a moderate amount of protein, accompanied by an appropriate exercise regimen, is the only way to gain muscle. Even body builders require small increases in protein intake over the recommendations for the general adult population. Runners can easily meet their slightly increased protein needs, particularly when adequate energy intake is met with a variety of food choices. Excessive protein intake contributes extra energy which is then stored as fat in the body.

A marathon runner who restricts energy intake to achieve a very lean body weight may inevitably increase protein breakdown for energy. The runner may therefore consume more protein to compensate for the increased turnover to ensure muscle growth due to an inadequate intake of carbohydrates. It may also be of concern that the quality of protein consumed may compromise the ultimate gain of protein in body. Certain athletes are keen to understand the structure and rate of protein availability or utilisation in order to take the right type of protein to modulate protein metabolism.

It is quite common to believe that strength athletes and bodybuilders require more protein than endurance athletes; however, Tarnopolsky et al. (1988) demonstrated a greater excretion of total daily urea in endurance athletes than in bodybuilders. The authors concluded that endurance athletes and bodybuilders should ingest 1.67 times and 1.12 times more daily protein respectively than sedentary controls in order to meet the needs of protein catabolism during exercise. The Report of the Scientific Committee on Food (2001) speculated that the higher intakes of protein required by endurance athletes compensate for the increased protein turnover.

Supplementation of amino acids is not uncommon among runners. However, it seems to be unnecessary as all the essential amino acids can be easily met through a balanced diet with great variety of foods. Amino acid supplementation and high protein intake are not recommended as high protein intake can increase calcium loss (Kerstetter et al., 2003; Massey, 2003) and put an extra burden on kidneys to filter excess protein metabolites. Consuming protein beyond the required amounts will be stored as fat and may increase the risk of hypohydration, which can be detrimental to running performance.

Plant and animal proteins

Another consideration is the choice of protein-containing food source. Plant protein sources are thought to have low biological value due to lower levels of one or more essential amino acids. Butterfield et al. (1992) suggested that protein needs of vegetarian athletes could be greater as their energy intake might be lower due to the high fibre vegetarian diet. In addition, plant proteins such as legumes are less easily digested than animal proteins. The National Research Council (1989) recommended that vegetarians consume an extra 10% protein. Plant proteins are more digestible after they are denatured by cooking. The digestibility of some plant proteins in humans is as good as animal proteins (Table 4). Despite many concerns about consuming plant proteins, a review by Young and Pellett (1994) claimed that sufficient protein requirements could be achieved and meet daily total energy requirements by consuming a combination of plant proteins from various sources.

Table 4 Values for the Digestibility of Proteins in Humans

Plant source	Digestibility relative to reference proteins	Animal source	Digestibility relative to reference proteins
Peanut butter	100	Egg	100
Rice, polished	93	Milk	100
Peas, mature	93	Fish	100
Wheat, whole	90	Cheese	100
Oatmeal	90		
Maize	89		
Beans	82		

Source: Energy and Protein Requirement FAO/WHO, 1985; Protein Quality Evaluation, FAO/WHO, 1991

Whey and casein

The aspects of "fast" and "slow" digestion and absorption exist in proteins as well as carbohydrates. Whey protein contains a higher level of essential amino acids and branched chain amino acids than casein. The digestion of whey protein is faster than that of casein; thus it is believed that the intake of whey leads to quicker repair or recovery of body proteins when compared with that of casein protein. Although the intake of whey protein appears to have a greater benefit on initial protein synthesis, casein protein appears to have a greater beneficial effect on protein synthesis after a prolonged intake

(Hoffman and Falvo, 2004). Thus, the authors agree that it is beneficial to include both whey and casein in a runner's diet. It is not necessary to consume either whey or casein supplements. Furthermore, the efficacy and purity of many protein-related supplements have not been completely tested or verified.

Adequate energy intake, predominantly from carbohydrate, can ensure a positive protein balance. Runners should be reminded that only proper training and exercise, together with sufficient protein intake, promotes positive changes in muscle mass.

Fat

The utilisation of free fatty acids can delay the onset of exhaustion during a marathon race.

Dietary fat intake is necessary to facilitate the absorption of fat-soluble vitamins (Vitamins A, D, E, and K) to provide essential fatty acids to promote growth and learning ability, and to maintain a normal immune system and reproductive functions in females. Insufficient fat intake disrupts the hormonal balance and menstrual cycle in female runners, leading to a negative impact on bone health and an increased risk of osteoporosis and bone fracture. On the other hand, male runners taking too little fat may inhibit the production of testosterone, which leads to a negative effect on muscle gain. Marathon runners should aim to consume the right types and amounts of fat to maximise the beneficial effects on health and overall performance without gaining unnecessary weight.

Biological needs

Generally, dietary fats can be categorised as essential fatty acids (EFAs) and non-essential fatty acids (NEFAs). Essential fatty acids cannot be synthesised sufficiently in the human body and need exogenous sources. Essential fatty acids are a component of phospholipids in body cell membranes and important for the production of prostaglandins and leukotrienes for normal immune functions. Essential fatty acids are generally polyunsaturated fatty acids. The recommended ratio for taking omega-6 vs. omega-3 fatty acids ranges between 4:1 (Scientific Review Committee, 1990) and 10:1 (FAO/ WHO, 1995). However, the current ratio in a typical Western diet is between 10:1 or even 25:1 (Simopoulos, 1991; Kris-Etherton et al., 2000). As marathon runners are more likely to have impaired immune function shortly after prolonged races, they should target adequate intake of EFAs during regular training and after prolonged races.

Table 5 Common Categories of Essential Fatty Acids and Food Sources

Group	Essential fatty acids	Food sources
Omega-3	Alpha-Linolenic acid (LNA)	Almond, flaxseed, and walnut
	Eicosapentaenoic acid (EPA) and docosahexaenoic acid (DHA)	Cold-water fish such as mackerel, salmon, sardine, and trout
Omega-6	Arachidonic acid (AA)	Meats such as pork and beef
	Linoleic acid (LA)	Corn, safflower, sesame, soybean, and sunflower oils
	Gamma-linolenic acid (GLA)	Black currant and evening primrose seed

Vitamins and Minerals

Vitamins and minerals have important roles in the human body, such as maintaining normal metabolism of macronutrients (e.g., carbohydrates, proteins, and fats) and muscle functions. It is commonly expected that the needs of vitamins and minerals increase with physical activities. Although there is no special recommended intake of vitamins and minerals for athletes, it is believed that any increased needs can be matched with increased energy intake via a wide variety of foods and a balanced diet.

Endurance exercises may compromise the immune system of athletes. Marathon runners, particularly female and/or vegan runners, are at a higher risk for insufficient intake of certain vitamins or minerals. Nevertheless, it should be noted that supplementation is not recommended unless the athletes are diagnosed with inadequacy or deficiency. There is no evidence that vitamin and mineral supplements enhance running performance. On the contrary, supplements can hinder the absorption of other nutrients and be detrimental to health when the intake of a single nutrient is in huge excess. In addition, the purity and the dosage of most supplements have not been completely tested or verified.

Water and Fluid

Water is the most important nutrient for athletes, despite the absence of energy, vitamins, and minerals. The intake of water and fluid is essential to keep the body well hydrated and at an optimal body temperature. Heat production in the body increases with exercise intensity and duration. Sweating not only facilitates heat dissipation to prevent heat stroke, but also leads to dehydration when fluid intake is inadequate. Hypohydration or dehydration has detrimental effects on motion coordination, muscle strength, and endurance. Even a mild dehydration by 2% of body weight can impair exercise performance. Severe dehydration can increase the risk of death. Runners should know their own rates of sweat loss in different environments and ensure an adequate fluid intake before, during, and after regular training and races. Details concerning fluid intake and replacement are discussed in Chapter 17.

Both macronutrients and micronutrients are essential for normal immune function and resistance to infection. Runners should take a variety of foods to optimise the intake of nutrients. Runners at a higher risk of energy and nutrient deficiencies should consult medical or nutritional professionals to prevent nutrient inadequacy or deficiency and to maintain or enhance running performance. Marathon runners should also bear in mind that both hypohydation and hyperhydration can jeopardise performance in a competition and even health or life.

Nutritional Needs for Competition

A poor diet strategy can make a top marathon runner become mediocre in a race.

An average well-nourished adult weighing 70 kg with 15% body fat has less than 0.5 kg carbohydrates in the body, stored primarily as muscle glycogen (~400 g), liver glycogen (90–110 g), and blood glucose (2–3 g). There are 12 kg of muscle protein and 12 kg of fat deposited mainly in subcutaneous tissues and stored within muscle fibres.

Carbohydrate and fat stored in the body are primary energy fuels. Energy contributed from carbohydrate and fat is mainly from glycogen stored in skeletal muscle, fatty acids from adipose tissue cells, and intramuscular triglycerides. Compared with the limited carbohydrate stored in the body, endogenous fat is the largest energy reserve. Despite the vast source of energy from fat, the use of body fat is limited due to its slow energy availability. Thus, carbohydrate remains the dominant substrate for energy during endurance exercise (Hawley et al., 2000).

Adequate availability of carbohydrates has a positive and beneficial effect on prolonged running performance, achievable through proper diet strategies adopted before, during, and after the marathon.

Eating for Race Preparation

Adequate intake of carbohydrates before a marathon maximises muscle glycogen reserves.

A good diet strategy before an endurance competition helps a participant maintain blood glucose levels; minimise the onset of hypoglycaemia, premature fatigue, and gastrointestinal upset; and maximise muscle glycogen stores. This helps to avoid hunger and, consequently, to enhance exercise performance (Hawley et al., 1997, Lambert and Goedecke 2003, Kiens 2001). It has been suggested by Lambert et al. (2001) that adopting a low carbohydrate and high fat diet will spare carbohydrates and increase the plasma free fatty acid level and the use of fat as energy. The digestion rate of dietary fat is rather slow and takes extra time before fat is readily available to contribute energy for use. Besides, high fat intake can cause gastrointestinal distress during prolonged exercise. Such dietary strategies reduce glycogen reserves and impair performance (Bergstrom et al., 1967; Galbo et al., 1979; Jansson and Kaijser, 1982). An ongoing supply of carbohydrates during endurance competitions is still the main and most important key for success.

Carbohydrate loading

How many runners believe the necessity of hitting the wall before gaining the award? "Hitting the wall" seems to be an idiom used by marathon runners to describe the phenomenon of running out of energy around the last five to ten km of a 42 km marathon. A top marathon runner, Dick Beardsley, said that hitting the wall felt like an elephant had jumped out of a tree onto his shoulders and made him carry it the rest of the way. Basically, hitting the wall is about running out of glycogen; energy then has to be obtained from fats (Stevinson and Biddle, 1998). Marathon runners may experience this phenomenon not only during the race, but also when applying an inappropriate strategy of carbohydrate loading.

It has been well established that a high intake of carbohydrates enhances the aerobic capacity of the muscles during endurance exercise (Christensen and Hansen, 1939). Scandinavian sports scientists developed a carbohydrate-loading protocol in the late 1960s to maximise glycogen reserves in muscles for athletes prior to their endurance competitions (Bergstrom et al., 1967; Bergstrom and Hultman, 1966; Hermansen et al., 1967). However, this protocol seems to push the runners to hit the wall before the onset of the race.

The classic carbohydrate-loading protocol involves a depletion period of three to four days, followed by a loading period three days prior to an endurance competition. Runners need to train extremely hard and adopt very low carbohydrate diets during the depletion phase. They then rest and adopt very high carbohydrate diets during the loading phase (Figure 1). These two phases are associated with accelerated glycogen synthase activity to increase the rate of glucose transport and the capacity of converting glucose into glycogen. The protocol can increase glycogen reserves from the normal range of 80–120 mmol per kg muscle (wet weight) to around 150–200 mmol per kg muscle (wet weight).

This classic protocol advises a marathon runner to take no more than 10% of energy from carbohydrates during the depletion phase. The runner then takes a very high carbohydrate diet, equivalent to 90% of energy, at the loading phase; this is almost ten times higher than during the depletion phase. A 60 kg runner requires around 2,400 kcal a day. For example, if a 60 kg runner requires around 2,400 kcal a day, the runner should take around 60 g of carbohydrates daily for the three days of the depletion phase, with a liberal intake of fat and protein to commit the energy requirement. The runner then drastically increases carbohydrate intake to nearly 540 g for the next three days of the loading phase.

It is not uncommon that runners following the classic protocol feel extremely tired, irritable, restless, disoriented, weak, and exhausted. The concern over this dietary protocol is that it increases the risk of injury before it offers opportunity to win the race. Furthermore, the drastic change in carbohydrate intake increases the risk of gastrointestinal distress, such as stomachaches, bloating, diarrhoea, or constipation.

In the early 1980s, a modified carbohydrate-loading protocol was developed by Sherman et al. (1981). Runners are still able to maximise muscle glycogen stores without less chances of hitting the wall. The modified protocol involves a tapering of training. Runners need to reduce 50% of their workout for three days, a week before an endurance competition, while adopting a moderate carbohydrate diet. They then enter a loading period for the next three days prior to the competition by further reducing 50% of their training volume and increasing carbohydrate intake to achieve supercompensation (Figure 1).

The modified protocol advises marathon runners to continue a moderate carbohydrate intake which provides 50% of total energy during the first three days of carbohydrate loading. The runners then increase energy contribution to 70% from carbohydrates for the following three days prior to the competition. The same 60 kg marathon runner mentioned above needs to manipulate his or her carbohydrate intake from 300 g to 420 g, i.e., from 50% to 70% of total energy of 2,400 kcal when following the modified protocol. Common carbohydrate-containing foods are shown in Table 2.

The modified carbohydrate-loading protocol is more practical, and it carries a smaller risk of exhaustion, fatigue, or gastrointestinal distress. Nevertheless, many marathon runners still undertake the rigid classic protocol since they believe the proverb, "no pain no gain." They believe they have to face the darkest hour before the dawn.

Figure 1 Graphic Demonstration of Classic and Modified Carbohydrate Loading
Protocols and Glycogen Supercompensation.

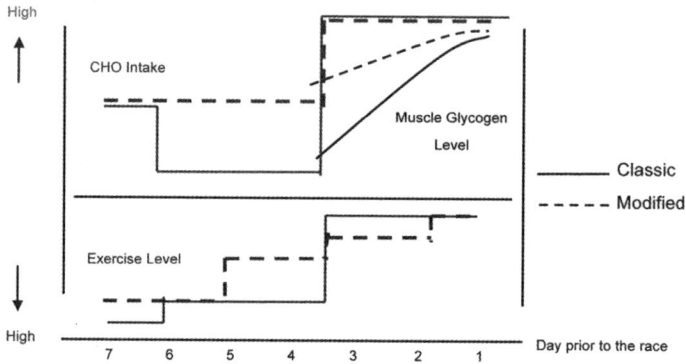

A good carbohydrate-loading strategy prior to a marathon will
help to:
- optimise key energy stores to prevent hypoglycaemia,
- reduce gastric discomfort or hunger during running,
- minimise weakness and postpone fatigue by ~20%, and
- enhance performance by 2%–3%.

Caffeine intake

Another area of interest to both researchers and marathon runners is the
influence of caffeine intake on performance. Runners tend to take caffeine
to improve endurance performance (Cox et al., 2002) as caffeine may
increase exogenous carbohydrate oxidation (Yeo et al., 2005) and alertness.
Nevertheless, there remains a discussion on whether caffeine should be
taken before an endurance competition. It is of concern that caffeine has a
diuretic effect which is associated with compromising hydration status.
Since the diuretic effect is mild and many runners are habitual coffee or tea
drinkers, sudden cessation of the intake of caffeine may possibly do more
harm. By and large, runners who are sensitive to caffeine should avoid its

consumption as caffeine can lead to certain side effects, including insomnia, irritability, nervousness, headaches, hand tremors, and palpitation. It should also be noted that caffeine's ergogenic benefits to performance still lack universal support.

Eating for the Run

A continuous supply of energy to delay the onset of fatigue is key for marathon success.

There are two factors of nutritional inadequacy that compromise endurance exercise performance: dehydration and hypoglycaemia. On the contrary, proper hydration and a continuous supply of glucose prevent or delay the onset of fatigue during a marathon.

Energy Supply Strategy

The contribution of glucose from muscle glycogen become less important as blood glucose contributes a greater percentage when running continues. It is well published that carbohydrate intake during endurance exercise delays the signs and symptoms of fatigue (Coyle et al., 1986; Coggan and Coyle, 1987). Many marathon races start at around 8:00 in the morning. Runners are encouraged to eat high carbohydrate breakfasts prior to the race. The purpose of a good pre-race meal is to replenish the liver glycogen stores depleted after an overnight fasting and to provide an ongoing release of glucose. Runners are also recommended to consume 1–4 g of carbohydrate per kg body weight from one to four hours before to the race in order to have enough time for digestion and absorption. However, there is a concern about the effect of high carbohydrate intake on the fluctuation of insulin levels. Some runners fear the surge of insulin that not only increases carbohydrate oxidation and reduces free fatty acid mobilisation (Coyle et al., 1985; Foster et al., 1979; Marmy-Conus et al., 1996; Sherman et al., 1989; Short et al., 1997), but also triggers the onset of hypoglycaemia shortly after the start of the race.

The purposes of consuming carbohydrates for performance are to provide energy for the run and to reduce the reliance on pre-race carbohydrate availability. It has been speculated that the ingestion of carbohydrates during endurance exercise results to less hypoglycaemic impact than prior to the race due to an increase in the permeability of muscle fibres during exercise that leads to a smaller secretion of insulin.

The maximum oxidation rate of exogenous single carbohydrate during exercise is around 0.8–1.1 g per minute (Hawley et al., 1992; Jeukendrup and Jentjens, 2000). Thus, the recommended goal of carbohydrate intake during running is around 30–60 g of carbohydrate per hour (Coggan and Coyle, 1991). Consuming carbohydrate in excess of the recommended levels does not further increase the exogenous oxidation rate, but it may provoke gastric discomfort during running. However, certain studies support the fact that exogenous carbohydrate oxidation rates can reach peak values of around 1.25–1.7 g per minute when combined carbohydrates are ingested (Jentjens et al., 2003, 2004a, 2004b, and 2004c; Jentjens and Jeukendrup, 2005).

Carbohydrate choices during the run

Foods and beverages such as bananas, chocolate, water, and sports drinks are usually supplied to marathon runners at stations along the route. The intake of moderate to high GI carbohydrates accelerates fuel availability. Bananas and chocolate are considered low to moderate GI while sports drinks are high GI. Sports drinks thus seem to be an ideal choice with the provision of carbohydrate and fluid at the same time. Although it is recommended to take high GI carbohydrates to speed up the availability of fuels, the monotonous flavour of sports drinks may not encourage continuous drinking. Sports drinks generally contain 6%–8% of carbohydrates, which are combinations of sucrose, glucose, and fructose. Runners may overload body fluid when attempting to achieve a sufficient intake of carbohydrate wholly from sports drinks. Moreover, bananas and chocolate are good alternative carbohydrate sources. Runners should take sufficient carbohydrates at earlier stages of an endurance run, rather than wait until the onset of fatigue. For the sake of safety, runners should also be considerate and dispose banana skins properly during the run.

Eating for Recovery

Replenishing muscle glycogen is the top priority during the post-race recovery period.

Recovery after a marathon focuses on replenishing depleted muscle and liver glycogen stores and restoring water and electrolyte balance. A rapid recovery is beneficial for runners to get back to regular training, work, or studies and to normalise impaired immune function. Runners should consume carbohydrates at early stages of recovery after a prolonged and exhaustive running competition.

Glycogen Replenishment Strategy

The timing and total amount of carbohydrates consumed after a marathon are the most critical factors for maximising muscle glycogen replenishment. Runners should consume high-carbohydrate foods as soon as possible after a prolonged race. The depleted glycogen reserve stimulates glycogen synthase activity, which is similar to the concept of carbohydrate loading during the depletion phase of the classic carbohydrate-loading protocol, and leads to an increase in the permeability of muscle cells to glucose and muscle sensitivity to insulin. The rate of glycogen storage becomes fastest at around 7–8 mmol per kg muscle (wet weight) per hour during the first two hours and then reduces to around 5 mmol per kg muscle (wet weight) per hour after a prolonged exercise (Blom et al., 1987; Ivy et al., 1988). As mentioned previously, the normal glycogen reserve ranges between 80–120 mmol per kg muscle (wet weight). Restoring depleted glycogen reserves, therefore, takes around 24 hours to reach normal values.

Burke et al. (1996) found no difference of the frequency or pattern of carbohydrate intake, whether nibbling or gorging, in the glycogen stores when sufficient carbohydrate intake over the day is met. Total carbohydrate intake should be 1–1.5 g per kg body weight in the first two hours and eventually reach 7–10 g per kg body weight within the first 24 hours after the race. Consuming carbohydrate greater than the recommendation in the first two-hour interval appears to have no additional benefit of accelerated muscle glycogen replenishment. Runners may experience gastric discomfort from the huge intake of carbohydrates. Furthermore, the form of ingested carbohydrates, whether as solid or liquid, is not a crucial factor for restoring glycogen stores after exhaustive exercise (Coggan and Swanson, 1992; Keizer et al., 1986; Reed et al., 1989). High GI carbohydrates appear to accelerate glycogen re-synthesis after exercise (Burke et al., 1993; Coyle, 1991; Walton and Rhodes, 1997). In addition, high GI foods generally are less bulky and more likely to be tolerated by runners when compared with low GI foods. Hence, runners may consider taking high-GI carbohydrate foods over low-GI carbohydrate foods as a main post-race dietary strategy for replenishment of muscle glycogen.

Other effects

Certain studies found a beneficial effect of taking protein with a carbohydrate-rich meal in order to accelerate the recovery of glycogen storage in the body and exercise capacity after a prolonged exercise (Betts, Duffy et al., 2005; Ivy et al., 2002; Zawadzki et al., 1992). However, this beneficial effect seems to be workable only when athletes have been exhausted. Besides, the benefit seems not to be proved in certain studies (Betts, Stevenson et al., 2005, 2006; Carrithers et al., 2000; Jentjens et al., 2001; Hall et al., 2000; Loon et al., 2000). Futher investigation is needed to see whether the beneficial effect of added protein in a post-race diet on accelerating glycogen replenishment is due to the subsequent increase in the concentration of circulating insulin, the extra supply of energy from protein which spares carbohydrates for storage, the promotion of muscle protein synthesis, or the additive effects of all of the above.

Nevertheless, the practical implementation of nutritional strategy is different from the scientific research, which is mainly focused on the investigation of single foods or drinks. Many naturally carbohydrate-rich foods such as bread, potatoes, and pastas contain certain amounts of protein. In addition, runners are most likely to consume meals with mixed foods after prolonged running. Runners actually ingest protein synchronously while following post-race dietary strategies.

Summary

Carbohydrate requirements increase with exercise intensity. Glycogen in muscle and liver cells are essential fuels for marathon races. The goals of nutritional strategies before, during, and after endurance exercise are to fuel up and restore muscle and liver glycogen, avoid hunger and gastrointestinal discomfort, reduce or delay the onset of fatigue so as to enhance exercise performance, return exercise capacity as soon as possible, and optimise the immune system. Diet strategies for marathon runners should practically meet the needs of personal preference and the availability of food sources during training and competition.

Table 6 Practical Summary of Carbohydrate Intake for Marathon Runners

Condition	Daily Carbohydrate Intake
Carbohydrate loading two to three days before marathon	8–10 g/kg body weight (BW)
One to four hours before marathon	1–4 g/kg BW
During the run	20–60 g/hr
Immediate recovery after marathon (0–4 hours)	1 g/kg BW
One-day recovery from marathon	7–12 g/kg BW

Ingestion of foods and fluids at appropriate times and in appropriate portions can provide marathon runners with a competitive advantage. A strategy of carbohydrate loading at a single pre-event or post-event meal cannot compensate for poor training regimens and training diets. Food preferences are very individualised. No single food works for all runners. Runners should experiment with food items and strategies during training, but they should not try any new foods or meal plans immediately prior to an important race.

References

American College of Sports Medicine, American Dietetic Association, Dietitians of Canada. 2000. Joint Position Statement: nutrition and athletic performance. American College of Sports Medicine, American Dietetic Association, and Dietitians of Canada. *Med Sci Sports Exerc* 32 (12): 2130–45.

Anderson RA, Bryden NA, Polansky MM, Thorp JW. 1991. Effects of carbohydrate loading and underwater exercise on circulating cortisol, insulin and urinary losses of chromium and zinc. *Eur J Appl Physiol Occup Physiol* 63 (2): 146–50.

Bergström J, Hermansen L, Hultman E, and Saltin B. 1967. Diet, muscle glycogen and physical performance. *Acta Physiol Scand* 71 (2): 140–50.

Bergström J and Hultman E. 1966. Muscle glycogen synthesis after exercise: an enhancing factor localized to the muscle cells in man. *Nature* 210 (5033): 309–310.

Blom PC, Høstmark AT, Vaage O, Kardel KR, Maehlum S. 1987. Effect of different post-exercise sugar diets on the rate of muscle glycogen synthesis. *Med Sci Sports Exerc* 19 (5): 491– 96.

Betts J, Duffy K, Gunner F, Williams C. 2005. Recovery of endurance running capacity following the ingestion of carbohydrate plus protein. *Med Sci Sports Exerc* 37 (5): S419.

Betts JA, Stevenson E, Williams C, Sheppard C, Grey E, Griffin J. 2005. Recovery of endurance running capacity: effect of carbohydrate-protein mixtures. *Int J Sport Nutr Exerc Metab* 15 (6): 590–609.

Betts J, Williams C, Tsintzas K, Boobis L. 2006. The effect of carbohydrate-protein mixtures on muscle glycogen resynthesis following prolonged treadmill running. *Med Sci Sports Exerc* 38 (5): S37.

Burgess ML, Robertson RJ, Davis JM, Norris JM. 1991. RPE, blood glucose, and carbohydrate oxidation during exercise: effects of glucose feedings. *Med Sci Sports Exerc* 23 (3): 353–59.

Burke LM, Collier GR, Davis PG, Fricker PA, Sanigorski AJ, Hargreaves M. 1996. Muscle glycogen storage after prolonged exercise: effect of the frequency of carbohydrate feedings. *Am J Clin Nutr* 64 (1): 115–19

Burke LM, Collier GR, Hargreaves M. 1993. Muscle glycogen storage after prolonged exercise: Effect of the glycaemic index of carbohydrate feedings. *J Appl Physiol* 75 (2): 1019–23.

Butterfield G, Cady C, Moynihan S. 1992. Effect of increasing protein intake on nitrogen balance in recreational weight lifters. *Med Sci Sports Exerc* 24 (5 Suppl): S71.

Carrithers JA, Williamson DL, Gallagher PM, Godard MP, Schulze KE, Trappe SW. 2000. Effects of postexercise carbohydrate-protein feedings on muscle glycogen restoration. *J Appl Physiol* 88 (6): 1976–82.

Christensen EH, Hansen O. 1939. Respiratorischen quotient und O2-aufisnahme. *Skandinavisches Archiv fur Physiologie* 81:180–89.

Coggan AR, Coyle EF. 1987. Reversal of fatigue during prolonged exercise by carbohydrate infusion or ingestion. *J Appl Physiol* 63 (6): 2388–89

Coggan AR, Coyle EF. 1991. Carbohydrate ingestion during prolonged exercise: effects on metabolism and performance. *Exerc Sport Sci Rev* 19:1–40.

Coggan AR, Swanson SC. 1992. Nutritional manipulations before and during endurance exercise: effects on performance. *Med Sci Sports Exerc* 24 (9 Suppl): S331–35.

Cox GR, Desbrow B, Montgomery PG, Anderson ME, Bruce CR, Macrides TA, et al. 2002. Effect of different protocols of caffeine intake on metabolism and endurance performance. *J Appl Physiol* 93 (3): 990–99.

Coyle EF. 1991. Timing and method of increased carbohydrate intake to cope with heavy training, competition and recovery. *J Sports Sci* 9 (Spec No:29–51): discussion 51–52.

Coyle EF, Coggan AR, Hemmert MK, Ivy JL. 1986. Muscle glycogen utilization during prolonged strenuous exercise when fed carbohydrate. *J Appl Physiol* 61 (1): 165–72.

Coyle EF, Coggan AR, Hemmert MK, Lowe RC and Walters TJ. 1985. Substrate usage during prolonged exercise following a preexercise meal. *J Appl Physiol* 59 (2): 429–33.

Deuster PA, Singh A, Hofmann A, Moses FM, Chrousos GC. 1992. Hormonal responses to ingesting water or a carbohydrate beverage during a 2 h run. *Med Sci Sports Exerc* 24 (1): 72–79.

FAO/WHO. 1985. Engery and Protein Requirements. Report of a Joint FAO/WHO/UNU Expert Consultation. *World Health Organ Tech Rep Ser* 724:1–206.

FAO/WHO. 1998. Carbohydrates in human nutrition. Report of a Joint FAO/WHO Expert Consultation. *FAO Food Nutr Pap* 66:1–140

FAO/WHO. 1991. Protein Quality Evaluation. Report of the Joint FAO/WHO Expert Consultation. *FAO Food Nutr Pap* 51:1–66.

FAO/WHO. 1995. Fats and oils in human nutrition. Report of a joint expert consultation. *Nutr Rev* 53 (7): 202–205.

Foster C, Costill DL, Fink WJ. 1979. Effects of pre-exercise feedings on endurance performance. *Med Sci Sports* 11 (1): 1–5.

Foster-Powell K, Holt SH, Brand-Miller JC. 2002. International table of glycemic index and glycemic load values: 2002. *Am J Clin Nutr* 76 (1): 5–56.

Foster-Powell K, Miller JB. 1995. International tables of glycemic index. *Am J Clin Nutr* 62 (4): 871S–890S.

Galbo H, Holst JJ, Christensen NJ. 1979. The effect of different diets and of insulin on the hormonal response to prolonged exercise. *Acta Physiol Scand* 107 (1): 19–32.

Hawley JA, Burke LM, Angus DJ, Fallon KE, Martin DT, Febbraio MA. 2000. Effect of altering substrate availability on metabolism and performance during intense exercise. *Br J Nutr* 84 (6): 829–38.

Hawley JA, Dennis SC, Noakes TD. 1992. Oxidation of carbohydrate ingested during prolonged endurance exercise. *Sports Med* 14 (1): 27–42.

Hawley JA, Schabort EJ, Noakes TD, Dennis SC. 1997. Carbohydrate-loading and exercise performance. An update. *Sports Med* 24 (2): 73–81.

Keizer HA, Kuipers H, van Kranenburg G, Geurten P. 1987. Influence of liquid and solid meals on muscle glycogen resynthesis, plasma fuel hormone response, and maximal physical working capacity. *Int J Sports Med* 8 (2): 99–104.

Hall G van, Shirreffs SM, Calbet JA. 2000. Muscle glycogen resynthesis during recovery from cycle exercise: no effect of additional protein ingestion. *J Appl Physiol* 88 (5): 1631–36.

Hermansen L, Hultman E, Saltin B. 1967. Muscle glycogen during prolonged severe exercise. *Acta Physiologies Scandinavica* 71 (2): 129–39.

Hoffman JR, Falvo MJ. 2004. Protein—Which is best? *J Sports Sci Med* 3:118–30.

Houtkooper LB, Going SB. 1994. Body composition: how should it be measured? Does it affect sport performance? *Sports Sci Exchange* 7:1–8.

Ivy JL, Goforth HW Jr, Damon BM, McCauley TR, Parsons EC, Price TB. 2002. Early postexercise muscle glycogen recovery is enhanced with a carbohydrate-protein supplement. *J Appl Physiol* 93 (4): 1337–44.

Ivy JL, Lee MC, Brozinick JT Jr, Reed MJ. 1988. Muscle glycogen storage after different amounts of carbohydrate ingestion. *J Appl Physiol* 65 (5): 2018–23.

Jansson E, Kaijser L. 1982. Effect of diet on the utilization of blood-borne and intramuscular substrates during exercise in man. *Acta Physiol Scand* 115 (1): 19–30.

Jenkins DJ, Wolever TM, Taylor RH, Barker H, Fielden H, Baldwin JM, et al. 1981. Glycemic index of foods: a physiological basis for carbohydrate exchange. *Am J Clin Nutr* 34 (3): 362–66.

Jentjens RL, Achten J, and Jeukendrup AE. 2004. High oxidation rates from combined carbohydrates ingested during exercise. *Med Sci Sports Exerc* 36 (9): 1551–58.

Jentjens RL, Cale C, Gutch C, Jeukendrup AE. 2003. Effects of pre-exercise ingestion of differing amounts of carbohydrate on subsequent metabolism and cycling performance. *Eur J Appl Physiol* 88 (4–5): 444–52.

Jentjens RL, Jeukendrup AE. 2005. High rates of exogenous carbohydrate oxidation from a mixture of glucose and fructose ingested during prolonged cycling exercise. *Br J Nutr* 93 (4): 485–92.

Jentjens RL, Loon LJ van, Mann CH, Wagenmakers AJ, Jeukendrup AE. 2001. Addition of protein and amino acids to carbohydrates does not enhance postexercise muscle glycogen synthesis. *J Appl Physiol* 91 (2): 839–46.

Jentjens RL, Moseley L, Waring RH, Harding LK, and Jeukendrup AE. 2004. Oxidation of combined ingestion of glucose and fructose during exercise. *J Appl Physiol* 96 (4): 1277–84.

Jentjens RL, Venables MC, Jeukendrup AE. 2004. Oxidation of exogenous glucose, sucrose, and maltose during prolonged cycling exercise. *J Appl Physiol* 96 (4): 1285–91.

Jeukendrup AE, Jentjens R. 2000. Oxidation of carbohydrate feedings during prolonged exercise: current thoughts, guidelines and directions for future research. *Sports Med* 29 (6): 407–24.

Kerstetter JE, O'Brien KO, Insogna KL. 2003. Dietary protein, calcium metabolism, and skeletal homeostasis revisited. *Am J Clin Nutr* 78 (3 Suppl): 584S–92S.

Kiens B. 2001. Diet and training in the week before competition. *Can J Appl Physiol* 26 Suppl:S56–63.

Kirwan JP, Costill DL, Houmard JA, Mitchell JB, Flynn MG, Fink WJ. 1990. Changes in selected blood measures during repeated days of intense training and carbohydrate control. *Int J Sports Med* 11 (5): 362–66.

Kris-Etherton PM, Taylor DS, Yu-Poth S, Huth P, Moriarty K, Fishell V, et al. 2000. Polyunsaturated fatty acids in the food chain in the United States. *Am J Clin Nutr* 71 (1 Suppl): 179S–88S.

Lambert EV, Goedecke JH. 2003. The role of dietary macronutrients in optimizing endurance performance. *Curr Sports Med Rep* 2 (4): 194–201.

Massey LK. 2003. Dietary animal and plant protein and human bone health: a whole foods approach. *J Nutr* 133 (3): 862S–65S.

Lambert EV, Goedecke JH, Zyle C, Murphy K, Hawley JA, Dennis SC, et al. 2001. High-fat diet versus habitual diet prior to carbohydrate loading: effects of exercise metabolism and cycling performance. *Int J Sport Nutr Exerc Metab* 11 (2): 209–25.

Lohman TG. 1992. *Basic Concepts in body composition assessment. Advances in body composition assessment.* Champaign, IL: Human Kinetics Publisher; 109–18.

Loon LJ van, Saris WH, Kruijshoop M, Wagenmakers AJ. 2000. Maximizing postexercise muscle glycogen synthesis: carbohydrate supplementation and the application of amino acid or protein hydrolysate mixtures. *Am J Clin Nutr* 72 (1): 106–11.

Marmy-Conus N, Fabris S, Proietto J, Hargreaves M. 1996. Preexercise glucose ingestion and glucose kinetics during exercise. *J Appl Physiol* 81 (2): 853–57.

Mitchell JB, Costill DL, Houmard JA, Flynn MG, Fink WJ, Beltz JD. 1990. Influence of carbohydrate ingestion on counterregulatory hormones during prolonged exercise. *Int J Sports Med* 11 (1): 33–36.

National Research Council. 1989. *Recommended Dietary Allowances (10th ed.).* Washington, DC: National Academy Press.

Reed MJ, Brozinick JT Jr, Lee MC, Ivy JL. 1989. Muscle glycogen storage postexercise: effect of mode of carbohydrate administration. *J Appl Physiol* 66 (2): 720–26.

Scientific Committee on Food, European Commission. 2001. *Report of the Scientific Committee on Food on composition and specification of food intended to meet the expenditure of intense muscular effort, especially for sportsmen.*

Scientific Review Committee. 1990. *Nutrition Recommendations.* Ottawa, ON: Minister of National Health and Welfare, Canada.

Sherman WM, Costill DL, Fink WJ, and Miller JM. 1981. Effect of exercise-diet manipulation on muscle glycogen and its subsequent utilization during performance. *Int J Sports Med* 2 (2): 114–18.

Sherman WM, Brodowicz G, Wright DA, Allen WK, Simonsen J, Dernbach A. 1989. Effects of 4 h preexercise carbohydrate feedings on cycling performance. *Med Sci Sports Exerc* 21 (5): 598–604.

Short KR, Sheffield-Moore M, Costill DL. 1997. Glycemic and insulinemic responses to multiple preexercise carbohydrate feedings. *Int J Sport Nutr* 7 (2): 128–37.

Simopoulos AP. 1991. Omega-3 fatty acids in health and disease and in growth and development. *Am J Clin Nutr* 54 (3): 438–63.

Sinning WE. 1996. Body composition in athletes. In Roche AF, Heymsfield SB, Lohman TG (Eds.), *Human body composition*. Champaign, IL: Human Kinetics Publishers; 257–73.

Stevinson CD, Biddle SJ. 1998. Cognitive orientations in marathon running and "hitting the wall". *Br J Sports Med* 32 (3): 229–34; discussion 234–35.

Walton P, Rhodes EC. 1997. Glycaemic index and optimal performance. *Sports Med* 23 (3): 164–72.

Tarnopolsky MA, MacDougall JD, Atkinson SA. 1988. Influence of protein intake and training status on nitrogen balance and lean body mass. *J Appl Physiol* 64 (1): 187–93.

Thomas DE, Brotherhood JR, Brand JC. 1991. Carbohydrate feeding before exercise: effect of glycemic index. *Int J Sports Med* 12 (2): 180–86.

Timmons BW, Bar-Or O. 2003. RPE during prolonged cycling with and without carbohydrate ingestion in boys and men. *Med Sci Sports Exerc* 35 (11): 1901–07.

Yeo SE, Jentjens RL, Wallis GA, Jeukendrup AE. 2005. Caffeine increases exogenous carbohydrate oxidation during exercise. *J Appl Physiol* 99 (3): 844–50.

Young VR, Pellett PL. 1994. Plant proteins in relation to human protein and amino acid nutrition. *Am J Clin Nutr* 59 (5 Suppl): 1203S–12S.

Zawadzki KM, Yaspelkis BB 3rd, Ivy JL. 1992. Carbohydrate-protein complex increases the rate of muscle glycogen storage after exercise. *J Appl Physiol* 72 (5): 1854–59.

Fluid Replacement and Hyponatremia for Athletes

Professor Stephen H. S. WONG & Mr. John O'REILLY

Introduction

Physical activity leads to an increase in body temperature. The process of cooling the body down to its normal temperature involves an increase in skin blood flow, which allows sweating to occur. This results in a loss of body water, which can be quite extreme in the case of some athletes, particularly those exercising in the heat. Dehydration is characterized by a condition in which the body contains an insufficient volume of water for normal functioning. Following the loss of body water during exercise, it is a constant challenge to both coaches and athletes to find the most suitable strategy of adequately replacing the fluid lost without compromising performance.

While the human body is composed predominantly of water, even small changes in its water content can impair physiological function.[1-3] Dehydration is a regular occurrence in athletes performing strenuous endurance exercise, but when the exercise is undertaken in hot and humid environmental conditions, the results of dehydration can pose a serious threat to health.[1,3,4] The negative impact of dehydration on physiological function and exercise performance is believed to be initiated at levels as small as 1% to 2% of body weight, and are more exaggerated when the water losses exceed 3%.[5,6]

Numerous studies[7-10] have demonstrated that consuming drinks containing various formulations of water, carbohydrates (CHO), and electrolytes result in improved endurance performance and/or attenuated physiological stress on an athlete's cardiovascular, central nervous, and muscular systems. However, since innumerable variations of physical stresses, environmental factors, acclimatization states, exercise duration, intensity, and individual characteristics exist, it is extremely challenging to establish universal practical recommendations for fluid replacement. As a result, various guidelines based on different research findings and expert opinions have been developed and advocated as the most appropriate method of fluid replacement for an endurance event such as the marathon. The purpose of this chapter, therefore, is to attempt to draw together practical suggestions on fluid replacement based on relevant studies found in the research literature.

Hydration before Exercise

Pre-exercise hydration is crucial to ensure proper physiological function at the onset of exercise. The latest American College of Sports Medicine (ACSM) Position Stand[6] on fluid replacement suggests that all athletes should ingest 5–7 ml/kg of body weight of fluid at least four hours before an event, and another 3.5 ml/kg two hours before, if urine is still dark in color. At mealtimes prior to exercise tasks, it is advisable to include small amounts of salted snacks or sodium-containing foods to stimulate thirst and retain the consumed fluid. This point was recently underlined when it was found that pre-exercise ingestion of a concentrated sodium beverage (164 mmol Na+/l) increased plasma volume, reduced thermoregulatory strain, and increased exercise capacity in females prior to endurance exercise when compared with a low-sodium beverage (10 mmol Na+/l).[11] In addition, athletes should consume a nutritionally balanced diet and fluids during the 24 hours before an exercise session in order to ensure that they begin exercise well hydrated with normal plasma electrolyte levels. It has been suggested that consuming energy drinks with high concentrations of CHO, i.e., >25 g per 8 ounces (approx 237 ml), may not enable the body to restore the fluid balance within a short period of time prior to exercise.[12,13] These types of energy drinks will slow the rate at which fluid is absorbed from the intestine into the blood, and consequently impede rehydration. As a result, such energy drinks are not suitable fluids for consumption before physical activity or during periods when replacement of sweat loss is important.

Inducing hyperhydration (overhydration), i.e., greater than normal body water content, has been suggested as a means by which the body's thermoregulatory function might be improved with consequent benefits for exercise performance in hot environmental conditions.[14] Pre-exercise hyperhydration has also been shown to improve endurance capacity and peak power output, and decrease heart rate and thirst sensation, when compared to commencing exercise in a euhydrated state.[15] Furthermore, recent data from a separate study found that combining creatine and glycerol during the week pre-exercise was an effective method of hyperhydration capable of reducing thermal and cardiovascular responses.[16] The arguments in favor of pre-exercise hyperhydration have been contradicted, however, by a recent study which found that, despite a body mass loss of ~3% due to dehydration, the core temperature of ironman triathletes averaged only ~1% above normal.[17] It may have been expected that expanding body water would reduce the cardiovascular and heat strain during exercise by expanding blood volume and reducing blood tonicity, thereby improving exercise performance. A negative effect of an increased body water level is the elevated risk of having to void during competition.[18,19]

Although an elevated hydration state is often reported with glycerol use, its contribution to exercise performance is still controversial. It has been shown that glycerol hyperhydration has no significant advantage over water hyperhydration on performance or thermoregulation during a one-hour, variable-intensity exercise performance.[20] In fact, hyperhydration can substantially dilute and lower plasma sodium levels and therefore increase risk of dilutional hypernatremia.[21] In a study examining the physiological responses to glycerol hyperhydration,[22] the increase in total body water during cold air exposure was found to be greater with glycerol hyperhydration than with water alone.

Fluid Replacement during Exercise

In 1996, the American College of Sports Medicine (ACSM)[23] recommended in its Position Stand that, "During exercise, athletes should start drinking early and at regular intervals in an attempt to consume fluids at a rate sufficient to replace all the water lost through sweating (body weight loss), or consume the maximal amount that can be tolerated." This opinion has been since updated due to a raised awareness of dilutional hypernatremia. The current ACSM Position Stands state that the amount and rate of fluid replacement depends on the individual sweating rates, exercise duration, and opportunities to drink.[6,24] It further indicated that, when large volumes of fluid are consumed during exercise, the most acceptable temperature for the fluid ranges from 15°C to 20°C.

Due to a large number of variables such as body size, type of activity, duration of activity, intensity of exercise, weather conditions, level of conditioning, and genotype, it is very difficult to make any broad-ranging general recommendations regarding fluid intake. For example, research has shown that the sweat rate in footballers performing intermittent exercise during practice was higher than that of athletes running continuously in the same environmental conditions.[2] With this in mind, the International Marathon Medical Directors Association (IMMDA) recommended a maximum (5 km) and minimum (1.6 km) distance at which fluid replacement stations should be apart during marathons.[25] This is with a view to encourage athletes to tailor fluid replacement strategies to their specific needs at all times. In order to customize fluid replacement as much as possible, it is recommended that individuals should monitor body weight changes following exercise to estimate their sweat loss. However, it is not universally agreed that body weight should be used as a measure for fluid regulation, as it has been claimed that during prolonged endurance exercise, there is a complex regulation of body fluid volume and distribution that is unrelated to the maintenance of body weight.[25]

Some investigators[7–10] have documented improved endurance performance, which is typically demonstrated by increased performance time from fatigue or by increased power output during the later stages of endurance exercise in athletes using CHO beverages, when compared with water or other placebo beverages. Since fatigue during intense endurance exercise is primarily due to the depletion of the body's CHO reserves and dehydration, the improvement of capacity and performance is likely to be achieved by preventing the occurrence of hypoglycemia and sparing muscle glycogen. The National Athletic Trainers' Association[5] has recommended that including 60 g of CHO in one liter of fluid provides an adequate supply of CHO during or while recovering from an exercise bout and the CHO concentration in the ideal fluid replacement solution should be in the range of 6%–8% (g/100 ml). The ACSM recommends that CHO levels should not exceed 8%, as anything above this rate would reduce gastric emptying. It is also suggested that caffeine consumption may help to sustain exercise performance without altering hydration status during exercise.[8,26] Considering the optimal gastric emptying and fluid absorption, it is generally recommended that athletes ingest 30–60 g CHO per hour during exercise that lasts more than one hour and elicits fatigue.[7]

When the environmental conditions are hot, however, the benefits of CHO in a solution on exercise performance and capacity are equivocal. Research has found that CHO availability is not the limiting factor during performance of intermittent running to fatigue in hot environmental conditions, i.e., 30°C.[14] However, ingesting a 6.5% CHO-electrolyte solution during exercise results in higher blood glucose and lower free fatty acid concentrations at the end of exercise, compared with flavored water or a taste placebo. The main benefits of CHO ingestion during an event such as the marathon are likely to be a delay in the onset of hypoglycemia and the sparing of limited muscle glycogen stores. In many cases, the limiting factor contributing to early fatigue during intermittent prolonged exercise in hot environments (where the exercise duration will be less than one hour) is probably hyperthermia and not CHO availability.

Ingestion of CHO during prolonged moderate-to-high-intensity exercise is crucial to maintain high rates of CHO oxidation late in exercise, and as a result is likely to postpone fatigue and improve exercise performance. Most studies examining CHO beverage supplementation during exercise have focused on a single CHO and demonstrated that CHO is oxidized at a peak rate of about 1 g per minute. However, a study on trained male cyclists[27] found that exogenous CHO oxidation rates were higher with peak values of 1.7 g per minute, and estimated endogenous CHO oxidation was reduced when a mixture of glucose, fructose, and sucrose was ingested compared with an iso-caloric amount of glucose, a fact endorsed by the ACSM.[6] Whether the increased exogenous CHO oxidation rates could contribute to the improvement of exercise performance is not yet known. This topic continues to generate investigation as it has been shown recently that, when compared to glucose alone, co-ingestion of glucose and caffeine causes an increase in exogenous CHO oxidation during sub-maximal endurance exercise,[28] while conflicting reports have argued for[29] and against[30] a combination of glucose and fructose increasing CHO oxidation when compared to ingesting glucose alone. Further study is needed to clarify this issue.

While it appears to be generally accepted that increasing CHO concentration above 8% in sports drinks will not produce additional performance benefits, it has been shown that the inclusion of small amounts of protein in CHO beverages may generate additional benefits when compared with CHO-only drinks.[22] A recent study has shown that a CHO-protein beverage consumed every 15 minutes of exercise resulted in improved cycling time to fatigue and an attenuation in muscle damage.[22] In fact, it has been argued that adding protein to CHO drinks is unlikely to have any demonstrable effect on the synthesis of muscle glycogen during recovery, compared to ingesting iso-caloric CHO alone, since protein is used as fuel in negligible amounts.[12] However, the addition of protein to a sports beverage (0.25 g · kg^{-1} · h^{-1}) does improve net protein balance before, during, and after endurance exercise.[31]

In addition to CHO, sodium (20–30 mEq/L) and potassium (~2.5 mEq/L) are also recommended to be included in beverages consumed during exercise. These elements help to replace electrolytes lost in sweat, while sodium also assists in the stimulation of thirst.[32] Indeed, replacement of sodium losses has been shown to maintain plasma volume and reduce dehydration during prolonged exercise of moderate intensity.[33]

Rehydration after Exercise

Post-exercise fluid replacement is crucial to correct any fluid loss accumulated during exercise. The generally accepted recommendations of fluid replacement suggest that athletes should consume fluids in volumes equivalent to 100%–150% of sweat losses.[2,34] When aiming to achieve rapid rehydration, additional fluid needs to be taken on board in order to compensate for increased urine production.[32] In addition, a rehydration fluid should contain water to restore hydration status, CHO to replenish glycogen stores, and electrolytes to speed up rehydration.[32] Guidelines have recommended that 50–75 g of CHO, which can be provided in drinks, should be consumed within 15–30 minutes after exercise.[35]

Ideally, replacement fluids will contain between 5%–10% CHO.[6] When used as part of a CHO-loading regimen, drinks containing sufficient CHO should be consumed during the first hour of recovery.[12] In addition, sodium and potassium may reduce or prevent cramping during and after exercise.[32] Research has been conducted comparing the restorative capacities of a high CHO-protein beverage containing electrolytes and a traditional 6%

CHO-electrolyte sports beverage (SB) after glycogen-depleting exercise,[36] with the results showing that time-to-exhaustion during a subsequent exercise bout at 85% VO2max was found to be 55% greater following post-exercise ingestion of the CHO-protein beverage than in the SB. Furthermore, it has been stated that ingesting a beverage with protein and CHO during recovery from aerobic exercise increased muscle synthesis and improved net protein balance, as compared to feeding strategies that provided CHO only.[37] As far as other ingredients, such as pyruvate, glutamine, branched-chain amino acids, and vitamins, are concerned (all stated ingredients in some sports drinks), no convincing evidence has demonstrated their beneficial effects on athletic performance.[12] Also, rehydration incorporating glycerol was shown to have little or no significant effect on fluid-regulating factors post endurance exercise.[38]

Athletes are generally advised to rehydrate as soon as possible after finishing exercise. Although a high rate of fluid replacement during the first two hours post-exercise is shown to increase plasma volume rapidly and significantly, it also results in substantial urine production. Comparisons have been made between the effects of high and low rates of fluid intake on post-exercise rehydration in eight well-trained cyclists.[39] As a conclusion, it was suggested that for maximum retention of fluid, "fluid replacement can be met by lower drink intake over a prolonged time period" and this would be an appropriate strategy where the recovery time to the next exercise session was substantial, rather than being ingested in large boluses.[39, 40]

Hyponatremia in Athletes

Hyponatremia is a disorder in fluid-electrolyte balance that results in an abnormally low plasma sodium concentration (<130 mmol/liter; normal = 136–142mmol/liter).[3] A sustained decrease in the plasma sodium concentration disrupts the osmotic balance across the blood-brain barrier, resulting in a rapid influx of water into the brain. The mechanism by which hyponatremia arises is that the intravascular and extracellular fluid has a lower solute load than the intracellular fluids, and water flows into the cells producing intracellular swelling causing neurologic and physiologic dysfunction.[41] On the basis of studies of elite athletes,[42] as well as on marathon runners who have collapsed,[43] dilutional hyponatremia is thought to occur mostly as a result of excessive hypotonic fluid intake. Isotonic hyponatremia, which results from the retention of sodium-free isotonic fluids, is quite rare and is more relevant to a clinical setting. Hypertonic hyponatremia occurs with severe hypoglycemia or with glycerol loading[44] when water retained in the vascular space is sufficient to temporarily reduce blood sodium concentrations.

There are four different hypotheses regarding the possible causes of hyponatremia. One hypothesis is the syndrome of inappropriate antidiuretic hormone (SIADH) as evidenced by a recent investigation.[45] This results in reduced urine production, often as a result of inappropriately secreted arginine vasopressin (AVP) during prolonged exercise, which increases urine osmolality, thus decreasing urine volume[46] and leading to greater retention of ingested fluid in the presence of fluid overload. A second hypothesis is the sequestering of water in the gut, which results in post-race dilution when the water is absorbed. Another hypothesis is the abuse of non-steroidal anti-inflammatory drugs (NSAIDs) which can alter kidney function and decrease urine production. Finally, it is thought that hyponatremia may be caused by abnormally high sodium losses in sweat. Increased ectopic production and pituitary secretion can also play a role in the onset of hyponatremia.[47]

Quite often, excessive consumption of fluids is the common denominator in each of the above scenarios.[3] This was most certainly the situation in each of the 40 cases of hyponatremia that occurred at a military training facility in Georgia in 1990, where it was found that every case was associated with excessive water intake.[48] Indeed, the reason is that the potential dangers of severe dehydration and the need to drink adequately during prolonged periods of exercise have been so well publicized that, as a result, some individuals may choose to ingest dangerously large volumes of fluid.[49] Generally, athletes suffering from hyponatremia present with a combination of disorientation, altered mental status, headaches, vomiting, lethargy, swelling of the extremities (hands and feet), pulmonary edema, cerebral edema, and seizures. In extreme cases, hyponatremia can result in death if not treated properly.[41]

Particularly at risk are those athletes that run slowly, are smaller, less lean, and ingest fluids heavily before, during, and after competition.[25] Recent research also suggests that losing >0.75 kg of body weight during a marathon is advisable in order to decrease the risk of exercise-associated hyponatremia.[50,51] Furthermore, some studies have suggested that slower, more inexperienced female athletes who heeded the upper limit of previous ACSM guidelines are at a greater risk of developing hyponatremia by ingesting more fluid than they could excrete over the course of an endurance activity.[52,53] As a result of this, the IMMDA lowered the recommended range of fluid ingestion to 400–800 mL/h with a view to protecting smaller athletes from overdrinking.[54] It has also been indicated that the placement of aid stations every five km during a standard marathon is associated with the absence of hyponatremia.[55] This is a move away from a previously issued position stand[35] which promoted a concept that it was a good idea for less well-conditioned athletes traveling at slow speeds (8–9 km/h) for prolonged periods (> 4.5 hours) "to drink as much as tolerable" during exercise. Other event-related risk factors, which can lead to the onset of hyponatremia, include the high availability of drinking fluids on the course,[56] unusually hot environmental conditions,[57] or exercise in extremely cold temperatures.[58] With a view to avoiding the onset of hyponatremia, many athletes attempt to replace sodium losses by ingesting sports drinks with sodium included. Recent findings have suggested that the contribution of the type of fluid is small as compared with the volume of fluid ingested.[52]

Although excessive sodium loss may not be the primary cause in the pathogenesis of exercise-associated hyponatremia,[59] any "salty sweater," particularly those who are unacclimatized, have a high sweat rate, and a low level of fitness, are at an increased risk for hyponatremia.[3] Marathon runners and similar athletes who take part in endurance events longer than four hours in duration[49] run the risk of suffering from hyponatremia. This point is clearly highlighted in a study on athletes participating in the Comrades Marathon in South Africa.[60] This study showed that each of the eight athletes that collapsed with hyponatremia was fluid overloaded by an amount ranging from 1.22 to 5.92 liters. The strongest single predictor of hyponatremia is weight gain during competition due to excessive fluid intake over an extended period of time.

Upon completion of a marathon, vomiting is the one sign that is significantly more common in runners with exercise-associated hyponatremia than other patients being treated in the medical tent post-race.[61] When an athlete is displaying symptoms of possible hyponatremia, it is essential to get an accurate diagnosis as early as possible. Treatments vary depending on the severity of the situation. Mild cases will only need to consume salty food and drinks to regain appropriate sodium levels, whereas in a more serious situation, an intravenous line should be placed to administer medication as needed and to increase sodium levels, induce diuresis, and control seizures.[41]

In order to assess fluid replacement strategies with a view to preventing the onset of hyponatremia, some common sense must be applied by the athletes. For example, when recording a 3% body weight loss after exercise, the athlete should be aware that fluid intake during exercise should have been greater. On the other hand, if an endurance athlete weighs 1% heavier than pre-exercise, he or she should cut back on fluid intake during the next exercise bout. This issue is particularly relevant in endurance events as studies have shown that fluid replacement at or above 100% does not seem to offer any performance benefits.[62]

Conclusion

Dehydration, which is common during prolonged or intense exercise, disturbs the physiological function and adversely affects exercise performance and capacity, especially in hot environments. To minimize the adverse consequences of dehydration on endurance exercise performance, several key points should be considered.

(1) Athletes should begin exercise sessions well hydrated. This can be achieved by ingesting 5–7 ml/kg body weight four hours before the event, and take in a nutritionally balanced diet and fluids during the 24 hours before an exercise session. It is important not to begin an exercise session in an over-hydrated state.[24]

(2) During exercise (provided that the athlete commences exercise in a euhydrated state), fluid replacement should approximate sweat and urine losses, which generally requires fluid intake of 0.4–0.8 liters or more per hour.[63] Apart from water and electrolytes, drinks producing an absorption rate of 30–80 g CHO per hour (i.e., approximately 5%–10% CHO, depending on consumption) will be beneficial to postpone fatigue and improve performance during exercise lasting more than one hour.[6]

(3) It is generally accepted that, for adequate fluid replacement during

the recovery period, athletes should consume fluids in volumes of 100% up to 150% of sweat losses.[2] In addition, a rehydration solution should contain water to restore hydration status, CHOs to replenish glycogen stores, and electrolytes to speed up rehydration.[6]

Hyponatremia is a disorder in fluid-electrolyte balance that results in an abnormally low plasma sodium concentration.

(1) It predominately affects endurance athletes (events lasting more than four hours) and usually is a result of excessive ingestion of hypotonic fluids before, during, and after competition. Particularly at risk are those athletes that run slowly, are smaller, less lean, have a high sweat-rate, and are less well conditioned.

(2) Athletes at risk need to revise hydration strategies and drink more conservatively during competition.

Despite these generally accepted key points of fluid replacement, it should be noted that an individual needs to develop his or her own strategy due to variations between the type of event undertaken and the environmental conditions in which such events take place.

References

1. Casa DJ, Clarkson PM, & Roberts WO. 2005. American College of Sports Medicine roundtable on hydration and physical activity: consensus statements. *Curr Sports Med Rep* 4 (3): 115–27.

2. Godek SF, Bartolozzi AR, Godek JJ. 2005. Sweat rate and fluid turnover in American football players compared with runners in a hot and humid environment. *Br J Sports Med* 39 (4): 205–11; discussion 205–11.

3. Murray B, Stofan J, Eichner RE. 2003. Hyponatremia in athletes. *Sports Science Exchange* 88: 16 (1)

4. Carter R 3rd, Cheuvront SN, Williams JO, Kolka MA, Stephenson LA, Sawka MN, et al. 2005. Epidemiology of hospitalizations and deaths from heat illness in soldiers. *Med Sci Sports Exerc* 37 (8): 1338–44.

5. Casa DJ, Armstrong LE, Hillman SK, Montain SJ, Reiff RV, Rich BS, et al. 2000. National Athletic Trainers' Association Position Statement: Fluid Replacement for Athletes. *J Athl Train* 35 (2): 212–24.

6. Sawka MN, Burke LM, Eichner ER, Maughan RJ, Montain SJ, Stachenfeld NS.

2007. American College of Sports Medicine position stand. Exercise and fluid replacement. *Med Sci Sports Exerc* 39 (2): 377–90.

7. Coyle EF. 1992. Fluid and fuel intake during exercise. *J Sports Sci* 22 (1): 39–55.

8. Coyle EF, Montain SJ. 1992. Carbohydrate and fluid ingestion during exercise: are there trade-offs? *Med Sci Sports Exerc* 24 (6): 671–78.

9. Jeukendrup AE. 2004. Carbohydrate intake during exercise and performance. *Nutrition* 20 (7–8): 669–77.

10. Welsh RS, Davis JM, Burke JR, Williams HG. 2002. Carbohydrates and physical/mental performance during intermittent exercise to fatigue. *Med Sci Sports Exerc* 34 (4): 723–31.

11. Sims ST, Rehrer NJ, Bell ML, Cotter JD. 2007. Preexercise sodium loading aids fluid balance and endurance for women exercising in the heat. *J Appl Physiol* 103 (2): 534–41.

12. Bonci L. 2002. "Energy" Drinks: Help, Harm, or Hype? *Gatorade Sports Science Exchange* 84 (15) no. 1.

13. Ryan AJ, Lambert GP, Shi X, Chang RT, Summers RW, Gisolfi CV. 1998. Effect of hypohydration on gastric emptying and intestinal absorption during exercise. *J Appl Physiol* 84 (5): 1581–88.

14. Morris JG, Nevill ME, Thompson D, Collie J, Williams C. 2003. The influence of a 6.5% carbohydrate-electrolyte solution on performance of prolonged intermittent high-intensity running at 30 degrees C. *J Sports Sci* 21 (5): 371–81.

15. Goulet ED, Rousseau SF, Lamboley CR, Plante GE, Dionne IJ. 2008. Pre-exercise hyperhydration delays dehydration and improves endurance capacity during 2 h of cycling in a temperate climate. *J Physiol Anthropol* 27 (5): 263–71.

16. Easton C, Turner S, Pitsiladis YP. 2007. Creatine and glycerol hyperhydration in trained subjects before exercise in the heat. *Int J Sport Nutr Exerc Metab* 17 (1): 70–91.

17. Laursen PB, Suriano R, Quod MJ, Lee H, Abbiss1 CR, Nosaka1 K, et al. 2006. Core temperature and hydration status during an Ironman triathlon. *Br J Sports Med* 40 (4): 320–25; discussion 325.

18. Freund BJ, Montain SJ, Young AJ, Sawka MN, DeLuca JP, Pandolf KB, et al. 1995. Glycerol hyperhydration: hormonal, renal, and vascular fluid responses. *J Appl Physiol* 79 (6): 2069–77.

19. O'Brien C, Freund BJ, Young AJ, Sawka MN. 2005. Glycerol hyperhydration: physiological responses during cold-air exposure. *J Appl Physiol* 99 (2): 515–21.

20. Marino FE, Kay D, Cannon J. 2003. Glycerol hyperhydration fails to improve endurance performance and thermoregulation in humans in a warm humid environment. *Pflügers Arch* 446 (4): 455–62.

21. Montain SJ, Cheuvront SN, Sawka MN. 2006. Exercise associated hyponatraemia: quantitative analysis to understand the aetiology. *Br J Sports Med* 40 (2): 98–105.

22. Saunders MJ, Kane MD, Todd MK. 2004. Effects of a carbohydrate-protein beverage on cycling endurance and muscle damage. *Med Sci Sports Exerc* 36 (7): 1233–38.

23. Convertino VA, Armstrong LE, Coyle EF, Mack GW, Sawka MN, Senay LC Jr, et al. 1996. American College of Sports Medicine position stand. Exercise and fluid replacement. *Med Sci Sports Exerc* 28 (1): i–vii.

24. American Dietetic Association, Dietitians of Canada, American College of Sports Medicine, Rodriguez NR, Di Marco NM, Langley S. 2009. American College of Sports Medicine position stand. Nutrition and athletic performance. *Med Sci Sports Exerc* 41 (3): 709–31.

25. Hew-Butler T, Verbalis JG, Noakes TD, International Marathon Medical Directors Association. 2006. Updated fluid recommendation: position statement from the International Marathon Medical Directors Association (IMMDA). *Clin J Sport Med* 16 (4): 283–92.

26. Cox GR, Desbrow B, Montgomery PG, Anderson ME, Bruce CR, Macrides TA, et al. 2002. Effect of different protocols of caffeine intake on metabolism and endurance performance. *J Appl Physiol* 93 (3): 990–99.

27. Jentjens RL, Achten J, Jeukendrup AE. 2004. High oxidation rates from combined carbohydrates ingested during exercise. *Med Sci Sports Exerc* 36 (9): 1551–58.

28. Yeo SE, Jentjens RL, Wallis GA, Jeukendrup AE. 2005. Caffeine increases exogenous carbohydrate oxidation during exercise. *J Appl Physiol* 99 (3): 844–50.

29. Jeukendrup AE, Moseley L, Mainwaring GI, Samuels S, Perry S, Mann CH. 2006. Exogenous carbohydrate oxidation during ultraendurance exercise. *J Appl Physiol* 100 (4): 1134–41.

30. Hulston CJ, Wallis GA, Jeukendrup AE. 2009. Exogenous CHO oxidation with glucose plus fructose intake during exercise. *Med Sci Sports Exerc* 41 (2): 357–63.

31. Koopman R, Pannemans DLE, Jeukendrup AE, Gijsen AP, Senden JMG, Halliday D, et al. 2004. Combined ingestion of protein and carbohydrate improves

protein balance during ultra-endurance exercise. *Am J Physiol Endocrinol Metab* 287 (4): E712–20.

32. Shirreffs SM, Armstrong LE, Cheuvront SN. 2004. Fluid and electrolyte needs for preparation and recovery from training and competition. *J Sports Sci* 22 (1): 57–63.

33. Sanders B, Noakes TD, Dennis SC. 2001. Sodium replacement and fluid shifts during prolonged exercise in humans. *Eur J Appl Physiol* 84 (5): 419–25.

34. Wong SH, Williams C. 2000. Influence of different amounts of carbohydrate on endurance running capacity following short term recovery. *Int J Sports Med* 21 (6): 444–52.

35. Position of the American Dietetic Association, Dietitians of Canada, and the American College of Sports Medicine: Nutrition and athletic performance. *J Am Diet Assoc* 100 (12): 1543–56.

36. Williams MB, Raven PB, Fogt DL, Ivy JL. 2003. Effects of recovery beverages on glycogen restoration and endurance exercise performance. *J Strength Cond Res* 17 (1): 12–19.

37. Howarth KR, Moreau NA, Phillips SM, Gibala MJ. 2009. Coingestion of protein with carbohydrate during recovery from endurance exercise stimulates skeletal muscle protein synthesis in humans. *J Appl Physiol* 106 (4): 1394–1402.

38. Kavouras SA, Armstrong LE, Maresh CM, Casa DJ, Herrera-Soto JA, Scheett TP, et al. 2006. Rehydration with glycerol: endocrine, cardiovascular, and thermoregulatory responses during exercise in the heat. *J Appl Physiol* 100 (2): 442–50.

39. Kovacs EM, Schmahl RM, Senden JM, Brouns F. 2002. Effect of high and low rates of fluid intake on post-exercise rehydration. *Int J Sport Nutr Exerc Metab* 12 (1): 14–23.

40. Wong SH, Williams C, Simpson M, Ogaki T. 1998. Influence of fluid intake pattern on short-term recovery from prolonged, submaximal running and subsequent exercise capacity. *J Sports Sci* 16 (2): 143–52.

41. Binkley HM, Beckett J, Casa DJ, Kleiner DM, Plummer PE. 2002. National Athletic Trainers' Association Position Statement: Exertional Heat Illnesses. *J Athl Train* 37 (3): 329–43.

42. Noakes TD, Sharwood K, Collins M, Perkins DR. 2004. The dipsomania of great distance: water intoxication in an Ironman triathlete. *Br J Sports Med* 38 (4): E16.

43. Davis DP, Videen JS, Marino A, Vilke GM, Dunford JV, Van Camp SP, et al.

2001. Exercise-associated hyponatremia in marathon runners: a two-year experience. *J Emerg Med* 21 (1): 47–57.

44. Frizzell RT, Lang GH, Lowance DC, Lathan SR. 1986. Hyponatremia and ultramarathon running. *JAMA* 255 (6): 772–74.

45. Siegel AJ, Verbalis JG, Clement S, Mendelson JH, Mello NK, Adner M, et al. 2007. Hyponatremia in marathon runners due to inappropriate arginine vasopressin secretion. *Am J Med* 120 (5): 461.e11–7.

46. Hew-Butler T, Jordaan E, Stuempfle KJ, Speedy DB, Siegel AJ, Noakes TD, et al. 2008. Osmotic and Nonosmotic Regulation of Arginine Vasopressin during Prolonged Endurance Exercise. *J Clin Endocrinol Metab* 93 (6): 2072–78.

47. Smellie WS, Heald A. 2007. Hyponatraemia and hypernatraemia: pitfalls in testing. *BMJ* 334 (7591): 473–76.

48. Gardner JW. 2002. Death by water intoxication. *Mil Med* 167 (5): 432–34.

49. Noakes TD, Speedy DB. 2006. Case proven: exercise associated hyponatraemia is due to overdrinking. So why did it take 20 years before the original evidence was accepted? *Br J Sports Med* 40 (7): 567–72.

50. Chorley J, Cianca J, Divine J. 2007. Risk factors for exercise-associated hyponatremia in non-elite marathon runners. *Clin J Sport Med* 17 (6): 471–77.

51. Maughan RJ, Shirreffs SM, Watson P. 2007. Exercise, Heat, Hydration and the Brain. *J Am Coll Nutr* 26 (suppl 5): 604S–612S.

52. Almond CS, Shin AY, Fortescue EB, Mannix RC, Wypij D, Binstadt BA, et al. 2005. Hyponatremia among runners in the Boston Marathon. *N Engl J Med* 352 (15): 1550–56.

53. Hew TD, Chorley JN, Cianca JC, Divine JG. 2003. The incidence, risk factors, and clinical manifestations of hyponatremia in marathon runners. *Clin J Sport Med* 13 (1): 41–47.

54. Noakes T. 2003. Fluid replacement during marathon running. *Clin J Sport Med* 13 (5): 309–18.

55. Reid SA, Speedy DB, Thompson JM, Noakes TD, Mulligan G, Page T, et al. 2004. Study of hematological and biochemical parameters in runners completing a standard marathon. *Clin J Sport Med* 14 (6): 344–53.

56. Wharam PC, Speedy DB, Noakes TD, Thompson JM, Reid SA, Holtzhausen LM. 2006. NSAID use increases the risk of developing hyponatremia during an Ironman triathlon. *Med Sci Sports Exerc* 38 (4): 618–22.

57. Goudie AM, Tunstall-Pedoe DS, Kerins M, Terris J. 2006. Exercise-associated hyponatraemia after a marathon: case series. *J R Soc Med* 99 (7): 363–67.

58. Stuempfle KJ, Lehmann DR, Case HS, Bailey S, Hughes SL, McKenzie J, et al. 2002. Hyponatremia in a cold weather ultraendurance race. *Alaska Med* 44 (3): 51–55.

59. Speedy DB, Rogers IR, Noakes TD, Wright S, Thompson JM, Campbell R, et al. 2000. Exercise-induced hyponatremia in ultradistance triathletes is caused by inappropriate fluid retention. *Clin J Sport Med* 10 (4): 272–78.

60. Irving RA, Noakes TD, Buck R, van Zyl Smit R, Raine E, Godlonton J, et al. 1991. Evaluation of renal function and fluid homeostasis during recovery from exercise-induced hyponatremia. *J Appl Physiol* 70 (1): 342–48.

61. Chorley JN. 2007. Hyponatraemia: identification and evaluation in the marathon medical area. *Sports Med* 37 (4–5): 451–54.

62. McConell GK, Burge CM, Skinner SL, Hargreaves M. 1997. Influence of ingested fluid volume on physiological responses during prolonged exercise. *Acta Physiol Scand* 160 (2): 149–56.

63. Cheuvront SN, Carter RI, Sawka MN. 2003. Fluid balance and endurance exercise performance. *Curr Sports Med Rep* 2 (4): 202–208.

Motivation and Psychological Preparation for Marathons

Mr. Johan NG & Dr. Chris LONSDALE

Introduction

The term *motivation* is used widely and frequently to describe and explain various human behaviors. Coaches and players often attribute success to "being very motivated" or relate failure to lack of motivation. Although no one would question the importance of motivation in enhancing performance, the term often represents a vague concept without a clear and precise definition. Indeed, motivation is sometimes used to represent ideas such as the desire to win, physiological arousal, or even rewards (Finch, 2002).

In psychology, motivation is defined by the initiation, direction, intensity, and persistence of effort (Vallerand and Rousseau, 2001). Motivation is a multifaceted construct that describes the "why," "how to," "how much," and "how long" of exerting effort in pursuit of a goal. In addition to motivation itself, Weiss and Ferrer-Caja (2002) suggested that knowledge of the antecedents and outcomes of motivation are also important in enhancing performance. By understanding the antecedents and outcomes of motivation, practitioners can structure the environment in order to achieve more beneficial motivational outcomes, such as better performance, greater adherence to training regimens, and enhanced well-being.

Marathon running represents a grueling challenge that requires athletes to output extreme physical effort over at least two hours (Dosil, 2006). Marathon training is also very taxing in terms of time and effort required. To attain optimal performance, a training program lasting six months of up to six sessions of tough training per week is required (Nerurkar, 2004). In spite of the hardships of races and trainings, the number of runners in marathon races around the globe has increased in recent years (e.g., Boston Athletic

Association, 2007; Hong Kong Amateur Athletic Association, n.d.). It is therefore interesting to know why more and more people are participating in this sport.

In this chapter, we review research on the participation motives of distance runners. Research comparing the motivation of various groups of runners (e.g., gender, experience) is also discussed. Two theories of motivation are presented, and the applications and implications of these theories are discussed. We conclude by offering suggestions regarding methods to enhance motivation for distance running.

The first studies investigating motivation in distance running were conducted in the 1980s. Studies specifically examining motivations for marathon running have been conducted in subsequent decades. These studies were designed to explore the reasons why people began and continued to participate in running as recreation or as a profession. Both quantitative (e.g., Masters, Ogles, and Jolton, 1993) and qualitative (e.g., Clerici, 2004) methodologies have been employed to gather data from runners, and the results of the studies suggested that runners had five broad types of participation motives including (a) physical health benefits, (b) mental health benefits, (c) social reasons, (d) achievement, and (e) enjoyment.

Physical health benefits

Distance running is an aerobic exercise that can help improve one's cardio-vascular fitness and control one's weight (Wilmore and Costill, 1999), and it is also considered one of the most convenient and economical types of exercise (Vitulli and DePace III, 1992). Not surprisingly, many studies have shown that enhancing health and physical fitness is rated as the most important motive for participating in distance running (Johnsgard, 1985a, 1985b; Vitulli, 1987; Vitulli and DePace III, 1992). Masters and Ogles (1995) have found that many beginning runners place health reasons as an important motive, suggesting that many runners may have started their training for such physical health-related reasons.

Apart from enhancing physical fitness and health, weight control was also found to be a salient reason for individuals to continue their running training programs (Johnsgard, 1985a, 1985b). Moreover, Ogles, Masters, and

Richardson (1995) found that women who competed in long distance races endorse weight concern as a more important motive than men do.

Mental health benefits

Physical activity has been shown to have psychological benefits such as reducing stress and anxiety (Scully, Kremer, Meade, Graham, and Dudgeon, 1998). Research has revealed that people run marathons in order to achieve these psychological health benefits. For example, in studies conducted by Johnsgard (1985a, 1985b), groups of dedicated distance runners reported that one of their reasons for running was to reduce tension and feel better about themselves. In another study investigating gender differences in motivation in a group of runners, Divine and colleagues (Divine, Chorley, Kohl, and Cianca, 1999) found that significantly more experienced female runners rated "to feel good about myself" as the most important motive to continue running. Past research has also demonstrated self-esteem and personal identity (Vitulli, 1987) as important motives to attain psychological benefits.

Social reasons

Research has also shown that people run for social reasons. One such reason is affiliating with others (Carmack and Martens, 1979). One study has suggested that affiliation is a more important motive in women than in men (Ogles et al., 1995). Furthermore, Ogles and Masters (2000) have reported evidence that, compared to younger runners, older marathon runners place more importance on social relationships.

Social recognition is another reason people participate in running. Clough, Shepherd, and Maughan (1989) have found that some runners run to acquire or maintain their social status. Masters and Ogles (1995) have also found that veteran marathon runners are generally more motivated by their social identity as a marathon runner than are beginner runners.

Achievement

The motive to achieve goals is also found to be an important motive for runners. Personal goal achievement has been reported as an important motive to run in various studies (e.g., Barrell, Holt, and MacKean, 1988; Hayashi and Weiss, 1994; Masters et al., 1993). Younger runners (Ogles and Masters, 2000) and beginner marathon runners (Masters and Ogles, 1995) have been found to endorse such motives more than older runners.

Runners are also motivated by the challenge in running marathons. In Johnsgard's (1985a, 1985b) studies, male runners have shown high motives to challenge and improve themselves. Clough and colleagues (1989) have also found that challenge is one of the prime motives for participation in running. Runners have reported that reasons such as the physical challenges and the ability to compete against oneself had strong influences in motivating them to run marathons. Elite runners in Clerici's (2004) study have also suggested that the enjoyment of winning and being able to challenge one's own goals are main reasons they participate in marathon running.

Enjoyment

Runners have also reported enjoyment as an important motive for their participation. This source of motivation refers to the enjoyment of the activity itself and differs from the enjoyment of winning or being with friends. A number of studies have revealed that runners continue for the enjoyment of running (e.g., Barrell et al., 1988; Summers, Machin, and Sargent, 1983). In particular, Clerici (2004) interviewed a number of elite marathon runners, and all of the respondents mentioned that they enjoyed running.

In summary, physical health and fitness benefits seem to be the most important motives for running (e.g, Vitulli, 1987) and running marathons specifically (e.g., Masters and Ogles, 1995). Enjoyment of running has also been found to be an important motive, especially in elite runners (Clerici, 2004). Much of the reviewed literature show that goal achievement is another important motive to run (e.g, Clough et al., 1989), whereas social reasons also motivated runners (Carmack and Martens, 1979).

The studies reviewed thus far are designed to investigate why people participate in marathons. While this descriptive research serves as a useful starting point, little, if any, research has been conducted to determine the antecedents and consequences of these different motives. For example, little is known about how significant others might influence the different motives of runners or how different motives would lead to various outcomes, such as adherence or enjoyment. This type of inferential research is important to broaden our understanding of the causes and effects of various factors, and it may assist practitioners to design interventions to motivate runners. In the following sections, two theoretical frameworks of motivation are introduced in an attempt to explain and predict runners' motivations. Suggestions for enhancing motivations are discussed in light of the theories.

Motivation Theories

Self-Determination Theory

According to self-determination theory (SDT) (Deci and Ryan, 1985; Ryan and Deci, 2002), humans have three basic psychological needs: competence, autonomy, and relatedness. SDT states that these needs are universal and innate. Optimal psychological health and well-being will be facilitated when these basic needs are satisfied.

The need for competence refers to our need for a sense of ability and achievement. The need is satisfied when one feels capable of performing a task or achieving a goal. Finishing a race within a targeted time or winning a race may provide a runner with positive information about his or her ability, thereby satisfying the need for competence. Autonomy refers to the perception of choice. Autonomous individuals will perceive what they are doing is due to their personal choice and that they are acting according to their own will. A less autonomous individual will feel that he or she is performing an act under pressure or other external force. The need for relatedness refers to the need of feeling connected to other individuals or certain social groups. This need can be satisfied when an individual feels a sense of belonging to a social group, such as running with a group of teammates.

Intrinsic and extrinsic motivation (Figure 1)

According to SDT, when the basic needs are satisfied while performing a certain act, intrinsic motivation toward the act will be facilitated or supported. Intrinsic motivation is defined as "the doing of an activity for its inherent satisfaction rather than for some separable consequence" (Ryan and Deci, 2000: 56). Intrinsically motivated runners typically run for the

Figure 1 Types of Extrinsic and Intrinsic Motivation According to Self-Determination Theory

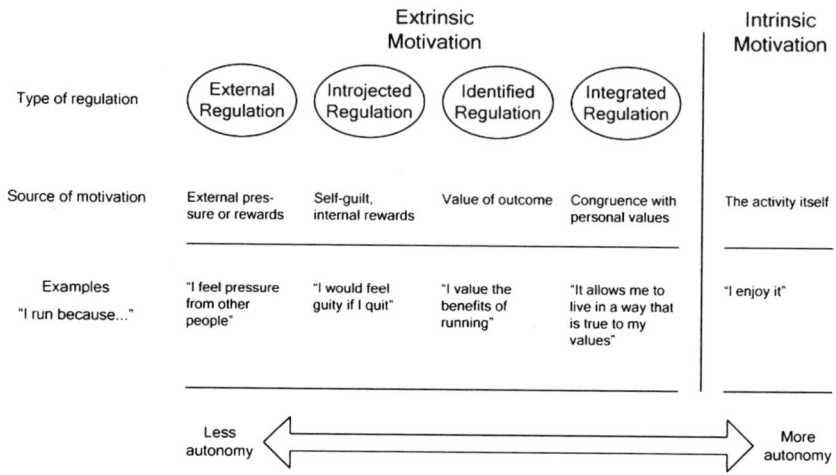

enjoyment of running. On the other hand, if an activity is done for other separable reasons and not the enjoyment of the activity itself, the motive to do the activity is referred as extrinsic motivation. Running in order to lose weight or to avoid feelings of guilt are examples of extrinsic motivation.

According to SDT, extrinsic motives can be divided into four categories, known as regulations. The four types of regulation lie along a continuum, according to the level of autonomy.

- External regulation is the least autonomous form, with motivation arising from external pressure or rewards such as money. An example is someone who runs a marathon in order to receive the prize money or sponsorships.
- Introjected regulation refers to motivation from guilt avoidance or ego-enhancement. A runner who runs to avoid guilt or to retain a sense of self-worth is classified under this type of regulation.
- Identified regulation occurs when an activity is pursued because the outcome of participation is valued. Running to maintain health may be one example.

- Integrated regulation is the type of regulation that results when behaviors are congruent with one's personally endorsed values, goals, and needs that are already part of the self (Ryan and Deci, 2002). This is the most autonomous form of extrinsic motivation. Actions underpinned by this type of motive may be carried out because the behavior is perceived as part of one's identity. An individual who runs because he or she believes that running is an important part of a healthy lifestyle is an example of an individual motivated by integrated regulation.

SDT predicts that having intrinsic motivation and more autonomous forms of extrinsic motivation towards an activity, such as identified or integrated regulations, will result in more volitional persistence, greater health and well-being, and more effective performance (Ryan and Deci, 2002). On the other hand, if an activity is motivated by the less autonomous forms of extrinsic motivation, such as external or introjected regulations, the perceived interest, value, or effort paid will be decreased (Ryan and Deci, 2000). In marathon running, for example, runners who think running is fun are predicted to persist longer in running and will run faster; whereas those who are coerced by health practitioners will perceive running as less interesting and will exert less effort.

Using SDT to interpret existing research

Our review of the literature involving marathon motivations has shown that many runners continue running for physical benefits. This group of runners may include those who run because they are forced by doctors or dietitians (external regulation) and those who value the physical benefits of running (identified regulation). Running to maintain self-esteem, a type of introjected regulation, has also been reported as a reason to run (Vitulli, 1987). Intrinsic motivation, or running for enjoyment, has been found to be a motive to compete in marathons (Clerici, 2004).

According to SDT, runners who adopt external or introjected regulated motives, such as people who are forced to run or who run only to maintain self image, are predicted to be more likely to drop out. On the other hand, runners who endorsed identified regulated motives, such as those who value the health benefits of running or who use running as a means to affiliate with certain social groups, are expected to continue participating. Ultimately, runners who enjoy running are the most likely to persist in running, to experience enhanced psychological well-being, and to achieve better performances.

Achievement Goal Theory

Achievement goal theory (AGT) (Ames, 1992; Nicholls, 1989) suggests that individuals have different ways of defining success which can be reflected in the achievement goals they adopt. When goals are met, individuals gain feelings of perceived competence. According to this theory, by understanding how success and failure are defined, changes in perceived competence and resultant achievement behaviors can be anticipated.

AGT proposes that achievement goals are differentiated into task-oriented goals and ego-oriented goals (Nicholls, 1989). Task-oriented goals, also known as mastery goals, are defined as self-referenced goals that aim at attaining self improvements (Ames, 1992). High task-oriented individuals, or those who endorse many task-oriented goals, measure success based on self-referenced performances or standards. They aim to challenge personal records or master difficult skills. For example, runners might set a task goal of finishing a marathon faster than the previous best time. When a task goal is not met, AGT suggests that the individual will more likely attribute the failure to the lack of effort rather than the lack of ability or competence. This attribution is expected to lead to increased effort and persistence in the future (Maehr and Nicholls, 1980). For instance, if a runner with a high task orientation finishes the race 10 minutes slower than his/her best time, he/she would likely feel that he/she has not tried his/her best, and will try harder in the next race.

Ego-orientated goals, or ego goals, are goals that aim at performing better than others. These goals are norm-referenced and are typically achieved by beating others (Nicholls, 1989). High ego-oriented individuals will be motivated to win races or finish races ahead of certain opponents. Such goals are based on comparisons with others, thus one may not be able to achieve ego-goals simply by giving more effort; rather, success is dependent on many other factors. Effort is not as prominent in reaching ego goals; therefore, individuals adopting these goals will likely perceive failure as a lack of ability and may lose motivation. According to AGT, these individuals tend to choose very easy or very hard goals to avoid feelings of failure (Maehr and Nicholls, 1980).

For example, an ego-oriented runner may set a goal of winning a race. However, if he/she finishes second, despite giving maximum effort and achieving a personal best time, he/she would still perceive a sense of failure. Over time, if the runner experiences many such failures, AGT predicts that his/her perceived ability, and motivation towards running, would decrease. As a result, he/she might eventually stop running altogether.

Researchers have demonstrated that task orientation and ego orientation are independent constructs (Duda and Nicholls, 1992; Nicholls, 1989). That is to say, one can be high in task and ego orientations or low in both (Hodge and Petlichkoff, 2000). In fact, evidence has shown that elite athletes who have adopted a high task and moderate-high ego orientation use more psychological skills, resulting in higher performances, as compared to groups of high-task, low-ego, and low-task, high-ego athletes (Harwood, Cumming, and Fletcher, 2004).

In the reviewed studies, motives such as enhancing physical health and fitness or improving oneself, are frequently reported. The success or failure of meeting the goals are judged by comparing self-performances. These goals are self-referenced, aiming at self-improvements, and thus might be considered task goals. Therefore, runners reporting these motives might have a high task orientation.

Elite runners have reported that, in addition to the enjoyment of running itself, they enjoyed the feeling of winning (Clerici, 2004). This finding suggests that elite runners also have at least moderate ego orientation. Harwood and colleagues (2004) have found that performances are greater in individuals who have high task and moderate-high ego orientations. However, moderate or high ego orientations do not always enhance performance or motivation. In fact, AGT predicts that having low task but high ego orientation would lead to higher dropout rates (Dweck, 1986).

According to AGT, high task-oriented runners who set goals such as improving personal best time or personal health are predicted to adhere longer and give more effort to running. Also, low-task, high ego-oriented runners are predicted to have higher tendencies of dropping out. However, high-task, moderate-high ego-oriented runners are anticipated to persist longer and might include competitive runners who aim at achieving higher performances.

In the preceding sections, we have utilized SDT and AGT frameworks to interpret the existing literature concerning motivation towards marathon running. In addition to understanding the nature of participation motivation, these theories may provide a framework to explain the mechanisms of how motivation is enhanced or thwarted. By utilizing these theories, a better understanding of training and race performance behaviors may also be gained. However, no research has tested the theories specifically within the context of marathon running. Research investigating the links between the different types of motivation as specified in SDT or the adoption of different goals in AGT, and outcomes such as training persistence and racing performance, may provide important evidence for those interested in promoting marathon participation and enhancing performance.

Enhancing Motivation

To conclude, we suggest a number of practical ways to help the enhancement of motivation in marathon training and races. These suggestions are based largely on existing research and the predictions of SDT and AGT. As previously noted, there is a need for more marathon-specific, theory-based motivation research.

Goal-setting to enhance perceived competence

Goal-setting has been found to be an effective way to enhance motivation in sport and exercise (Gould, 2006; Weinberg, Burton, Yukelson, and Weigand, 1993). By setting clear goals for training and races, runners can direct attention and effort to aspects which may have been overlooked, such as stride lengths and pace during runs. By meeting goals they have set, runners can see improvements explicitly and enhance their own feelings of competence, thus promoting intrinsic motivation.

To maximize the effectiveness of goal setting, there are some guidelines that runners should note. First, according to AGT, the use of task goals is recommended to strengthen the persistence of effort and avoid feelings of incompetence (Weinberg, 1996). Goals such as finishing a distance faster than an improved time would be common for runners. Some runners may set ego goals, such as finishing in the top 10 in the race. They may see such goals as an extra boost to their motivation and performance in races. However, runners should be careful not to see such goals as their primary focus, but just as an additional bonus if achieved.

Another point to note is that some runners tend to set too many or too difficult goals (Weinberg and Gould, 2003). On the other hand, goals should not be too easy either, as achieving easy goals may require very little or no effort (Weinberg, 1996) and will result in little enhancement of competence perceptions. Thus, runners should attempt to set a modest number (i.e., two or three) of challenging, but not too difficult, goals (Locke, Shaw, Saari, and Latham, 1981).

Goals should also be specific and measurable (Weinberg, 1996). Goals such as "to improve" are too vague, making it difficult to determine whether or not the goal has been reached. Objective measures such as time and distance can be utilized to provide concrete and measurable goals. It is also important that goals are self-set (Smith, 1994), as runners will adhere to goals set themselves more than to those set by coaches, parents, etc.

Goals can also be categorized as short-term and long-term goals. Short-term goals are to be met within a short period of time, such as during a particular training session. Long-term goals are those to be met after a longer period, such as one year later. The use of a series of short-term goals in order to meet a long-term goal is encouraged (Kyllo and Landers, 1995). Long-term goals help to set up a clear target for the future, while short-term goals help to reach the more difficult long-term goals one step at a time.

Athletes often overlook the importance of writing out and recording their goals (Weinberg, 1996). Writing out goals will help athletes define and remember their goals more easily, and can provide them with clear information of whether the goals have been met. Goals, especially long-term goals, should be flexible and adjustable. Goals should be set so that they can be adjusted according to the changes of environmental factors, progress of improvement or other factors that are unknown at the time the goals are set.

Supporting autonomy

As indicated in SDT, intrinsic motivation towards a behavior can be supported by perceptions of autonomy. By promoting more autonomous forms of motivation, higher persistence, well-being, and performance are more likely to be achieved (Ryan & Deci, 2002). Supporting autonomy does not mean the athlete is allowed to take full control of their training sessions. Instead, it concerns providing guidance with choice within the limits and rules set by the coach.

Mageau and Vallerand (2003) have provided criteria for autonomy-supportive behaviors. They suggest that the following autonomy-supportive behaviors should be encouraged:

- provide as many choices as possible within the limits set;
- provide a rationale for tasks;
- acknowledge athletes' feelings; and
- provide athletes with opportunities to take initiatives.

Mallett (2005) has suggested a few behaviors that may be autonomy-supportive. To provide perception of personal choice, coaches might allow athletes decide on training content, training times, and training venues. By holding formal meetings, the rationale for decisions made by the coach can be communicated. Actively seeking for suggestions and opinions might allow athletes' voices to be heard. Finally, runners may be given the opportunity to take initiative on deciding matters such as the choice of team uniform. Autonomy-supportive behaviors will not only improve athletes' perception of autonomy, but they may foster trust and perceptions of relatedness between individual athletes and the coach or team. Hence, such behaviors are predicted to be effective in promoting runners' intrinsic motivation.

Cognitive strategies

In running, researchers have focused on two types of cognitive strategies: namely association and dissociation. Association refers to the cognitive strategy of focusing on one's body sensations in order to maintain a physical awareness that is critical to performance (Weinberg, Smith, Jackson, and Gould, 1984). Runners who use this type of strategy will monitor and control their breathing and other bodily sensations. They can make adjustments to their pace or stride according to physiological feedback.

Dissociation, on the other hand, refers to attempts to distract oneself from bodily sensations while running (Weinberg et al., 1984). Runners who employ such a strategy may focus on the music to which they are listening or on the environment in which they are running.

Association and dissociation strategies have advantages and disadvantages. As the former is related to monitoring sensations and physiological feedback, runners who associate may become accustomed to withstanding higher levels of pain but are more vulnerable to injuries (Masters and Ogles, 1998b). However, studies have shown that the use of association might lead to faster running, and it is more commonly used by elite athletes (Masters and Ogles, 1998a). Conversely, dissociation has been found to be related to slower running, but it is also found to be positively related to persistence, as runners who employ this type of strategy can reduce the monotony of training (Masters and Ogles, 1998a, 1998b).

Given the outcomes of using different strategies, it is suggested that dissociation might be adopted during training sessions, as the means to decrease boredom and enhance motivation. During races, elite runners are recommended to use association in order to improve their performances. However, leisure runners whose main aim is to finish the marathon are still advised to use dissociation strategies (Masters and Ogles, 1998b).

Finding partners

Higdon (1998) has suggested that it is easy to lose the motivation to train during the last months of preparation for a marathon. He suggests that runners should seek regular training partners to train together. For those who have difficulties starting a training program, it is also wise to find someone to train together, as the initiation is often the hardest step to take. These suggestions are in line with SDT, as having training partners can fulfill the need for relatedness and may enhance intrinsic motivation.

Conclusion

In this chapter, we have reviewed some of the evidence regarding motivation for marathon running. Marathon training and competition represent particularly grueling endeavors in which one must be highly motivated in order to succeed. Motivation refers not only to the amount of effort that is expended, but also to the reasons why an individual chooses to pursue a particular activity. The available evidence on marathon motives is limited to descriptive studies in which different reasons for marathon running have been identified. These motives include running for physical and psychological health benefits. Social motives, as well as feelings of enjoyment and achievement, also motivate people to participate in marathons.

There is a clear need for theory-based research in which methods for promoting more adaptive forms of motivation are identified and the specific outcomes of different forms of motivation are observed. Keeping in mind the paucity of marathon-specific research, we have attempted to provide suggestions for enhancing marathon runners' motivation. A variety of methods are suggested, but the major principles behind these recommendations are that individuals should focus mostly on self-referenced goals and that social-environmental factors that promote more self-determined forms of motivation will likely prove to be the most beneficial.

References

1. Ames C. 1992. Classrooms: goals, structures, and student motivation. *J Educ Psychol* 84 (3): 261–71.
2. Barrell GV, Holt D, MacKean JM. 1988. A comparison of the reasons for marathon participation of British and Australian non-elite runners. In E. F. Broom, R. Clumpner, B. Pendleton & C. A. Pooley (Eds.), *Comparative physical education and sport, Volume 5* (pp. 131–48). Champaign, IL: Human Kinetics Publishers.
3. Boston Athletic Association. 2007. *Boston marathon: Participation through the years*. Retrieved 14 March, 2007, from http://www.baa.org/BostonMarathon/Participation.asp.
4. Carmack MA, Martens R. 1979. Measuring commitment to running: a survey of runners' attitudes and mental states. *J Sport Psychol* 1:25–42.
5. Clerici P. 2004. The whys and the wherefores: Why in the world would anyone want to run 26 miles? There are as many reasons as marathoners. *Marathon & Beyond* 8:77–86; 88–90; 92.
6. Clough P, Shepherd J, Maughan R. 1989. Motives for participation in recreational running. *J Leisure Res* 21:297–309.
7. Deci EL, Ryan RM. 1985. *Intrinsic motivation and self-determination in human behavior*. New York: Plenum Press.
8. Divine J, Chorley J, Kohl H, Cianca J. 1999. Motivation for starting a marathon

traning program: Running experience and gender differences. *Med Sci Sports Exerc* 31 (5): S93.

9. Dosil J. 2006. The psychology of athletics. In J. Dosil (Ed.), *The sport psychologist's handbook: A guide for sport-specific performance enhancement* (pp. 265–84). Chichester, England: John Wiley & Sons Ltd.

10. Duda JL, Nicholls JG. 1992. Dimensions of achievement motivation in school-work and sport. *J Educ Psychol* 84 (3): 290–99.

11. Dweck CS. 1986. Motivational processes affecting learning. *American Psychologist*, 41 (10): 1040–48.

12. Finch L. 2002. Understanding individual motivation in sport. In J. M. Silva & D. E. Stevens (Eds.), *Psychological Foundations of Sport* (pp. 66–79). Boston: Allyn & Bacon.

13. Gould D. 2006. Goal setting for peak performance. In J. M. Williams (Ed.), *Applied sport psychology: Personal growth to peak performance* (5th ed., pp. 240–59). New York: McGraw-Hill.

14. Harwood C, Cumming J, Fletcher D. 2004. Motivational profiles and psychological skills use within elite youth sport. *J Appl Sport Psychol* 16 (4): 318–32.

15. Hayashi CT, Weiss MR. 1994. A cross-cultural analysis of achievement motivation in Anglo-American and Japanese marathon runners. *Int J Sport Psychol* 25:187–202.

16. Higdon H. 1998. *Hal Higdon's smart running: Expert advice on training, motivation, injury prevention, nutrition, and good health for runners of any age and ability.* Emmaus, Pa.: Rodale Press.

17. Hodge K, Petlichkoff L. 2000. Goal profiles in sport motivation: A cluster analysis. *J Sport Exercise Psy* 22:256–72.

18. Hong Kong Amateur Athletic Association. (n.d.). *Hong Kong Standard Chartered Marathon 2007: Event history.* Retrieved 14 March, 2007, from http://hkmarathon.esdlife.com/marathon/eng/mcorner/history.jsp.

19. Johnsgard K. 1985a. The motivation of the long distance runner: I. *J Sports Med* 25:135–39.

20. Johnsgard K. 1985b. The motivation of the long distance runner: II. *J Sports Med* 25:140–43.

21. Kyllo LB, Landers DM. 1995. Goal setting in sport and exercise: A research synthesis to resolve the controversy. *J Sport Exercise Psy* 17:117–37.

22. Locke EA, Shaw KN, Saari LM, Latham GP. 1981. Goal setting and task performance. *Psychol Bull* 90:125–52.

23. Maehr ML, Nicholls JG. 1980. Culture and achievement motivation: A second book. In N. Warren (Ed.), *Studies in cross-cultural psychology* (pp. 221–67). New York: Academic Press.

24. Mageau GA, Vallerand RJ. 2003. The coach-athlete relationship: A motivational model. *J Sports Sci* 21:883–904.

25. Mallett CJ. 2005. Self-Determination Theory: a case study of evidence-based coaching. *Sport Psychol* 19:417–29.

26. Masters KS, Ogles BM. 1995. An investigation of the different motivations of marathon runners with varying degrees of experience. *J Sport Behav* 18:69–79.

27. Masters KS, Ogles BM. 1998a. Associative and dissociative cognitive strategies in exercise and running: 20 years later, what do we know? *Sport Psychol* 12:253–70.

28. Masters KS, Ogles BM. 1998b. The relationships of cognitive strategies with injury, motivation, and performance among marathon runners: results from two studies. *J Appl Sport Psychol* 10:281–96.

29. Masters KS, Ogles BM, Jolton JA. 1993. The development of an instrument to measure motivation for marathon running: The Motivations of Marathoners Scales (MOMS). *Res Q Exerc Sport* 64 (2): 134–43.

30. Nerurkar R. 2004. *Marathon running: From beginner to elite (2nd ed.)*. London: A & C Black.

31. Nicholls JG. 1989. *The competitive ethos and democratic education*. Cambridge, Mass: Harvard University Press.

32. Ogles BM, Masters KS. 2000. Older vs. younger adult male marathon runners: participative motives and training habits. *J Sport Behav* 23:130–43.

33. Ogles, BM, Masters KS, Richardson SA. 1995. Obligatory running and gender: An analysis of participative motives and training habits. *Int J Sport Psychol* 26:233–48.

34. Ryan RM, Deci EL. 2000. Intrinsic and extrinsic motivations: Classic definitions and new directions. *Contemp Educ Psychol* 25:54–67.

35. Ryan RM, Deci EL. 2002. An overview of self-determination theory: An organismic-dialectical perspective. In E. L. Deci & R. M. Ryan (Eds.), *Handbook of self-determination research* (pp. 3–33). Rochester: The University of Rochester Press.

36. Scully D, Kremer J, Meade MM, Graham R, Dudgeon K. 1998. Physical exercise and psychological well being: a critical review. *Br J Sports Med* 32:111–20.

37. Smith HW. 1994. *The 10 natural laws of successful time and life management: Proven strategies for increased productivity and inner peace.* New York: Warner.

38. Summers JJ, Machin VJ, Sargent GI. 1983. Psychosocial factors related to marathon running. *J Sport Psychol* 5:314–31.

39. Vallerand RJ, Rousseau FL. 2001. Intrinsic and extrinsic motivation in sport and exercise: A review using the hierarchical model of intrinsic and extrinsic motivation. In R. N. Singer, H. A. Hausenblas & C. M. Janelle (Eds.), *Handbook of sport psychology* (pp. 389–416). New York: John Wiley and Sons, Inc.

40. Vitulli WF. 1987. Manifest reasons for jogging. *Percept Motor Skill* 64:650.

41. Vitulli WF, DePace III AN. 1992. Manifest reasons for jogging and not jogging. *Percept Motor Skill* 75:111–14.

42. Weinberg RS. 1996. Goal setting in sport and exercise: Research to practice. In J. L. Van Raalte & B. W. Brewer (Eds.), *Exploring sport and exercise psychology* (1st ed., pp. 3–24). Washington, DC: American Psychological Association.

43. Weinberg RS, Burton D, Yukelson D, Weigand D. 1993. Goal setting in competitve sport: An exploratory investigation of practices of collegiate athletes. *Sport Psychol* 7:275–89.

44. Weinberg RS, Gould D. 2003. *Foundations of sport and exercise psychology (3rd ed.).* Champaign, IL: Human Kinetics.

45. Weinberg RS, Smith J, Jackson A, Gould D. 1984. Effect of association, dissociation and positive self-talk strategies on endurance performance. *Can J Appl Sport Sci* 9 (1): 25–32.

46. Weiss MR, Ferrer-Caja E. 2002. Motivational orientations and sport behavior. In T. S. Horn (Ed.), *Advances in sport psychology* (pp. 101–83). Champaign, IL: Human Kinetics.

47. Wilmore JH, Costill DL. 1999. *Physiology of sport and exercise (2nd ed.).* Champaign, IL: Human Kinetics.

Marathon Training

Dr. CHAN Kwok-Ki

Each marathon runner has his or her own goals. Some of them may just want to complete the race, while others may aim to finish the race within a particular time limit. As a result of differences in fitness levels, racing experiences, and goals among athletes, they have different training strategies. Runners should have a basic understanding of the science behind training so that they can design and monitor their own training program according to their specific requirements. The aim of this chapter is to highlight important principles of training and their applications in marathon training.

Basic Principles of Training

1. Overloading

Overloading means to place a demand on the body greater than that to which it is accustomed.[1] In the training response, this refers to the stress that causes fatigue with a temporary decrease in exercise ability followed by improved performance after recovery. However, after the adaptation, the same training stimulus will not elicit further improvement. A higher training stimulus is then required. Overloading can be accomplished by an increase in training volume, training intensity, or a combination of the two.[2]

2. Adaptation

Adaptation refers to the phenomenon of when the body adjusts and finally adapts to training stress.[1] If the training stress is appropriate, adaptation will occur and lead to an improvement in bodily function (e.g., improvement in cardiorespiratory function resulting in an improvement in exercise endurance).

3. Specificity

Specificity refers to training in a specific manner in order to produce a specific adaptation or training outcome.[1] For example, individuals who train with long-distance running improve in running more than cycling, although both are endurance exercises that train the cardiovascular system.[3]

4. Progression and periodization

The body adapts well to increasing training overloads only if there is a proper rate of progression. These may include the number of training sessions per week, the percentage of low and high intensity training per week, and the periodization pattern for a given training cycle. Progression of training should not merely be a gradual increase in training intensity and volume. Periodization is necessary so that there is overloading of the body for a few weeks, followed by decreased training volume and intensity for a week or so. This process helps the body to gradually build up with adequate recovery. The cycle is then repeated with a progression of training volume and intensity, and the body will then train up to a higher fitness level.

Elements of Training

1. Training maximal oxygen consumption

Maximal oxygen consumption (VO_{2max}) is the highest amount of oxygen the body can consume during exercise for the aerobic production of Adenosine Triphosphate (ATP).[4] As oxygen consumption is directly related to energy expenditure, VO_{2max} is an indication of an individual's capacity to do aerobic work.

There are two main strategies for training VO_{2max}. The first is aerobic conditioning training with moderate intensity exercises of long duration. In highly trained runners, further improvement in VO_{2max} will not occur with this type of training.[5,6]

Interval training is another strategy to further improve VO_{2max}, especially when VO_{2max} cannot be further improved by moderate intensity exercises. This can be defined as repeated bouts of short to moderate duration exercise (10 seconds to five minutes) completed at an intensity greater than the anaerobic threshold. These exercise bouts are separated by a brief period of low-intensity exercise or rest so that a partial recovery can occur.[7] Using this training strategy, the athlete will be able to train at a high intensity for a greater amount of time than could be accomplished in a single exercise session on a continuous basis. The benefits of this kind of exercise include improvement in both VO_{2max} and anaerobic metabolism.[8,9]

Interval training may be more effective in increasing VO_{2max}, as this permits greater volumes of high intensity work to be performed.[10,11] This strategy has long been used by coaches in training elite endurance athletes.[12] In general, their training programs usually consist of an early aerobic base component with submaximal continuous training, complemented by high-intensity interval training sessions nearer to the competitive season.[7]

2. Training lactate threshold

Lactate threshold is the balance point where lactic acid is produced at the same rate as it is being cleared by the body. This can be defined as the exercise intensity above which blood lactate level will rise disproportionally in relation to oxygen consumption, meaning the onset of anaerobic metabolism and lactate accumulation.[13] In practice, the lactate threshold is the point of maximum sustainable exercise intensity. Therefore, a runner with a higher lactate threshold will run at a higher sustainable speed than runners with lower lactate thresholds, assuming other attributes are the equal.

With training, improvement in lactate threshold is slower than VO_{2max}. Development of a lactate threshold also requires a different training strategy. It involves interval training near one's lactate threshold.[14,15]

3. Training running economy

Another important determinant of running performance is running economy.

A runner with a better running economy means that he or she can run at a faster speed at the same energy cost.[16,17] It is found that running economy improves with the mileage that one has been running.[18] Therefore, one way to improve running economy is to increase mileage over time. Another strategy is the use of anaerobic capacity training, with repeated intervals of fast running over short distances.[19] This can improve neuromuscular coordination, eliminate unnecessary movements, and maintain control at high speed, contributing to improved running economy.

4. Other training strategies

a. Flexibility training

Flexibility is the range of motion in a joint or a series of joints that reflects the ability of the muscles and tendons concerned to elongate within the physical limits of the joint.[20] Running does not demand high flexibility. However, running strengthens and tightens muscle groups such as the hamstrings, hip flexors, and calf muscles. This causes imbalances in muscle strength and flexibility between antagonistic muscle groups, which can limit performance and increase injury risks. Therefore, stretching exercises should be incorporated in the training program to balance the flexibility of different muscle groups, improve running techniques, and reduce injury risks. Stretching exercises should be done before and after the run.[15,21]

b. Resistance training

Resistance training can be used to correct muscle imbalances. It can also reduce the risk of injury by strengthening the connective tissue, including tendons and ligaments. Core stability training is a specific form of resistance training. For marathon runners, exercises are designed to strengthen the abdomen, lower back, hip, and gluteal muscles. This can correct muscle imbalances, thus reducing the risk of injuries and improving running economy.[15]

c. Cross-training

Cross-training refers to training in different ways with the aim of developing or maintaining cardiovascular fitness.[1] In marathon training, this means running can be supplemented with other aerobic activities such as cycling and swimming. The primary reason to cross-train is to provide additional cardiovascular training without increasing the repetitive wear and tear from running, thus reducing the risk of injury. This form of training is commonly used during injury rehabilitation in order to maintain fitness while allowing the injury to recover. Cross-training may also be used during recovery runs to hasten recovery without further increasing impact forces on the body.[22]

Exercise Intensity

The intensity of exercise is one of the most important elements in the design and implementation of training programs. Heart rate during exercise is commonly used to determine exercise intensity.

Maximum heart rate (MHR)

The most accurate way to find one's own MHR is to measure the highest heart rate achieved during a maximal exercise stress test on a treadmill. A simple method to estimate MHR is: estimated MHR = 220 – age.

Training zones

With the use of the percentage of MHR during exercise, one can estimate the intensity of exercise. Different training intensities produce different adaptations in the body that cannot be duplicated at a lower or higher intensity. Training zones can generally be divided as follows:[21,23,24]

a. Recovery training zone

This is training below 60% MHR. This is commonly used during the cooldown phase immediately after exercise or during the days following a competition or hard workout. Recovery training encourages recovery and reduces muscle lactate levels faster than complete rest. There is also a beneficial psychological effect by enhancing relaxation.

b. Aerobic conditioning training zone

This is training at about 70%–80% MHR. This is the level at which all long endurance running should be done. Training at this level improves the aerobic energy system and free fatty acid utilization. However, too much training at this intensity may preclude more optimal adaptations that occur with lower intensity, especially for serious endurance athletes. Therefore, it has been suggested that training at 60%–70% MHR may be a better alternative.

c. Lactate threshold (anaerobic conditioning) training zone

This is training at about 80%–90% MHR. Lactate threshold training should be done close to the pace that one could race for one hour or at the half-marathon pace (for experienced runners). A typical training strategy should be 20–40 minutes of tempo run or broken down into two to five repetitions at lactate threshold pace with two to three minutes of slow running in between. Training at this level improves both the aerobic and anaerobic energy system, which delays the onset of lactic acid accumulation, thus increasing the lactate threshold.

d. Aerobic capacity training zone

This is training above 90% to 95% of MHR. This corresponds to the race pace for 3000 m to 5000 m. Running intervals at this intensity is an efficient way to improve VO_2 max. Typically, each interval lasts between two to eight minutes. The work to rest ratio is about 1:1, and the total workout time is 10 to 21 minutes of exercise. The rest interval should be done at fairly light exercise to assist full recovery.

e. Anaerobic capacity training zone

This refers to very intense training at or close to 100% of MHR. The primary goal of anaerobic capacity training is to improve short-distance racing speed and strength. Therefore, this kind of training may be of less importance for marathon training, but is of more importance to middle-distance runners.

Training Program Design

1. Basic structure of exercise programs

Every exercise program consists of the following elements, which form the basis of training program design:[25]

a) Frequency of training—This refers to the number of exercise sessions per week. The recommended frequency should be at least three times per week. Training fewer than two times per week does not generally result in any improvement in fitness.

b) Intensity of training—This refers to the intensity of exercise during each training session. Depending on the specific training goal, intensity can vary from below 60% to approaching 100% of MHR.

c) Duration of training—This refers to the duration of exercise during each exercise session.

d) Mode of activity—This refers to the type of exercise used for training. For long-distance runners, running is the prime mode of exercise. Other forms of exercise, such as flexibility training, resistance training, or cross–training, with different exercise modes can also be used to supplement running.

2. Warm-up and cool down

This is necessary for each exercise session. Warm-ups can increase the connective tissue extensibility, improve the range of motion and function of joints, and enhance muscular performance. All of these can help to reduce the risks of injury.[26]

On the other hand, after each exercise session, it is recommended to have cool-down activities in the form of easy jogging and stretching. Cool-down activities can hasten the removal of lactic acid and enhance muscle recovery.

3. Progression of training

Progression of training, in terms of both training volume and intensity, should be slow. A general guideline is that one should not increase more than 10% of mileage each week.[27] One should build up a strong aerobic base in terms of moderate intensity training first. Speed work can then be gradually added into the training program.

4. Rest

Rest is an integral part of any training program. Performance will not improve, and it may even deteriorate, without adequate rest. One should consider rest after a hard training day, for example, after a long run, or after high-intensity interval training. Rest can either be passive (i.e., no exercise) or active rest in the form of recovery training.

Tapering

Tapering is the gradual reduction in training before important competitions so as to allow the body to recover from previous training, maintain physiological conditioning, and improve performance.[1] In general, if training volume is reduced and training intensity is maintained, physical performance is maintained or even improved after a taper period of 7–21 days.[28,29] The exact type of taper depends on the length, type, and importance of the event, and from past experience with tapering. Therefore, the optimal duration and method of tapering is different for each runner.

General guidelines for tapering:

1. Reduce the total training mileage during the two-week period just before the marathon. Consider taking an additional rest day in order to reduce the mileage. The exact amount of training reduction is different for each runner. A general rule is to cut total mileage by at least 50%.
2. Consider having a complete leg rest one or two days before the race.
3. Take more rest if physically or mentally tired.
4. Do more stretching exercises.

5. Reduce caloric intake during tapering, except the week before the race (carbohydrate loading), as there is less energy expenditure due to reduced training.

Program Monitoring

Program monitoring is an important measure in the prevention of overtraining. Once a training program is designed, one should record what exactly has been performed and its effect on the body. One can then analyze the results and modify the training program according to changes in performance and stress on the body. A typical training log may include the following:[23,24]

1. **Week**
This is the week number of the training program.

2. **Day**
This is the day number of the week's training.

3. **Training time and method**
This is the mode of exercise used. This should include warm-up and cool-down activities, stretching exercises, running or other cross-training, resistance training, or any other exercise activities. One should also record whether the prescribed training was completed successfully.

4. **Training intensity**
This may be the actual training heart rate or a general remark with a self-derived scale of perceived intensity.

5. **Feeling**
One may use a self-designed scale for the general feeling about the difficulty of a particular day's training.

6. **Resting heart rate**
One should measure the resting heart rate before getting out of bed each day in the morning.

7. **Body weight**
One should measure body weight in the morning before eating breakfast. A sudden drop in body weight may indicate dehydration.

8. **Quality of sleep**
One should record the quality of sleep each night.

A well-kept training log can give an indication of any trends in body changes. If there is persistent tiredness or difficulty in completing the training, sudden changes in resting heart rate, or a poor quality of sleep, it may indicate an over-aggressive training program and be an indication of overtraining. One should then modify the training program to reduce training volume or intensity or take the day off. On the other hand, one may discover a particular training pattern that leads to an improvement in performance. This can then be used as a guide to construct a personalized training program in the future.

The training log can also indicate whether the training program can fit into one's own schedule. If there is persistent difficulty in meeting the training goal, one should consider modifying the training schedule. It is unadvisable to increase the training load for the rest of the week in order to compensate for missed training days, as this can easily lead to overtraining and injury.

References

1. Plowman SA, Smith DL. 2003. *Exercise Physiology for Health, Fitness, and Performance*, 2–21. San Francisco: Benjamin Cummings.
2. Lehmann M, Netzer N, Steinacker JM, Opitz-Gress A. 1998. Physiological responses to short and long term overtraining in endurance athletes. In R. B. Kreider, A. C. Fry, and M. L. O'Toole (Eds.), *Overtraining in Sport*, 19–46. Champaign, IL: Human Kinetics.
3. Roberts JA, Alspaugh JW. 1972. Specificity of training effects resulting from programs of treadmill running and bicycle ergometer riding. *Med Sci Sports*, 4 (1): 6–10.
4. Anshel MH, Freedson P, Hamill J, Haywood K, Horvat M, Plowman SA. 1991. *Dictionary of the Sport and Exercise Sciences*. Champaign, IL: Human Kinetics.
5. Hickson RC, Hagberg JM, Ehsani AA, Holloszy JO. 1981. Time course of the adaptive responses of aerobic power and heart rate to training. *Med Sci Sports Exerc* 13 (1): 17–20.
6. Londeree BR. 1997. Effect of training on lactate/ventilatory thresholds: a meta-analysis. *Med Sci Sports Exerc* 29 (6): 837–43.
7. Laursen PB, Jenkins DG. 2002. The scientific basis for high-intensity interval training: optimising training programmes and maximising performance in

highly trained endurance athletes. *Sports Med* 32 (1): 53–73.

8. Baquet G, Berthoin S, Gerbeaux M, Van Praagh E. 2001. High intensity aerobic training during a 10 week one-hour physical education cycle: effects on physical fitness of adolescents aged 11 to 16. *Int J Sports Med* 22 (4): 295–300.

9. Tabata I, Nishimura K, Kouzaki M, Hirai Y, Ogita F, Miyachi M, Yamamoto K. 1996. Effects of moderate-intensity endurance and high-intensity intermittent training on anaerobic capacity and VO$_2$max. *Med Sci Sports Exerc* 28 (10): 1327–30.

10. Hurley BF, Seals DR, Ehsani AA, Cartier LJ, Dalsky GP, Hagberg JM, Holloszy JO. 1984. Effects of high-intensity strength training on cardiovascular function. *Med Sci Sports Exerc* 16 (5): 483–88.

11. MacDougall D, Sale D. 1981. Continuous vs. interval training: a review for the athlete and coach. *Can J Appl Sport Sci* 6 (2): 93–97.

12. Hawley JA, Myburgh KH, Noakes TD, Dennis SC. 1997. Training techniques to improve fatigue resistance and enhance endurance performance. *J Sports Sci* 15 (3): 325–33.

13. Wasserman K, Whipp BJ, Koyl SN, Beaver WL. 1973. Anaerobic threshold and respiratory gas exchange during exercise. *J Appl Physiol* 35 (2): 236–43.

14. Janssen P. 2001. *Lactate Threshold Training*. Champaign, IL: Human Kinetics.

15. Pfitzinger P, Douglas S. 2001. *Advanced Marathoning*. Champaign IL: Human Kinetics.

16. Daniels J, Daniels N. 1992. Running economy of elite male and elite female distance runners. *Med Sci Sports Exerc* 24 (4): 483–89.

17. Morgan D, Craib M. 1992. Physiological aspects of running economy. *Med Sci Sports Exerc* 24 (4): 456–61.

18. Scrimgeour AG, Noakes TD, Adams B, Myburgh K. 1986. The influence of weekly training distance on fractional utilization of maximum aerobic capacity in marathon and ultramarathon runners. *Eur J Appl Physiol* 55 (2): 202–209.

19. Daniels J. 1985. A physiologist's view of running economy. *Med Sci Sports Exerc* 17 (3): 332–38.

20. Hubley-Kozey CL. 1991. Testing flexibility. In J. D. MacDougall, H. A. Wenger, and H. J. Green (Eds.), *Physiological Testing of the High-Performance Athlete*. Champaign, IL: Human Kinetics.

21. Martin DE, Coe PN. 1997. *Better Training for Distance Runners*. Champaign, IL: Human Kinetics.

22. Kibler WB, Chandler TJ. 1994. Sport-specific conditioning. *Am J Sports Med*

22:424–32.

23. Evans M. 1997. *Endurance Athlete's Edge*. Champaign, IL: Human Kinetics.

24. Sleamaker R, Browning R. 1996. *Serious Training for Endurance Athletes*. Champaign, IL: Human Kinetics.

25. Franklin BA, Whaley MH. 2000. General principles of exercise prescription. ACSM's guidelines for exercise testing and prescription. *American College of Sports Medicine*. Philadelphia: Lippincott Williams & Wilkins, 137–64.

26. Pollock ML, Gaesser GA, Butcher JD. 1998. The recommended quantity and quality of exercise for developing and maintaining cardiorespiratory and muscular fitness, and flexibility in healthy adults. *Med Sci Sports Exerc* 30:975–91.

27. *Burfoot A. 1999. Runner's World Complete Book of Running : Everything You Need to Know to Run for Fun, Fitness and Competition. Emmaus, Pa.: Rodale Books.*

28. Houmard JA, Costill DL, Mitchell JB, Park SH, Hickner RC, Roemmich JN. 1990. Reduced training maintains performance in distance runners. *Int J Sports Med* 11 (1): 46–52.

29. Shepley B, MacDougall JD, Cipriano N, Suton JR, Coates G, Tarnopolsky M. 1992. Physiological effects of tapering in highly trained athletes. *J Appl Physiol* 72 (2); 706–11.

Injuries in Marathon Running

Dr. Albert LIT

Introduction

Over the years, there has been a progressive and significant increase in the number of marathon participants in Hong Kong. At the same time, there has also been a similar increasing trend in the number of injuries or medical conditions associated with the event.

The injury and illness rates vary among different events. The incident rate range is wide among different studies, ranging from 2.5% to around 20%.[1,2] Such a wide range is likely due to different environmental conditions and inclusion criteria.

Types of Marathon Injuries

The vast majority—90%—of medical encounters, including injuries and illnesses, are generally mild and self-limiting.[3]

In the Twin Cities Marathon (TCM) from 1983 to 1994, skin abrasions and blisters accounted for about 20%, muscle strain and cramps accounted for around 20%, and exercise-associated collapse accounted for around 60%.[3]

In a local study of the Hong Kong International Marathon at the Tsing Ma Bridge in May 1997, muscle cramp was the most common condition presented to the Auxiliary Medical Service support stations. Most of the injuries seen were of the lower limbs. At the same time, muscle strain was the most common problem encountered at the physiotherapy station.[4]

During the Hong Kong International Marathon in February 2006, there were around 5,000 requests for medical assistance (including 4,800 due to muscle strain/cramp), representing 12.8% of all entrants. The majority of injuries encountered were also minor injuries with muscle strain/cramp accounting for 95% of cases, and superficial skin or soft tissue injuries accounting for another 4.6% (statistics with kind permission of the Auxiliary Medical Service of Hong Kong).

On the whole, a majority of injuries encountered during marathons are minor injuries, and most of them are of the lower limbs.[5,6,7] During the 1994 New York City Marathon,[8] common lower-extremity injuries included blisters, corns and calluses, muscle cramps, acute knee and ankle injuries, plantar fasciitis, and metatarsalgia.

In addition to acute injuries, stress fracture and chronic overuse injuries have also been reported.

Musculoskeletal Injuries

Both soft-tissue and bone injury may occur during marathon running. The gross majority of these injuries are minor. Serious ligament and bone injuries are relatively uncommon. Common injuries include the following:

1. **Muscle cramps**

   Muscle cramps are sudden painful spasms in muscles. They are related to an electrolyte imbalance due to salt and water loss as a result of sweating. These cramps usually affect the calf or thigh muscles.

   Prevention is achieved by maintaining a proper fluid and electrolyte balance and by ensuring adequate physical training before the race. Treatment of established muscle cramps is performed by stretching and massaging the affected muscles and correcting fluid and electrolyte imbalances.

2. **Plantar fasciitis**

   This is relatively common among marathon runners and can be quite troublesome. The plantar fascia is a ligamentous structure on the underside of the foot, and it is connected to the calcaneum. Undue strain of this attachment results in inflammation, causing pain.

   Soft heel pads and oral analgesics may help to relieve pain. Soft heel pads and a small heel raise are used to prevent the injury.

3. **Metatarsalgia**

   This results from repeated stress on the metatarsal bones in the foot. It is more common in runners with a prominent metatarsal head. It causes pain in the forefoot, especially when bearing weight.

Soft insoles and oral analgesic may help to relieve pain, and prevention is achieved by using proper footwear with good insoles.

4. **Lower limb sprain**

This is usually minor and most commonly involves the ankle. Sprain injuries are due to abnormal or excessive movement of joints that disrupt (complete or partial) the supporting ligament(s). A sprained joint might be swollen and bruised. It is painful, especially during movement and weight bearing. Movement of the joint might also be limited.

Minor sprain injuries will improve gradually, though pain and swelling will generally subside after two to three weeks. Simple measures such as RICE therapy (Rest, Immobilization, Cold Therapy, and Elevation) will be sufficient for the majority of minor sprains.

- Rest—Rest the injured joint to prevent further injury and to promote healing.

- Immobilization—The affected joint should be immobilized to prevent further injury and progressive swelling. Commercial braces or crepe bandages might be used to support and immobilize the affected joint. It is important to ensure that the immobilization device is not too tight, as distal circulation will be compromised if it is. The distal end of the affected limb should be exposed for observation of circulation.

- Cold Therapy—Coldness can cause vasoconstriction and help reduce swelling. It may also help to reduce pain and muscle spasms. A cold compress might be applied for about 15 minutes every two to four hours during the initial acute stage. However, ice should not be allowed to be in direct contact with the skin. Use a towel to wrap the ice pack before applying it to the affected region.

- Elevation—Elevation of the affected limb helps to reduce swelling. The limb should be elevated in a comfortable position when sitting or lying down.

Analgesics may sometimes be necessary to reduce pain. It is necessary to investigate further under the following circumstances:

- difficulty bearing weight or walking immediately or shortly after the injury
- persistent or increasing pain and/or restriction of movement after a few days
- numbness or pallor over the injured site or distal part to the sprained joint

5. **Other acute knee and ankle injuries**

In a study of a six-day track race (ultramarathon), it was found that Achilles tendonitis, patellofemoral pain, and tendonitis of the foot dorsiflexors were the three most common injuries.[9] Meniscal tears have also been reported in marathon runners.[10]

Management is mainly by resting the affected part. Analgesics may help to alleviate the pain, but immobilization/braces might be necessary in certain cases. For refractory or complicated cases, specialist advice might be necessary.

Besides acute injuries, chronic overuse injuries and stress fractures have also been reported in marathon runners. These result from repeated undue stress on the involved body part, leading to either soft-tissue injuries or bone fractures. They will result in potentially chronic pain.

Stress fractures are rare conditions. They are relatively more common among endurance athletes and military recruits. Stress fractures have been reported in the tarsal bone, tibia,[11] femur,[12,13] femoral neck,[14,15,16] pelvis,[17] and sacrum.[18]

Skin Injuries

Most skin injuries are due to local friction. Common skin injuries include blisters, corns, calluses, subungual hematoma, dermatitis, and nipple abrasion.[19]

1. **Blisters**

They are some of the most common complaints among marathon runners. They are due to local friction and commonly involve the tips of toes, metatarsal heads, and the posterior heel.[20] They are predisposed by poor-fitting shoes and excessive or unaccustomed exercises.[21]

They may be prevented by wearing appropriate and well-fitting shoes, keeping the feet dry, and applying petroleum jelly over the pressure points. Painful blisters may be pierced with a needle under aseptic condition. Particular attention should be paid to keep it clean and prevent infection.

2. **Calluses and corns**

   Calluses and corns are hypertrophic skin lesions over bony prominences. They are commonly found over the metatarsal heads and the medial side of the big toe. If necessary, they might be treated by paring and the application of topical salicylic acid.

3. **Subungual hematoma (*jogger's toe*)**

   Subungual hematoma of the toe results from repetitive hitting of the toe against the toebox of the shoe. Improper footwear predisposes it, especially when running downhill. It is relatively common among marathon runners. According to one study of the 1979 New York City Marathon, this condition occurred in about 2.5% of runners.[22]

   Prevention is by wearing proper footwear with a spacious toebox and by cutting toenails straight and close to skin.

4. **Dermatitis (*chafing*)**

   Superficial dermatitis may occur over skin areas that rub together, especially where they are subjected to increased moisture.[23] It may be prevented by applying petroleum jelly and keeping the skin dry. If necessary, a topical steroid may help.

5. **Nipple abrasions (*jogger's nipples*)**

   Repeated friction with clothing may result in painful erosions of the nipples and the surrounding area (areola). It is predisposed by wearing shirts made of coarse materials. It is more common in women who run without bras.

   Prevention is by applying nipple patches or topical petroleum jelly. Painful lesions may be treated by applying petroleum jelly or antibiotic ointment.

6. **Exercise-induced purpura**

   Erythematous, purpuric, or urticarial lesions may occur over the lower legs after unusual or strenuous physical activities. This is related to venous stasis resulting from acute failure of the calf muscle pump and thermoregulation decompensation. Areas compressed by socks are usually spared.[24]

This is relatively more common during hot weather. It may result in itchiness, burning sensations, or pain. It is generally self-limiting and will disappear after a few days. Prevention is by local compression, local steroid application, and venoactive drugs.24

Heat-related Injuries

A lot of heat is generated during marathon running. About two-thirds of the energy produced from metabolism during endurance exercise is in the form of heat.[25] Hence, heat-related injuries might occur in marathon runners, especially under hot and humid conditions. Concomitant use of certain medications, such as antihistamines containing cough mixture, might impair heat loss and predispose to its development.[26] Dehydration compromises exercise heat loss and will increase thermal strain.[27]

It was found that post-marathon rectal temperatures are commonly and consistently high in marathon runners.[27] However, a severe form of heat-related illness that is potentially life-threatening is relatively uncommon. Post-race rectal temperature was not statistically correlated with finishing times in the 1982 Aberdeen Marathon. However, it was significantly correlated with the time taken to complete the second half of the race.[28]

Basically, heat-related illness is preventable. Good fluid balance is important to prevent heat-related illness.

Heat-related illnesses vary in degree and significance. They include:

1. **Heat stroke**

    Heat stroke is a true medical emergency and can be life-threatening. The patient has a very high core temperature (generally higher than 40°C) resulting from a failure of the body to properly regulate temperature.

    The patient typically has an altered mental status (semi-conscious or unconscious). The heart and breathing rates are high. A significant proportion of patients also have hypotension. Heat stroke may be complicated by rhabdomyolysis (damage of skeletal muscle cells) with resultant acute kidney failure.

    Rapid and aggressive cooling is of paramount importance. The body temperature should be lowered as soon as possible. Intravenous fluid and electrolyte replacement is essential, and the patient should be sent to the hospital as soon as possible.

2. **Heat exhaustion**

   The core temperature of the patient is generally high. Symptoms, which include malaise, nausea, vomiting, and dizziness, are generally nonspecific. Patients may have fast heart and breathing rates, and they may sweat profusely. Postural hypotension (low blood pressure during an erect position) may also occur.

   Heat exhaustion has the potential to progress into more serious and life-threatening heat stroke if not managed adequately. Rest, cooling, and replacement of fluids and electrolytes are the mainstays of treatment.

3. **Heat syncope**

   Heat syncope is more common in runners poorly acclimatized to hot conditions and the elderly. It is due to fluid depletion and decreased blood vessel (vasomotor) tone as a result of dilatation of blood vessels.

   The patient may lose consciousness transiently. He or she may also develop postural hypotension. Other potentially serious causes of syncope should be excluded. Treatment consists of rest and fluid replacement.

4. **Heat cramps**

   Heat cramps are painful muscle spasms. They generally affect the lower limbs and are due to low blood sodium concentration resulting from inadequate salt replacement (dilutional hyponatremia). Patients may have high or normal core temperatures. Treatment consists of rest together with salt and water replacement.

5. **Heat tetany**

   Heat tetany is due to respiratory alkalosis as a result of hyperventilation. Resultant paresthesia of extremities, circumoral paresthesia, and carpopedal spasms may be present. Treatment involves removal from the heat stress, cooling, and reassurance. Rebreathing through a paper bag may sometimes be necessary.

6. **Heat rash**

   Heat rash is maculopapular eruption of the skin. It usually occurs over areas covered by clothes. It is due to inflammation and obstruction of sweat glands. It is initially itchy. Treatment includes antibiotics and local application of 1% salicylic acid.

Death Associated with Marathon Running

Although most medical conditions encountered in marathon runners are minor, there are occasional reports of death.

In fact, the relationship between vigorous exercise and sudden death has long been recognized.[29] Death from marathon running dates back to 490 BC. Phidippides dropped dead after running to Athens to deliver news of victory over the Persians at Marathon. Marathon-related deaths may occur during or immediately after the race.[30,31]

However, it must be stressed that the risk of sudden death associated with marathon running is **exceedingly small** (generally around 0.001%–0.002%).

Among the 215,413 endurance runners competing in the 42-km Marine Corps Marathon from 1976 to 1994 (Washington DC, 1976–1994) and the Twin Cities Marathon from 1982 to 1994 (Minneapolis-St. Paul, Minnesota, 1982–1994),[30] there were four exercise-related sudden deaths (1 in 50,000, or 0.002%). It was subsequently found that all of the deceased had serious underlying cardiac problems (three were due to [coronary heart disease] CHD (two or three vessel disease) and one was due to anomalous origin of [left anterior descending coronary artery] LAD from the right sinus of Valsalva.)

The mortality rate in the combined New York City and London marathon races through the mid-1990s was around 1 in 100,000 finishers (~0.001%).[32] Among men alone, the incidence was slightly higher, around 1 in 15,000–18,000, during jogging and other vigorous exercise (0.006%–0.007%).[33,35] According to the American College of Cardiology, the risk is 1/100th of the annual overall risk associated with the activity of daily living, either with or without heart disease.[30]

Extension of the above-mentioned review involving runners of the Marine Corps Marathon (Washington DC, 1976–2004) and the Twin Cities Marathon (Minneapolis-St. Paul, Minnesota, 1982–2004) until 2004 showed that the incidence of sudden death associated with marathon running seemed to have decreased over the past decade.[31] From 1976–1994, there were four deaths and one nonfatal cardiac arrest. From 1995–2004, there was one death and three nonfatal cardiac arrests. It was revealed that the combined prevalence of sudden death and nonfatal cardiac arrest decreased slightly during the past decade from 1 in 44,000 to 1 in 55,000 (0.0022% to 0.0018%). The actual death rate has decreased even more significantly from 1 in 55,000 (0.0018%) between 1976–1994 to 1 in 220,000 (0.00045%) between 1995–2004.

A large number of studies of sudden death, including studies of exercise-related death, have shown that nearly all victims of sudden death during exercise have a serious disease, usually of the heart, that can adequately explain the death. Unfortunately, these people were usually unaware of the underlying problem prior to the tragedy.[34]

The most common cause of sudden death during exercise among those aged 40 or older in the West is coronary artery disease. For those younger than 40, hypertrophic cardiomyopathy is the more usual underlying heart problem.[34] Other less common causes of sudden death during exercise include congenital anomalies of the coronary arteries, right ventricular dysplasia, aortic rupture associated with Marfan's syndrome, coronary artery dissection, myocarditis, and conduction disturbances related to pathological changes of the conduction pathways of the heart.[34]

It should be noted that none of these potentially life-threatening cardiac conditions is caused by exercise, and there is also no evidence that exercise accelerates their progression.[34] Runners who die suddenly have advanced cardiac disease, and they are therefore at high risk of dying suddenly, whether they exercise or not. For these people, the chance of a tragedy is always present, although the catastrophic event is more likely to occur when they are exercising.[34,35,36]

Detection of some of these conditions in asymptomatic athletes is difficult and may need sophisticated investigation rather than routine physical examination or basic investigation (such as routine blood tests or resting [electrocardiagram] ECG). Besides, some athletes might have a 30%–60% noncritical lesion that does not produce any ST-segment changes or angina during exercise testing.[34] In fact, evidence has shown that most acute coronary events occur due to rapid progression of disease at sites where a critical lesion was not previously present.[34]

Practically, detection can be difficult, if not impossible.[34] This is because the incidence of these predisposing diseases in the athletic population is extremely low, possibly of the order of 1 per 10,000 to 200,000 athletes (0.01% to 0.0005%).

With the above limitations, and given the extremely low incidence of sudden death associated with marathon running (generally around 0.001%–0.002%), it does not seem to be reasonable or realistic to require routine pre-participation medical screening in asymptomatic runners. Of course, it might be appropriate for runners with symptoms, a known history of significant underlying medical conditions, or a known family history of sudden death to undergo extensive medical assessment before they embark on strenuous exercise such as the marathon.

However, it must be emphasized that the overall net effect of habitual vigorous exercise is favorable, and clinically healthy individuals should not be discouraged to participate in vigorous exercise.[35,36] A community-based study involving 133 male patients who experienced sudden cardiac deaths without a prior history of cardiac disease has shown that habitual participation in exercise is associated with an overall reduction in the risk of sudden cardiac death.[35] Likewise, several other epidemiological studies have suggested that regular habitual exercise is associated with decreased cardiovascular morbidity and mortality and a reduced risk of sudden cardiac death.[34,36]

References

1. Crouse B, Beattie K. 1996. Marathon medical services: strategies to reduce runner morbidity. *Med Sci Sports Exerc* 28 (9): 1093–96.

2. Jones BH, Roberts WO. 1991. Medical management of endurance events. In R. C. Cantu and L. J. Micheli (Eds.), *ACSM: Guidelines for the Team Physician*. Philadelphia: Lea & Febiger, 266–86.

3. Roberts WO. 2000. A 12-yr profile of medical injury and illness for the Twin Cities Marathon. *Med Sci Sports Exerc* 32 (9): 1549–55.

4. Wong TW, Yeung SSM, Lit CH. 1999. A Report of two mass sports events at the Tsing Ma Bridge. *Pre-hospital Immediate Care* 3:2–4.

5. Nicholl JP, Williams BT. 1982. Popular marathons: forecasting casualties. *Br Med J* (Clin Res Ed) 285:1464–65.

6. Kretsch A, Grogan R, Duras P, Allen F, Sumner J, Gillam I. 1984. 1980 Melbourne marathon study. *Med J Aust* 141 (12–13): 809–14.

7. Satterthwaite P, Larmer P, Gardiner J, Norton R. 1996. Incidence of injuries and other health problems in the Auckland Citibank marathon, 1993. *Br J Sports Med* 30 (4): 324–26.

8. Caselli MA, Longobardi SJ. 1997. Lower extremity injuries at the New York City Marathon. *J Am Podiatr Med Assoc* 87 (1): 34–37.

9. Bishop GW, Fallon KE. 1999. Musculoskeletal injuries in a six-day track race: ultramarathoner's ankle. *Clin J Sport Med* 9 (4): 216–20.

10. Tersegno MM. 1992. Meniscal tears in marathon runners. *AJR Am J Roentgenol* 159 (2): 434.

11. Clayer M, Krishnan J, Lee W, Tamblyn P. 1992. Longitudinal stress fracture of the tibia: two cases. *Clinical Radiology* 46 (6): 401–404.

12. Weishaar MD, McMillian DJ, Moore JH. 2005. Identification and management of 2 femoral shaft stress injuries. *J Orthop Sports Phys Ther* 35 (10): 665–73.

13. Dugowson CE, Drinkwater BL, Clark JM. 1991. Nontraumatic femur fracture in an oligomenorrheic athlete. *Med Sci Sports Exerc* 23 (12): 1323–25.

14. Baer S, Shakespeare D. 1984. Stress fracture of the femoral neck in a marathon runner. *Br J Sports Med* 18 (1): 42–43.

15. Scott MPF, Davis JT. 1999. Femoral neck stress fracture. *Arch Phys Med Rehabil* 80 (2): 236–38.

16. Kerr PS, Johnson DP. 1995. Displaced femoral neck stress fracture in a marathon runner. *Injury* 26 (7): 491–93.

17. Eren OT, Holtby R. 1998. Straddle pelvic stress fracture in a female marathon runner. A case report. *Am J Sports Med* 26 (6): 850–51.

18. Bono CM. 2004. Low-back pain in athletes. *J Bone Joint Surg Am* 86A (2): 382–96.

19. Mailler EA, Adams BB. 2004. The wear and tear of 26.2: Dermatological injuries reported on marathon day. *Br J Sports Med* 38 (4): 498–501.

20. King MJ. 1997. Dermatologic problems in podiatric sports medicine. *Clin Podiatr Med Surg* 14 (3): 511–24.

21. Knapik JJ, Reynolds KL, Duplantis KL, Jones BH. 1995. Friction blisters: pathophysiology, prevention and treatment. *Sports Med* 20 (3): 136–47.

22. Bird N, Andreola V, Galli L. 1980. Medical care in the New York City Marathon. *New York Running News* 24:72.

23. Eiland G, Ridley D. 1996. Dermatologic problems in the athlete. *J Orthop*

Sports Phys Ther 23:388–402.

24. Ramelet AA. 2004. Exercise-induced purpura. *Dermatology* 208 (4): 293–96.

25. Noakes T. 2003. Fluid replacement during marathon running. *Clin J Sport Med* 13 (5): 309–18.

26. Weaving EA, Berro VE, Kew MC. 1980. Heat stroke during a "run for fun": A case report. *S Afr Med J* 57 (18): 753–54.

27. Cheuvront SN, Haymes EM. 2001. Thermoregulation and marathon running: biological and environmental influences. *Sports Med* 31 (10): 743–62.

28. Maughan RJ. 1985. Thermoregulation in marathon competition at low ambient temperature. *Int J Sports Med* 6 (1): 15–19.

29. Siscovick DS, Weiss NS, Fletcher RH, Lasky T. 1984. The incidence of primary cardiac arrest during vigorous exercise. *N Engl J Med* 311 (14): 874–77.

30. Maron BJ, Poliac LC, Roberts WO. 1996. Risk for sudden cardiac death associated with marathon running. *J Am Coll Cardiol* 28 (2): 428–31.

31. Roberts WO, Maron BJ. 2005. Evidence for decreasing occurrence of sudden cardiac death associated with the marathon. *J Am Coll Cardiol* 46 (7): 1373–74.

32. Pedoe DT. 2000. Sudden Cardiac death in Sport—Spectre or preventable risk? *Br J Sports Med* 34: 137–40.

33. Thompson PD, Funk EJ, Carleton RA, Sturner WQ. 1982. The Incidence of death during jogging in Rhode Island from 1975 through 1980. *JAMA* 247: 2535–38.

34. Noakes TD. 1998. Sudden death and exercise. *Encyclopedia of Sports Medicine and Science*. Retrieved October 20, 2009, from http://sportsci.org/encyc/suddendeath/suddendeath.html

35. Siscovick DS, Weiss NS, Fletcher RH, Lasky T. 1984. The incidence of primary cardiac arrest during vigorous exercise. *N Engl J Med* 311 (14): 874–77.

36. Siscovick DS, Weiss NS, Hallstrom AP, Inui TS, Peterson DR. 1982. Physical activity and primary cardiac arrest. *JAMA* 248 (23): 3113–17.

Sports Injuries Encountered During Marathon Preparations

Dr. YUNG Shu-Hang Patrick

Introduction

Have you ever thought about how many footsteps it takes to finish a marathon? It has been estimated that one takes approximately 30,000 to 50,000 steps to run a marathon. However, for an athlete training for six months in preparation for a marathon, can you imagine how many times the body repeats that simple step?

A runner training for a marathon, regularly running 60 km a week, can easily strike the ground well over a million times per leg over six months. Every time the foot hits the ground, a stress three to four times the body weight is absorbed via the ankles, knees, hips, and then the back. Thus, it is no surprise that most runners will eventually suffer certain injuries during training. In fact, much research has shown that injury strikes a quarter to half of all runners each year, and a majority happen during training rather than during the race. It has been shown that 30 to 53 percent of runners develop injuries during training, four to ten times more than running a marathon.

Most of the injuries occur to the feet and knees, followed by the shins and hips. The pre-marathon injury rate increases with the frequency, intensity, mode, and duration of training. Of course, there are many other factors that contribute to injuries during training, such as pre-existing anatomical abnormalities, medical problems, the training programme and technique, distribution of training and rest, and how the body adapts to wear and tear, equipment and environmental conditions, etc. Thus, to minimize morbidity during training, detailed knowledge and anticipation of potential problems are of paramount importance for all marathon runners.

After an Injury, What to Do Next?

Many runners approach injuries like an ostrich, burying their heads in the sand and hoping that the problem will soon go away. Certainly, that is not the way it will work, and indeed many injuries are minor at the onset and become more complicated and difficult to treat with time and repeated injury.

Some athletes are experienced enough and understand how to treat acute injuries, for example applying the principle of " RICE " (Rest, Ice, Compression and Elevation) or " PRICE " (Protection, Rest, Ice, Compression, and Elevation). This helps to decrease inflammation, swelling, and pain in the early stages of injuries, and it probably enables athletes to get back to training earlier. It is very true that resting a few days or a week can relieve flaring symptoms arising from overuse or acute injuries. However, if the cause of the injuries, such as biomechanical inefficiency or inappropriate footwear, is not identified and the runner goes back to running, the problem may happen again and complicate the process of recovery. Simply taking some time off from running does not solve the underlying cause of most overuse injuries in running. One should identify the cause of injury to prevent recurrence; otherwise, relapse is almost certain. In fact, about half of all running injuries are recurrences.

When a runner encounters red flag signs after an injury, such as gross swelling and redness, limited range of joint motion, deformity of limbs, pain even when resting, persistent symptoms that last longer than a week or in case of doubt, one should consult a sports medicine specialist as soon as possible as the injury may be more complicated. A sports medicine specialist can be a general practitioner experienced in taking care of athletes, a podiatrist, an orthopaedic surgeon, or a physiotherapist. Who to consult really depends on the problem or on word of mouth from other running specialists, training partners, and coaches. Most importantly, runners need a specialist who is familiar with treating running injuries and not those with qualifications only.

Athletes have always faced the dilemma, after an injury, of whether they should continue to "train through" an injury with a lowered intensity or have a complete rest. There is no easy answer to this problem, and a runner always has to balance the benefits of "training through" (e.g., maintaining cardiovascular and muscle fitness) against the problems (e.g., continuous trauma to the injured part). However, certain cross-training, such as swimming and cycling, is probably a good compromise after an injury.

Commonly Encountered Musculoskeletal Injuries In Marathon Training

This chapter aims to cover the most commonly encountered musculoskeletal sports injuries during the marathon training. The non-musculoskeletal illnesses, such as heat-related illness, cardiac and pulmonary problems, and electrolyte imbalance, are covered in other chapters. Most sports injuries occur in the feet and knees, followed by the shins and hips.

The foot and ankle unit is one of the most commonly injured site among running athletes, whether it results in a seemingly benign blister or a serious stress fracture. This should not come as a surprise since the feet and ankles absorb the brunt of stress through repeated running steps during marathon training.

Overuse Injuries of the Foot and Ankle

Acute foot and ankle injuries from marathon training include fracture, joint dislocations, ligament sprain, and muscle strain. These occur when tissues are directly impacted or stressed beyond their normal elasticity. Overuse foot and ankle injuries are more common than acute injuries among running athletes in preparation for a marathon, and they include plantar fasciitis, stress fractures, tendonitis, and bursitis. They usually result from repeated stress over normal tissue or, more commonly, because of other intrinsic abnormalities of the foot, such as anatomical abnormalities, strength and flexibility deficits, and unfit footwear.

1. **Plantar Fasciitis**

    Plantar fasciitis is an inflammation of the plantar fascia, which is a thick fibrous tissue covering the whole length of the foot from the calcaneum to the forefoot. Onset of pain is usually gradual. Often, the athlete can still run even for weeks after the onset of symptoms. The pain usually starts at the inner side of the sole, and maximally over the medial aspect of the heel pad. Pain is more severe after inactivity; for example, the first step in the morning when one gets out of bed or after sitting for a long while. Pain is diminished with rest, but becomes intensified with weight-bearing activities, even during normal walking.

Causes:

When the athlete repeatedly needs to push off during running or jumping, this stretches the fascia, creating microtrauma at its insertion point over the calcaneum. There are several predisposing factors:

a.   increasing body weight

b.   over-pronated foot

c.   tightness or weakness of Achilles tendon

d.   shoes with inadequate arch supports

e.   over-stiff shoes

f.   over-worn-out shoes

Treatment:

a.   Discontinue intensive running and start cross-training with nonimpact activities (e.g., stationary bicycle, swimming, water running).

b.   Ice and massage the sole regularly.

c.   Use a well-cushioned heel pad inside the shoes to relieve the stress.

d.   Avoid walking on bare feet since this places excessive stress on the inside of the feet

e.   Stretch the calf muscles and plantar fascia regularly.

f.   Get a sports medicine specialist to assess the biomechanics of running and see if there is a predisposing factor that can be controlled, such as orthotics to control over-pronated feet, if necessary.

g.   Anti-inflammatory agents are useful to relieve pain and control inflammation.

h.   A night splint is sometimes useful.

i.   Very rarely, the doctor may recommend giving a short dose of steroid injections in resistant cases. However, this increases the risk of potential complications.

j.   Physiotherapists can offer some relief of symptoms with physical modalities such as ultrasound. The recent introduction of shockwave therapy has shown to be quite promising in the treatment of resistant cases.

k.   Surgery is very rarely indicated in the treatment of plantar fasciitis.

When to start running again?

Most cases require at least four to six weeks of relative rest and treatment before athletes can resume full training. Start running on soft ground or grass and avoid hills and speed training.

2. **Blisters**

Blisters are portions of skin that become irritated from friction with shoes or socks, causing them to fill with clear fluid, blood, or pus when infected. They usually occur at pressure points of the feet. They commonly affect running athletes at the beginning of the season after a long rest, at the beginning of a new program of training, or when they wear a new pair of shoes.

Treatment:

Athlete should always remember the real potential for infection if a blister is mismanaged. The surface of the blister should be kept intact as it acts as a protective barrier against bacteria. Never try to break the blister deliberately. On the other hand, one should try to protect it by wearing a doughnut pad to avoid further friction. Most blisters resolve gradually without complication.

Even though many people have taught athletes how to properly pierce a blister, athletes are not recommended to treat the problem themselves because infected blisters will create many more complications. Have medical personnel tackle the problem with aseptic techniques.

Prevention:

Keep the feet dry and wear properly fitted shoes and socks. Cover sore spots with a moleskin or petroleum jelly to reduce friction. Most importantly, try to identify and avoid predisposing factors that might lead to blisters.

3. **Calluses:**

   A callus is a thickening of skin caused by repetitive friction between the skin and the shoes, thus causing pain while running. It may be caused by shoes that are too tight or too narrow or an anatomical abnormality such as hallux valgus, hammer toes, or flat feet. The most commonly affected regions include the back of the heel, the metatarsal heads, the medial side of the first metatarsal head, and the interphalangeal joints of lesser toes.

   Treatment:

   Early calluses can be treated by soaking the foot in warm water to soften the callus or by applying lanolin over it to soften the skin. Wear a doughnut pad over the callus, choose a properly fitted shoe, and treat any underlying causes. With chronic thick calluses, a keratolytic agent such as salicylic acid (5%–10%) can be applied at night and peeled off in the morning. A podiatrist will always be helpful in resistant cases.

4. **Subungual Hematoma**

   Repetitive impact to the front of the big toe can cause bleeding beneath the nail of the big toe. It is not uncommon in long-distance runners, especially among those who wear shoes that are too tight or those who run downhill a lot, causing the nail to be pried upward with each step. When the nail becomes separated from the underlying nail bed, bleeding occurs and is pooled into a confined area, resulting in pain. With time, the nail will fall off.

   Prevention:

   This can be prevented by wearing shoes that provide enough room for the big toes and by avoiding downhill running too much. Padding over the nail of the big toe may also help to prevent the nail from being pried upward.

5. **Stress Fracture of the foot**

   A stress fracture is a series of microfractures that develop in a bone which is subjected to rhythmic, repetitive, sub-threshold impact, such as experienced in marathon runners. 95% of stress fractures occur in the lower limbs. The bones of the foot most commonly affected include the metatarsals, navicular, and calcaneum. The vast majority are found in the metatarsals, dubbed "march fractures" because they were first diagnosed in a group of soldiers forced to march vigorously every day.

Causes:

Classical overtraining (i.e., running too much or too fast when the body is not conditioned appropriately) is usually defined as a sudden increase in the frequency, duration, and intensity of training and is a typical cause of stress fractures. Contributing factors include running on hard surfaces, worn-out shoes, an irregular menstrual cycle in women, poor nutrition, biomechanical disadvantages (e.g., flat feet, Morton's foot), and poor running techniques.

Symptoms:

The symptoms are usually gradual, subtle, and occult from the very beginning. The athlete usually complains of pain over the affected bone (mostly metatarsals) during activity—initially subtle and gradual—but then it become sharp, intense, and localized. With time, the associated swelling may become obvious, and the pain is so severe that one must stop running immediately.

Investigations:

X-rays of the bone usually do not reveal stress fractures until four to eight weeks after symptoms occur; thus, diagnosing stress fracture can be difficult, and we cannot rely on plain radiographs alone. Bone scans and MRIs are both useful and reliable in detecting stress fractures even at very early stages.

Treatment:

The injured athlete should stop running once a stress fracture is diagnosed. Analgesics can be prescribed for pain relief, but the athlete should always be aware of the mask effect of analgesics. He or she should not think that the problem has resolved once the pain decreases. The athlete is also advised to engage in protective weight-bearing walking (i.e., wear a cushioned boot, or Aircast) during the acute phase to relieve the stress. One can start non-weight-bearing cross-training, such as swimming, to maintain cardiovascular fitness. With time—usually after about six to eight weeks—the pain will subside and the athlete can gradually start weight-bearing exercise training, first on soft ground until he or she is pain free without swelling, and then resume normal training. Moreover, any pre-existing anatomical abnormalities which might lead to the problem should be identified, and, if so, they should be addressed before resuming running.

6. **Achilles Tendonitis**

   Achilles tendonitis is an inflammation of the strong tendon connecting the calf muscle to the calcaneum. It is a response to a series of microtears in the tendon, caused by repeated stretching during running, and it is a common problem among long-distance runners. Very often, athletes will try to "run through" the early stages of pain. However, because of the limited blood supply to the tendon near its insertion to the calcaneum, the normal inflammatory healing process after an injury is easily compromised. This leads to long-term problems with a likely recurrence of symptoms. In time, an inflexible scar tissue may form in the area and rupture if one continues to work on it. Achilles tendonitis is especially common in runners older than thirty because of natural degenerative changes which make the tendon tighter and weaker. Moreover, athletes with pronated feet are more prone to develop this problem.

   Symptoms:

   The onset of symptoms is usually gradual, with pain during and after running and a bit of swelling around the heel region. As conditions worsen, there may be redness and an increase in warmth over the tender region. The calf muscle will be stiff, resulting in relatively inflexible ankle movement. The symptoms may get worse during uphill walking or simply walking upstairs.

   Treatment:

   Achilles problems must be treated early before excessive tearing or scarring occurs. Because the blood supply to the Achilles tendon is limited, it can be difficult to heal. Ignoring symptoms in the early stages can worsen the condition, leading to scarring and rupture.

   One must cease running and start ice massage over the region to control inflammation. Non-steroidal anti-inflammatory agents

(NSAID) are helpful to relieve early symptoms of pain and swelling. Physiotherapists can advise on appropriate stretching, eccentric strengthening exercise of the calf muscle, and flexibility training after the acute inflammatory phase. Shoes with a half-inch heel wedge can relieve tension over the tendon. Athletes can also start cross-training such as swimming or cycling to maintain cardiovascular fitness. Preexisting anatomical abnormalities leading to the problem also need to be identified, and they should be addressed before resuming running. Corticosteroid injections are not recommended for Achilles tendonitis, as they can weaken the tendon and lead to rupture.

Lower Leg Injuries

"Shin Splints—An Outdated Diagnosis"

The term "shin splints" has been traditionally used to describe any chronic, exercise-related lower leg pain, encompassing inflammation of the tissue over the distal tibia, stress fractures of the lower leg, and compartment syndrome. Even though many athletes and sports therapists still use the term, doctors do not use this vague term because the symptoms, causes, diagnosis, treatment, and rehabilitation of each condition differ considerably.

1. **Stress fracture of tibia**

   According to a study from Watanabe, the most commonly seen stress fractures among runners happen in the tibia (34%), with 19% over the upper mid-tibia, 4% over the mid-tibia, and 11% over the distal tibia.

   Causes:

   This arises from running too much or too fast when the body is not conditioned appropriately and is usually associated with a sudden increase in frequency, duration, and intensity of training. Contributing factors include running on hard surfaces, wearing worn-out shoes, an irregular menstrual cycle in women, poor nutrition, biomechanical disadvantages (e.g., flat feet, Morton's foot), and poor running techniques.

Symptoms:

Symptoms are usually gradual, subtle, and occult from the very beginning. Usually, athletes complain of mild pain over the leg during activities, which then become sharp, intense, and localized. With time, the associated swelling may become obvious and the pain so severe that one must stop running immediately.

Treatment (see "Stress fracture of the foot" in the previous section)

2. **Compartment syndrome**

   The muscles in the lower leg are encased in four different compartments, surrounded by a thick fascial wall. Excessive training can induce muscle swelling inside the compartment, which may compress the muscles and nerves and produce the characteristic symptoms of compartment syndrome, which most commonly occurs in the anterior compartment of the leg, although it can happen in all four compartments.

Symptoms:

Onset of symptoms is usually gradual, but it can increase with an ache, sharp pain, or pressure in the anterior-lateral aspect of the lower leg or numbness and tingling in the lower leg during running. The symptoms completely abate when the activity is stopped. When the conditions deteriorate, there may be weakness when trying to dorsiflex the foot and toes upward, and there is pain when the foot and toes are flexed passively. Numbness over the dorsum of the foot and between the big and second toes are common complaints in later stages. The athlete will be unable to exercise once the symptoms appear.

Treatment:

One should cease running once the diagnosis is confirmed. It is important to identify predisposing factors and to modify training regimens, paying particular attention to training surfaces, footwear, and running techniques.

However, most cases will recur once the athlete resumes running. Once the diagnosis is confirmed and conservative treatment has failed, doctors will usually advise on surgery (fasciotomy) if the athlete wishes to continue running.

3. **Medial tibial pain syndrome (tibial periostitis)**

   Medial tibial pain syndrome has replaced the old term of "shin splints" and is characterized by pain over the medial side of the distal tibia, resulting from inflammation of the tissue overlying the medial aspect of the distal tibia, with inflammation of the periosteum. It is thus called tibial periostitis. Diagnosis should be reached with care to rule out compartment syndrome and a stress fracture of the tibia.

   Causes:

   This is commonly caused in marathon runners by overtraining, with predisposing factors very similar to those of stress fractures, including tight calf muscles, over-pronated feet, training on hard surfaces, and worn-out shoes.

   Treatment:

   Treatment includes stopping running while continuing cross-training such as swimming or cycling to maintain cardiovascular fitness. It is important to identify predisposing factors and to modify training regimens, paying particular attention to training surfaces, footwear, and running techniques. The pain will subside in about four to six weeks, and the athlete can gradually resume running, first on soft ground until he or she is totally pain free without swelling.

Knee and Hip Injuries

In this section, we discuss those sports injuries of the knee and hip regions that commonly result from overuse during marathon training. Other injuries around the knee, like meniscus and ligament injuries, though important, do not commonly result from marathon training, and will not be covered.

1. **Patellofemoral pain syndrome (runner's knee)**

   The affliction of runner's knee has also been called chondromalacia patella. It is now more commonly described as Patellofemoral Pain Syndrome (PFS). It is most commonly associated with running, and it occurs when the patella tracking is not on the right way, causing pain over the anterior aspect of the knee.

Symptoms:

The onset of symptoms is usually gradual, with pain in front of the knee. The pain intensifies during sports activity, particularly during uphill running or when walking upstairs. Usually, there is crepitation over the anterior aspect of the knee during examinations, and there may be associated anatomical abnormalities.

Causes:

Causes usually include a biomechanical problem, with patella malalignment brought on by various types of anatomical abnormalities or deficits in strength and flexibility. These include excessive femoral anteversion, patella alta, shallow trochlear groove, weak vasta medialis muscle, tight lateral retinaculum of the knee, increasing Q angle or valgus knee, tight hamstring and calf muscle, and overpronated feet. There is the so-called "Miserable Malalignment syndrome" for runners with anterior knee pain which includes an internally rotated hip, knock-knee, and flat feet.

Treatment:

Treatment needs to tackle the underlying cause of the patella maltracking directly, and this usually starts with non-operative treatment, including the use of orthotics to correct limb malalignments, strengthening weak muscles, stretching tight structures to realign the patella, and maintaining cardiovascular endurance with other cross-training methods. However, in about 10% of cases, conservative treatment will fail and operative treatment may be needed, which ranges from minimally invasive surgery, such as knee arthroscopy, to realignment surgery to restore the correct biomechanics.

2. **Iliotibial Band syndrome**

The iliotibial band (ITB) is a thick fibrous band running from the outer rims of the pelvis down to the lateral aspect of the proximal tibia. In marathon runners, excessive friction injuries can occur at points where the band rubs against bony prominences such as the lateral epicondyle of the distal femur, causing inflammation of the underlying bursa and resulting in iliotibial band syndrome.

Symptoms:

The onset of symptoms is gradual, with tightness felt over the lateral aspect of the distal thigh and knee. There will be increasing pain while running, worse during downhill running or movement downstairs. The discomfort subsides when running stops. In worse conditions, the pain will force the athlete to walk with the injured leg fully extended to relieve the friction of the ITB over the lateral epicondyle of the knee.

Causes:

Causes include repetitive flexion and extension of the knee. Athletes running on a slanted or downhill surface are at risk, as are those who do not warm up or cool down properly. This causes tightness and decreased flexibility of the iliotibial band. Athletes with anatomical abnormalities like hip abductor weakness, underpronated feet, and bow legs are prone to this problem as well.

Treatment:

Affected persons should reduce training intensity and put ice on the affected sites. Taking NSAID will help relieve the acute symptoms. Caution should be taken when cross-training, as activities such as cycling or rowing also cause irritations to the ITB over the lateral aspect of the knee. Swimming while the legs are immobilized is one of the suggested cross-training modalities. Shoes should be evaluated, and consultation with a sports medicine specialist on a biomechanical evaluation of running patterns is also useful. Physiotherapy is helpful to relieve pain over the trigger point, stretch the tight lateral structures, strengthen the weak muscle, and encourage flexibility. Surgery is rarely needed.

3. **Trochanteric Bursitis**

   Trochanteric bursitis is an inflammation of the bursa overlying the greater trochanter of the hip joint. This is caused by friction of the iliotibial band over the greater trochanter region, which happens with repeated flexion and extension of the hip, like during marathon training.

   ### Symptoms:

   Pain is gradual and felt over the greater trochanter region of the hip, and it worsens when attempting hip abduction. Sometimes, a snapping sensation over the hip, known as "snapping hip syndrome," may be felt. The pain may radiate down the lateral aspect of the thigh.

Causes:

It results from repetitive flexion and extension of the hip, such as that experienced during marathon training. There is increased risk in athletes with wide pelvises, excessive pronation of the feet, and leg length discrepancies.

Treatment:

Athletes should cease running or reduce the intensity of training. Ice and NSAID are used to reduce the inflammation. If the condition is caused by excessive foot pronation, then shoe inserts will be helpful. Physiotherapy will be helpful to relieve the pain over the trigger point, stretch the tight lateral structures, strengthen the weak muscle, and encourage flexibility. Surgery is rarely needed.

Conclusion

Running injuries are common during marathon training. The correct attitude is to face this situation and tackle it with knowledge once an injury occurs. Patients are always guided to think of this in two distinct ways:

1. Heal the actual trauma so that one can return to activity without pain.
2. Determine the underlying causes of the injury so as to prevent recurrence.

Most runners ignore the second point, and thus relapse is almost certain in most cases. Management should not be stopped once pain has subsided with medication or ice. Patients should continue the detective work to identify the cause and tackle it with the help of a sports medicine specialist. Only knowing the science and anticipating potential sports injuries associated with marathon training can allow us to play wise, to play smart, and not to become a statistic of recurrence.

References

General

1.   Fredericson M, Misra AK. 2007. Epidemiology and aetiology of marathon running injuries. *Sports Med* 37 (4–5): 437–39.

2.   Taunton JE, Ryan MB, Clement DB, McKenzie DC, Lloyd-Smith DR, Zumbo BD. 2002. A retrospective case-control analysis of 2002 running injuries. *Br J Sports Med* 36 (2): 95–101.

3.   McKean KA, Manson NA, Stanish WD. 2006. Musculoskeletal injury in the masters runners. *Clin J Sport Med* 16 (2): 149–54.

4.   Taunton JE, Ryan MB, Clement DB, McKenzie DC, Lloyd-Smith DR, Zumbo BD. 2003. A prospective study of running injuries: the Vancouver Sun Run "In Training" clinics. *Br J Sports Med* 37 (3): 239–44.

Ilial-Tibial Band Syndrome

5.   Messier SP, Edwards DG, Martin DF, Lowery RB, Cannon DW, James MK, et al. 1995. Etiology of iliotibial band friction syndrome in distance runners. *Med Sci Sports Exerc* 27 (7): 951–60.

6.   Fredericson M, Cookingham CL, Chaudhari AM, Dowdell BC, Oestreicher N, Sahrmann SA. 2000. Hip abductor weakness in distance runners with iliotibial band syndrome. *Clin J Sport Med* 10 (3): 169–75.

Runners' Knee

7.   Fredericson M, Yoon K. 2006. Physical examination and patellofemoral pain syndrome. *Am J Phys Med Rehabil* 85 (3): 234–43.

8.   Messier SP, Davis SE, Curl WW, Lowery RB, Pack RJ. 1991. Etiologic factors associated with patellofemoral pain in runners. *Med Sci Sports Exerc* 23 (9): 1008–15.

Shin splint and tibia stress fractures

9.   Bates P. 1985. Shin splints—a literature review. *Br J Sports Med* 19 (3): 132–37.

10. Batt ME. 1995. Shin splints—a review of terminology. *Clin J Sport Med* 5 (1): 53–57.

11. Pell RF, Khanuja HS, Cooley GR. 2004. Leg pain in the running athlete. *J Am Acad Orthop Surg* 12 (6): 396–404.

12. Wall J, Feller JF. 2006. Imaging of stress fractures in runners. *Clin Sports Med* 25 (4): 781–802.

Compartment Syndrome

13. Edwards PH, Wright ML, Hartman JF. 2005. A practical approach for the differential diagnosis of chronic leg pain in the athlete. *Am J Sports Med* 33 (8): 1241–49.

14. Abramowitz AJ, Schepsis AA. 1994. Chronic exertional compartment syndrome of the lower legs. *Orthop Rev* 23 (3): 219–25.

Achilles Tendonitis

15. Furia JP. 2006. High-energy extracorporeal shock wave therapy as a treatment for insertional Achilles tendinopathy. *Am J Sports Med* 34 (5): 733–40.

16. McCrory JL, Martin DF, Lowery RB, Cannon DW, Curl WW, Read HM Jr, et al. 1999. Etiologic factors associated with Achilles tendinitis in runners. *Med Sci Sports Exerc* 31 (10): 1374–81.

Stress Fracture of foot

17. Tuan K, Wu S, Sennett B. 2004. Stress fractures in athletes: risk factors, diagnosis, and management. *Orthopedics* 27 (6): 583–91; quiz 592–93.

18. Wall J, Feller JF. 2006. Imaging of stress fractures in runners. *Clin Sports Med* 25 (4): 781–802.

19. Monteleone GP. 1995. Stress fractures in the athlete. *Orthop Clin North Am* 26 (3): 423–32.

Plantar Fasciitis

20. Warren BL. 1984. Anatomical factors associated with predicting plantar fasciitis in long-distance runners. *Med Sci Sports Exerc* 16 (1): 60–63.

21. Riddle DL, Pulisic M, Pidcoe P, Johnson RE. 2003. Risk factors for Plantar fasciitis: a matched case-control study. *J Bone Joint Surg Am* 85-A (5): 872–77.21.

Physiotherapy for Marathon Runners

Mr. Elton NG

Introduction

We have been providing voluntary physiotherapy service to the Standard Chartered Marathon for a number of years. In the first few years, runners just treated us as people who could provide free massage services. But, as time went by, people began to recognize that we had more to offer. Physiotherapists could in fact make differential diagnoses for acute injuries with the aim of providing immediate treatment or referral to advanced medical care or hospitalization. We could even provide advice to runners regarding injury management, injury prevention, and specialized training methods.

Physiotherapy services are not limited to onsite acute injury management. If a runner is serious about running, it is highly desirable for him/her to seek the advice of a sports physiotherapist six months prior to a major event, so that he/she could learn about his/her foot type, running posture, and physical condition. Sports physiotherapists also design a specialized training program which can maximize a runner's performance and minimize the chances of injury. Physiotherapists also prescribe therapeutic exercise and advice on shoe and insole selection (according to running posture and potential).

As a sports physiotherapist and multi-sports athlete for over a decade, I will discuss in this chapter the three most common marathon injuries and share some simple self-treatment methods. A brief discussion on shoe selection for different foot types is followed by a running posture demonstration. I will also talk about functional training for injury prevention and speed development, so that you can get a basic idea of thorough preparation from a sports physiotherapist's point of view.

The Three Most Common Injuries among Marathon Runners

The three most common injuries among marathon runners are patellofemoral pain syndrome (PFPS), iliotibial band friction syndrome (ITBFS), and plantar fasciitis. According to British research (Taunton et al, 2002), most running injuries are in the knee and ankle. The most common injury is PFPS and the second most common injury is ITBFS.

Table 1 Ten Common Running Injuries

Common Injury	Men (No.)	Women (No.)	Total
Patellofemoral pain syndrome (PFPS)	124	207	331
Iliotibial band friction syndrome (ITBFS)	63	105	168
Plantar fasciitis	85	73	158
Meniscal injuries	69	31	100
Tibial stress syndrome	43	56	99
Patella tendinitis	55	41	96
Achilles tendinitis	56	40	96
Gluteus medius injuries	17	53	70
Stress fracture—tibia	27	40	67
Spinal injuries	24	23	47
Total	563	669	1,232

Source: Statistics of common running injuries (adapted from Taunton JE et al., 2002.)

Although there are no systematic injury statistics from the Hong Kong running events, my experience indicates that the number of athletes suffering from ITBFS may even outnumber those with PFPS. My explanation is that most long-distance running competitions in Hong Kong, including the Standard Chartered Marathon, have total climbs for nearly 200 meters, and this involves much greater altitude differences which are uncommon among marathons worldwide. In addition, abnormal feet shapes are more common among Asians. Moreover, busy lifestyles, which may curtail preparation and training, may also contribute to the injuries.

I. Patellofemoral Pain Syndrome (PFPS)

PFPS is a common condition characterized by diffused pain in the anterior knee or retropatellar region which is exacerbated by daily activities such as stair climbing, prolonged sitting, squatting, kneeling, etc. Many young athletes have pain under the knee cap after squatting on the ground, climbing or descending stairs, or prolonged sitting though they have no obvious injuries such as a ligamentous tear. Most of them think the pain is the result of exhausted trainings or an unavoidable degenerative phenomenon, but in fact they may suffer from PFPS. It is one of the most common knee conditions among young athletes, especially in the events with repetitive lower limb loading (Van Mechelen, 1992; Taunton et al., 2002). The etiology of PFPS is not well understood, but the most commonly accepted hypothesis is the abnormal lateral tracking of the patella within the trochlear groove which will increase the uneven stress and articular cartilage wear causing pain. (Wise et al., 1984; Schutzer et al., 1986; Fulkerson and Shea, 1990; Grabiner et al., 1994; McConnell, 1986, 1996).

In knee extensor mechanisms, four components of quadriceps (vastus medialis, vastus lateralis (VL), vastus intermedius, and rectus femoris) act together to produce movements. Each component generates tension with a particular magnitude and direction (Figure 1). The resultant knee extension force vector tends to displace the patella laterally, attributing to the pull of VL (Hughston et al., 1984). This lateral displacement is resisted by passive constraints, for example congruency of the lateral aspect of the patella, lateral femoral condyle, and medial retinaculum, whereas vastus medialis obliquus (VMO) has no contribution to the knee extension torque but is the only dynamic medial stabilizer believed to be important in resisting lateral patellar displacement (Hughston et al., 1984). Therefore, imbalance in the activity of

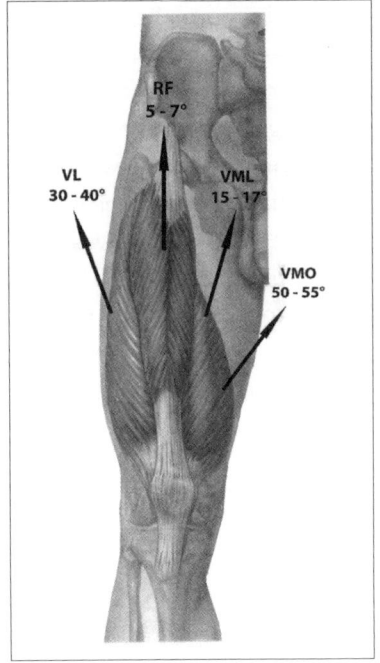

Figure 1 illustrated diagram of quadriceps insertion (Wilk et al., 1998).

VMO relative to VL was proposed for abnormal patellar tracking, and is a main contributing factor of patellofemoral pain syndrome (PFPS) (Insall, 1982; Voight and Weider, 1991; Brukner and Khan, 2000).

In addition to the imbalanced active structures, structural abnormalities such as tight lateral retinaculum, lax medial retinaculum, increased femoral anteversion, genu valgum, genu recurvatum, internal tibial torsion, patella alta, hypoplasia of the femoral groove, increased Q angle, and hyperpronation have been reported to alter lateral tracking of the patella (Wise et al., 1984; Schutzer et al., 1986; Cox, 1990; Grabiner et al., 1994; Fulkerson and Hungerford, 1997).

Clinically, physiotherapy treatments for PFPS vary from acupuncture, ice, and electrical modalities to stretching exercises to increase the flexibility of tight structures; however, tight lateral retinaculum and maligned patella are ineffective to stretch to restore normal alignment. From my experience, there are still some sports tapping techniques, myofascial release techniques, and patellar mobilization techniques that are shown to be effective for instant pain relief.

To treat the cause, the objective is to restore equilibrium of patella tracking by normalizing passive structures, muscles, and the neuromotor control systems. As the passive structures may not be easily altered, muscle activation patterns are often addressed in clinical practice by selectively activating VMO in functional positions.

During the past two decades, numerous electromyographic (EMG) studies have investigated the relationship between VMO and VL. Though there are many controversies, current trends have gradually developed consensus in some areas. Witvrouw et al. (1996), Cowan and Bennell, et al. (2001), and Cowan and Hodges, et al. (2001) have discovered that the reflex response time of VMO would be significantly shorter than that of VL in normal subjects but delayed onset of EMG activity of VMO relative to VL in PFPS subjects. Beside the onset timing, abnormal VMO:VL ratio may also be a biomechanical factor that leads to PFPS (Souza and Gross, 1991; Lam and Ng, 2001). A recent study by Neptune et al. (2000) demonstrated the functional significance of such a timing difference that a 5-ms delay in VMO would be associated with a significant increase in lateral patellofemoral joint (PFJ) loading. Summary of different training comparisons and some therapeutic exercises are suggested below.

Opened kinetic chains (OKC) and closed kinetic chains (CKC) exercise

CKC exercises are performed with the foot on a surface and the entire limb loaded while the OKC exercise is performed with the distal part of the lower limb free from the ground (Bynum et al., 1995). Patellofemoral Joint Compressive Force (PFJCF) is described as the compression of patella against femur depending on the angle of knee and muscle tension (Bentley and Dowd, 1984). First of all, the patellofemoral contact area is increased with knee flexion. During OKC exercises, when the knee is gradually extended, the quadriceps force will be increased while the contact area is decreased, contributing to greater PFJCF (Hungerford and Barry, 1979). During CKC exercises, the quadriceps force increases with knee flexion range though the patella contact area increases. Therefore, the PFJCF will be greater when the knee is flexed. Hence, we may avoid excessive knee extension during OKC exercises and excessive flexion range during CKC exercises to minimize the PFJCF.

In addition to PFJCF, we should also consider the patellar congruence concerning the stress and patellar stability. Doucette and Child (1996) have suggested that patellar congruence is increased from 0° to 40° of knee flexion in CKC and OKC exercises. During 0° to 20° knee flexion, there is less lateral tracking of the patella in CKC exercises compared with OKC exercises. To sum up, Wilk and Reinold (2001) have suggested that OKC exercises should be performed in 90° to 40° of knee flexion, as the patellofemoral contact area is larger while the PFJCF is lowered. Moreover, CKC exercises can be done with initially 0° to 30° of knee flexion and then progressing to 0° to 60°.

Hip abduction and external rotation

The gluteus medius is the prime mover of hip abductors. During CKC exercises, the gluteus medius will contract eccentrically to control internal rotation of the hip in order to avoid the lateral tracking of the patella, thus assisting activation of VMO. External rotation of the hip also decreases the lateral pull of tensor fascia lata and stretches the VMO. However, research results are still controversial. Sykes and Wong (2003) have suggested increased VMO activity during straight leg raise (SLR) exercises with the hip in an externally rotated position.

Hip adduction

Hanten and Schulthies (1990) have found greater VMO activity during maximal isometric hip adduction. Hodges and Richardson (1993a, 1993b) have discovered increased VMO activity, compared with VL, during simultaneous hip adduction and knee extension in a CKC semi-squatting exercise. Miller et al (1997) have also suggested selective VMO activation during step-down exercises.

Besides adducting the thigh, adductors magnus will transfer a physiological stretch to VMO, altering the length tension properties of VMO and enhancing the force production. Hodges and Richardson (1993a, 1993b) have suggested some fibers of VMO originated from adductor groups, so that contraction of adductors provides a stable base for VMO contraction.

Hip internal rotation

Fredericson and Power (2002) have suggested that internal rotation of the femur may rotate the trochlear groove beneath the patella, placing the patella relatively lateral and in a position possible to assist the activation of VMO. However, research results are still controversial.

Ankle dorsiflexion and plantarflexion

It is observed that knee extension exercises with ankle dorsiflexion would decrease patellofemoral pain. Zakaria et al. (1997) have reported a 20% increase of VMO and VL activities during knee extension exercises with ankle dorsiflexion. Tepperman et al. (1986) have found that the EMG output of VMO, VL, and rectus femoris in dorsiflexed and plantarflexed position would be superior to the neutral position during isometric hip and knee extension in a supine position. It is suggested that reduction of flexor withdrawal reflex and stretch of gastrocnemius will aid the hamstrings, keeping the knee slightly flexed and reducing pain.

Suggested therapeutic exercises:

Gluteus Medius Recruitment Training

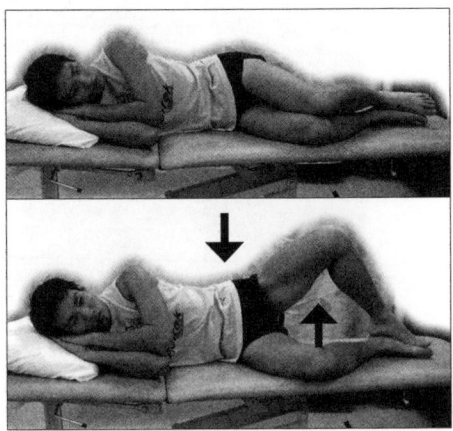

1. Lie on one side and bend the knees 90°.
2. Raise the upper thigh slowly (separating your knees).
3. Keep the spine in neutral and hold this position for 3 to 5 seconds; repeat action 20 to 30 times.

CKC Semi-Squat Exercise With Isomeric Hip Adduction against a Ball

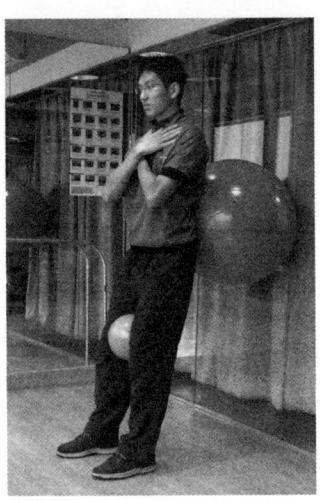

1. Stand straight with a ball at the back and place the feet parallel to the shoulder.
2. Keep squeezing a ball between the knees. Slowly squat down and keep vision and toes straight ahead.

3. The knee should not go further to the toes; hold for 3 to 5 seconds.
4. Repeat the action 20 to 30 times.

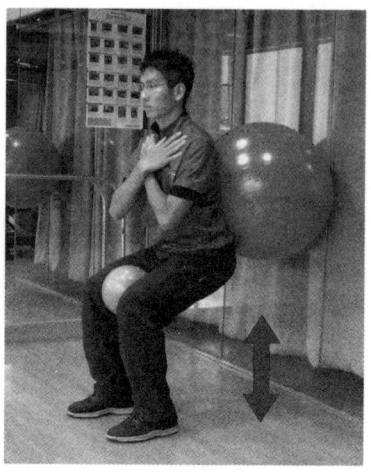

Isomeric Gluteus Recruitment Training with Knee Extension

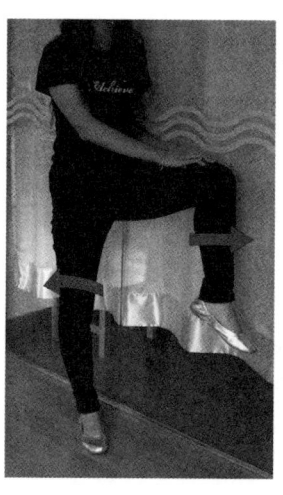

1. Raise one leg and push it against a wall.
2. Standing on the other leg, keep the spine in neutral and with knee bent at 5°.
3. Tighten the buttock muscles by turning the standing leg outward isomerically.
4. Hold this position for around a minute and repeat the action for 3 to 5 sets.

Other treatment approaches

Patellar taping was originally developed by McConnell (1986). The purported aim is to create a mechanical realignment of the patella, thus centralizing it within the trochlear groove and improving patellar tracking that may enhance the activation and/or timing of the VMO relative to the VL. For an immediate effect, McConnell (1986) has supported the idea that the

McConnell's taping procedures

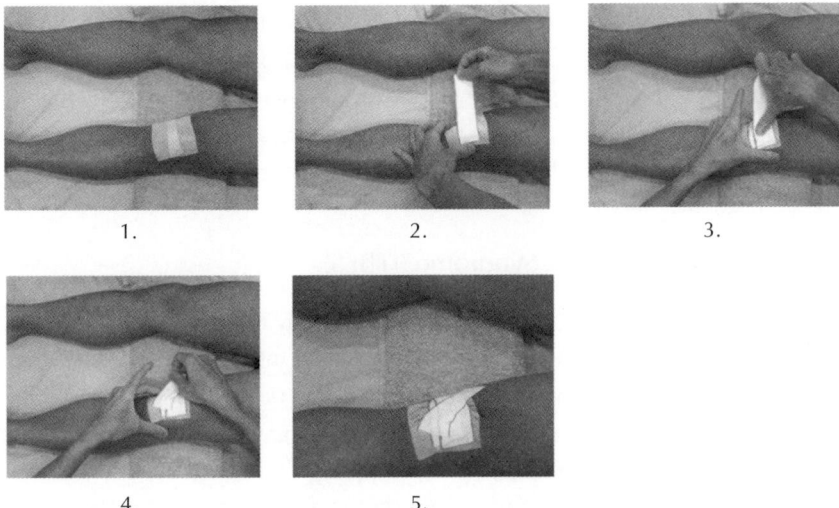

1.   2.   3.

   4.   5.

1. Cover dressing sheet on area where tapes will be applied to reduce skin irritation.
2. Use rigid tape to provide medial glide for correcting patella malignment.
3. Second tape corrects patella tilting.
4. Third tape corrects rotation deficit.
5. Finish up.

application of tapes would increase the amplitude of VMO EMG activity. For temporal control of VMO, Gilleard et al. (1998) have found that the onset timing of VMO occurs earlier during stair stepping tasks after taping. However, research results are controversial in other practical application aspects. From my experience, patellar taping is effective in relieving pain instantly and is important for restarting initial pain-free knee muscle training. Unfortunately, we cannot use this effective technique for patients who are allergic to taping materials.

Orthotics are prescribed if there is excessive foot pronation which is believed to aggravate the pain, particularly for patients with PFPS who are unable or too fatigued to control a good (neutral) lower limb alignment when exercising. On the other hand, modifications of training or daily activities, such as swimming, cycling and slow jogging on grass, also help to ease the pain in the early stages. Exercises may increase the impact on the knee cap and aggravate the condition. Thus, bunny hops, running, and stair climbing should be avoided. If the condition persists or worsens, it is highly advisable to consult sports surgeons and sports physiotherapists to perform an in-depth biomechanical analysis of running posture.

II. Iliotibial Band Friction Syndrome (ITBFS)

ITBFS is the most common lateral knee pain and may easily trigger other types of knee pain. Clinically, ITBFS sufferers have difficulty flexing the knee and experience extreme pain while descending a slope or flight of stairs. A penetrating dull ache on the outer thigh and knee may gradually aggravate in the middle of training or competition, without apparent injuries (Kirk et al., 2000). In the early stages, it is only a light pain on the outer side of the knee which usually occurs after exercising and can be soothed by resting or applying ice. However, the pain may extend to the anterolateral tibia, fibula head, and patella. Swelling and pain may persist even after resting for a few weeks.

The iliotibial band (ITB) itself is a thickened inelastic strip of fascia that extends from the tubercle of the iliac crest and provides the insertion for the tensor fascia lata and gluteus maximus muscles. The ITB continues down the lateral side of the leg and, in conjunction with the patellar retinaculum, ultimately attaches onto the lateral tubercle of the tibia (Gerdy's tubercle) and lateral proximal fibular head. Mercer et al. (1998) have explained that, although ITB is free over the lateral aspects of the hip and knee joints, it is firmly attached to the linea aspera of the femur via the lateral intermuscular septum. Zachazewski (1996) has suggested that when the ITB becomes tight, repetitive knee bending and increased rubbing at the femoral lateral epicondyle will make it

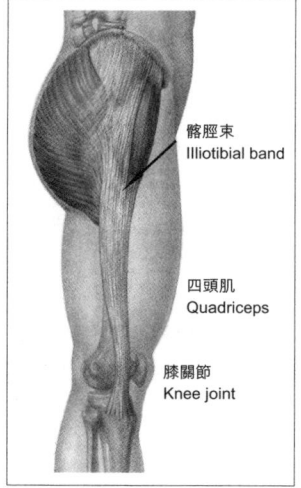

髂脛束
Illiotibial band

四頭肌
Quadriceps

膝關節
Knee joint

Figure 2 Origin and insertion of ITB.

swell and cause inflammation of this band. If the case worsens, it will alter the smooth movement of the patella inside the femoral groove and trigger pain in the patella as well. Therefore, it is common to see ITBFS sufferers walking in a "locked" knee position to avoid flexing the knee and to reduce the rubbing of the inflamed ITB.

Taunton et al. (2002) and Kirk et al. (2000) have concluded from their reviews that pathobiomechanics (such as abnormal tibia and femur alignment, flat feet, leg length discrepancy, and large Q angle) would increase friction on the ITB and surrounding tissues. Moreover, weak or incompatible hip adductors, vastus medialis, and gluteus medius muscles would aggravate abnormal running patterns (such as overpronation and over or under bending of knee) and worsen the case. In addition, hard ground, too many hill descents and stepped ascents, and a lack of training also contribute to the cause of pain. Orchard et al. (1996) have found that single plane movement repetitive sports (such as long-distance running) increase inflammation possibilities more than multi-plane or quick sport activities (such as short runs or basketball).

There are various ways to cure and prevent ITBFS. Acupuncture, ice and electrical modalities, and taking non-steroid anti-inflammatory drugs (NSAIDs) can help to ease inflammation. However, to really cure the disease, the best way is to reduce the friction and stress at the ITB. From my experience, ITB stretching exercises are not as effective as expected, whereas muscle relaxation and trigger-point release techniques along the ITB are more effective at releasing the tightened ITB.

Demonstration of trigger point release techniques along the ITB

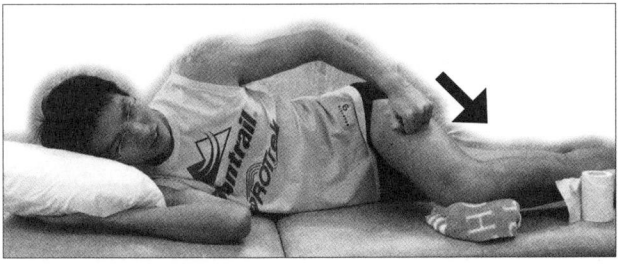

1. Lie on your side and keep your leg bent.
2. Apply oil on your thigh.
3. Massage the muscle from your thigh to your knee.

In view of functional anatomy analysis, Mercer et al. (1998) have suggested that it is still useful to stretch the vastus lateralis (VL) and vastus intermedius (VI) (two muscle groups of the quadriceps), but not the ITB, as the ITB is too inelastic to stretch. However, since the ITB is adhered with VL and VI, stretching VL and VI may indirectly increase the flexibility of the ITB.

Effective Hurdle Stretch for vastus lateralis (VL) and vastus intermedius (VI)

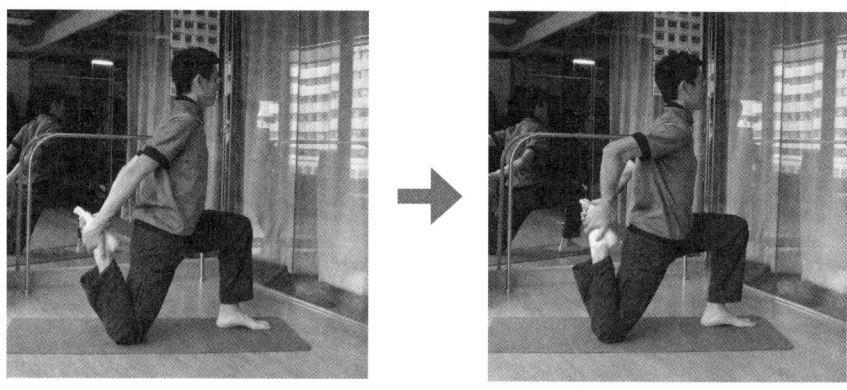

1. Kneel down and keep the back straight. Place one thigh farther behind in the neutral position.
2. Lift the lower leg up to stretch the thigh muscles.
3. Maintain posterior pelvic tilt and hold for 10 to 30 seconds; repeat the stretch 3 to 4 times.

On the other hand, from a biomechanical point of view, ITB can be treated through muscle reeducation and conditioning, especially those muscles involved in pelvic and lower extremity control. Strengthening the quadriceps, vastus medialis oblique, gluteus maximus, and gluteus medius can improve abnormal running postures (such as overpronation). Strengthening of hip abductors for gait correction inhibit the tensor fasciae latae (TFL). The TFL internally rotates the hip and is also a synergistic hip abductor with the gluteus medius during stance phase. Therefore, if the TFL develops over-activity, the gluteus medius can potentially become inhibited. As a result of the hyperactivity of TFL, the lower limbs will be "forced" into an internally rotated position. This will in turn trigger possible pronation of the foot. This biomechanical fault will be amplified as a result of intrinsic foot muscle fatigue after prolonged standing or running. Therefore, some authors have suggested that trigger-point release therapy on TFL is also effective to relieve

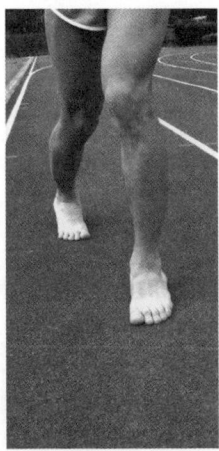

Figure 3 Poor leg alignment and early intrinsic foot muscle fatigue exaggerate the internal rotation, and thus increase tension on the ITB.

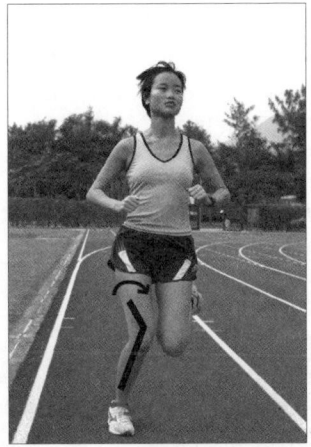

Figure 4 Demonstration of an incorrect running posture

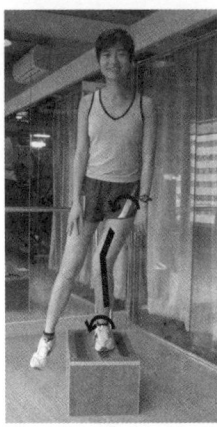

Figure 5 Demonstration of an incorrect step-descending posture

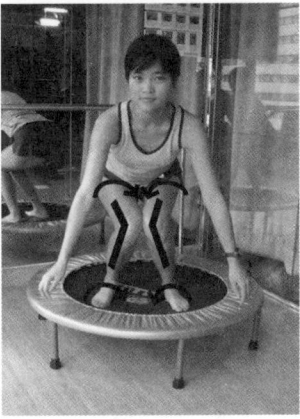

Figure 6 Demonstration of an incorrect squatting posture

tension on the ITB. Moreover, insole or low-dye sports taping techniques (shown below in plantar fasciitis) can also help to reduce intrinsic muscle fatigue in the foot as well as internal rotation in the lower limb, and thus reduce the tension on ITB biomechanically.

As an endurance adventure racer, I have been caught by this syndrome a few times because of tough races. From my self-treatment experience, acupuncture is an excellent way to control the inflammation. Some acupoints, which are close to the fibrous connective tissue and the capsular extension near the knee joint, have more obvious effects than that of the "fengshi" (GB31) acu-point as suggested by most classic reference books.

Agility exercise for reeducating leg external rotation

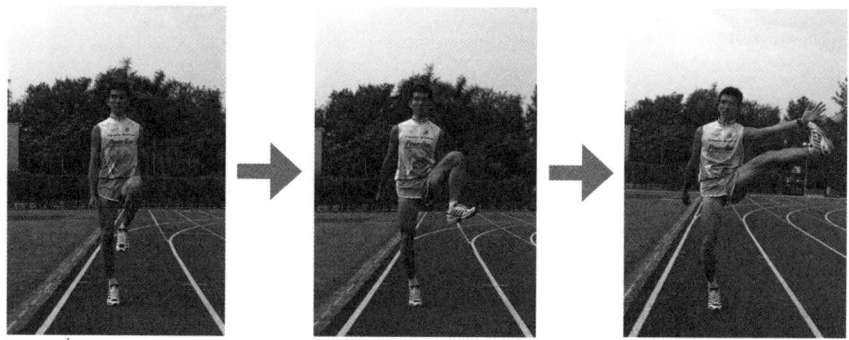

Agility training: Butt kicking—Essential for speed development and good for ITB rehabilitative training

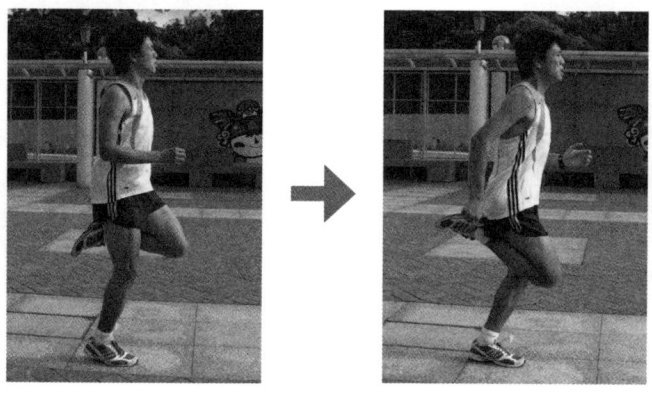

Nemeth and Sanders (1996) and Costa et al. (2004) have found that some patients would not only have inflammation of the ITB, but also in the cysts and synovial recess of knee joints. Thus, applying acupuncture on these tissues may be an additional treatment method.

While the key to healing is to intensively control swelling and inflammation and to monitor the retraining program carefully and precisely since symptoms often reappear at similar mileage during the initial stages. Rehabilitation training such as jogging on lawns, swimming, running in water, and cycling are used to replace ordinary sports training in the acute phase. Affected runners should avoid jumping, sprinting, downhill running, and stair climbing which will put a lot of stress on the ITB. Mileage and high-impact training (e.g., downhill run, intervals) should proceed gradually with respect to the symptoms. Some agility exercises with straight knees, such as running backward, running sideways, etc., can be tried first.

Recent research has analyzed the specific force, joint angle, and frequency one could train to benefit the ITBFS. Orchard et al. (1996) have suggested one should restart training with a few bouts of quicker movements in multi-plane—rather than routine—long, slow jogging. A few bouts of butt-kicking exercises and interval training are more preferable. Most of all, we should constantly be aware of our running postures.

III. Plantar Fasciitis

Plantar fasciitis commonly causes inferior heel pain and occurs in up to 10% of the U.S. population (Cole et al., 2005). Plantar fasciitis is an inflammation of the plantar fascia which is usually caused by microtears near its attachment to the heel from repetitive trauma. However, many have confused heel spurs and plantar fasciitis. Plantar fascia is the thick fibrous tissue that runs from the heel to the heads of metatarsals. It supports the joints and soft tissues underneath and creates a rigid lever for push-off. It also helps to maintain the longitudinal foot arch.

Pain associated with plantar fasciitis may be throbbing or piercing, especially with the first few steps in the morning or after periods of inactivity. The condition normally improves after warm-up activities or further ambulation as the shortened plantar fascia is gradually stretched out, but it worsens again with continued activity. Walking barefoot, on toes, or up stairs may also exacerbate the pain. Many patients usually have tenderness around the medial calcaneal tuberosity at the plantar aponeurosis (American College of Foot and Ankle Surgeons, 2001). The longer the inflammation lasts, the greater the possibility osteophytes on the anterior calcaneus (i.e., heel spurs) will develop. However, the presence or absence of heel spurs is not helpful in diagnosing plantar fasciitis. Radiography may show heel spurs or calcifications in the soft tissues, but 50% of patients with plantar fasciitis and up to 19% of patients without plantar fasciitis have heel spurs (DiMarcangelo and Yu, 1997).

A sudden increase in mileage or training frequency over a short period of time, inadequate recovery time, running on surfaces that are too hard or soft, or running upslope may easily cause injury to the plantar fascia. Moreover, plantar fasciitis is also related to the lack of strength and flexibility of the calf. Good strength of peroneus longus and tibialis posterior muscles is also important in maintaining the longitudinal foot arch, and thus less stressful to the plantar fascia. Lower limb biomechanical problems such as genu varus, genu valgus, tibial torsion, leg length discrepancy, and flat feet pose a higher risk of causing plantar fasciitis (Kibler et al., 1991).

Stretching exercises, electrophysical therapy, and acupuncture can be used to reduce pain. However, DiGiovanni et al. (2003) discovered that stretching the plantar fascia is more effective than calf stretching and should be recommended for all patients with pain.

Stretching exercise of the plantar fascia

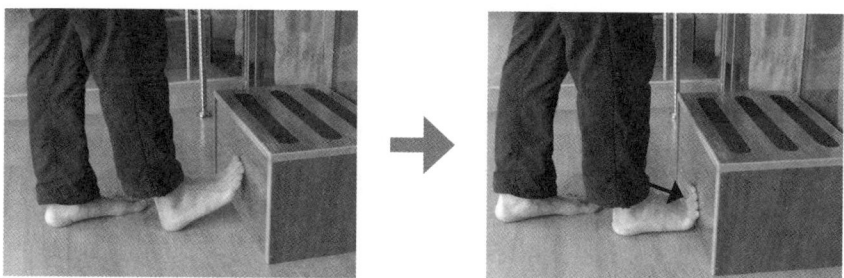

1. Raise up toes by pressing again the wall and weight bear on it.
2. Hold the stretch over the sole of foot for 10 to 30 seconds and repeat 3 to 4 times.

Many authors agree that the most effective intervention is to take active rest by decreasing mileage by 25% to 75%, minimizing running uphill and repetitive high-impact sports such as sprinting. Manual therapy to subtalar joints, talonavicular joints, and the first ray may improve foot mechanics, but a thorough physical examination and mechanics analysis is needed for deciding treatment approaches.

For the active component, strengthening exercises of calves, tibialis posterior, and peronaeus longus muscles can be started at early rehabilitation phase. Clinically, intrinsic muscle recruitment training, balance training, and reeducation exercises for leg alignment and running posture are essential to reduce stress on plantar fascia.

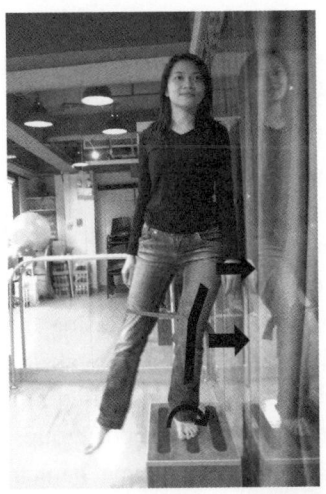

An example of training for improving descending posture

1. lean against the wall or tie up the leg with a resistance bend to facilitate the outer-side of the leg muscle to work more.
2. Keep the supporting leg straight

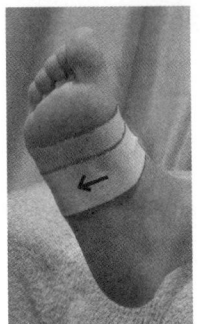 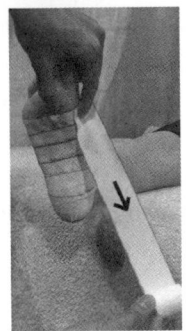 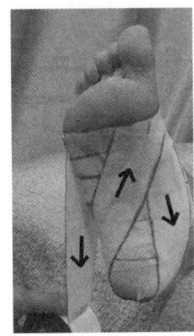 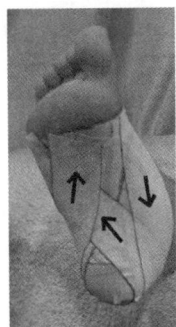

Fig 7 Sports taping method for plantar fasciitis

Though no studies have adequately evaluated the effectiveness of taping or strapping for managing plantar fasciitis (Cole et al,. 2005), some sport taping methods (e.g., low dye taping) are effective for subjective pain relief and aid early retraining programs. This is because the taping temporarily supports the arch and obviously decreases the stress on the plantar fascia.

Some features of orthotics also achieve similar functions. Heel lift reduces heel contact pressure as well as shortening plantar fascia. Heel cups act as a cushion and a kind of heel lift. Arch support slows down and reduces foot pronation and decreases stress on plantar fascia. The heel counter limits subtalar joints for excessive shearing and reduces stress around the plantar fascia insertion. A supportive shank of orthotics or shoes limits the over-elongation/dorsiflexion of midfoot so as to also decrease plantar fascia stretch.

Clinically, foot orthotics have a positive effect on treating various musculoskeletal disorders for alleviating symptoms, preventing deformity, and enhancing performance. Many literature reviews support it and report that, on average, 70% to 80% respond positively to orthotic treatment (Gross et al., 1991), including the use of foot orthoses for treating plantar fasciitis and shin splints. Ferguson et al (1991) assessed 40 patients complaining of plantar fasciitis/heel spur syndrome. Thirty-four out of 40 felt that their symp-toms improved with foot orthoses. A well-controlled study assessing the effects of functional orthoses on plantar fasciitis was compared with the effects of conventional treatments (Lynch et al., 1998). One hundred and three subjects were randomly assigned to one of three treatment groups: anti-inflammatory, accommodative (viscoelastic heel cup), or mechanical (taping and orthotics). The results showed that patients in the mechanical group had significantly decreased pain levels and improved functional activities.

Few well-controlled studies have investigated the mechanism of orthotic use and efficacy in injury prevention. Moreover, we do not have much evidence or many guidelines for prescribing orthoses and applying sport taping. Nonetheless, we should always keep joints in neutral alignment and in neutral geometry and angle of functions, according to joint kinetics and kinematics.

When conventional treatment is not effective for severe cases, custom-made night splints can be considered to relieve plantar heel pain. Crawford and Thomson (2003) have recommended that corticosteroid injections should only be considered for short-term relief of plantar heel pain if initial therapy fails. Physicians should be cautious about administering this treatment, because corticosteroid injections are associated with plantar fascia rupture, which may cause long-term discomfort (Acevedo and Beskin, 1998). Boddeker et al. (2001) have found that extracorporeal shock wave therapy is not effective and should only be used to treat runners with chronic heel pain.

Runners with plantar fasciitis need to control the inflammation seriously and progress their treatment and exercise load slowly and carefully. The most critical factor for minimizing the chance of relapse and recurrence is how and when the athlete resumes training. When acute inflammatory symptoms subside, one may try to resume training with lower mileage, shorter duration, and lower impact. A useful guideline for a safe progression is the "10% rule": only progress mileage about 10% each week when the condition does not worsen. If the condition relapses, try to remain in the same training for one more week for delayed adaptation of training. If it continues to worsen, training should be stepped down or even halted.

Running Shoe Advice

There are no perfect running shoes; only those that are appropriate and suitable. Strictly speaking, different feet require different shoe types, depending on the type of sport, activity duration, climate and weather, ground situation, and performance level of the athletes. More information can be found in books and research written by authorities such as Clark (1989), Nigg (1986, 2001) and Subotnick (1999).

During the 1960s, though there were many systematic studies by specialists concentrated on the mechanics of running shoes. In the 70s and 80s, scientists turned running shoes into an important "cushioning" tool. The air cushion invented by Nike is a classic example. In the last decade, experts no longer considered cushioning the most important element.

Recent research has pointed out that cushioning materials which are too thick will interfere with the feet from feeling the surface and, thus, runners are more likely to twist. Nigg (2001) and Wit et al. (2000) have suggested a new idea that sensory input in barefoot running will induce an active adaptation strategy that lowers the peak heel pressure, and this is even better than shoe running. However, it may not be practical to run barefoot. The usual guideline for the thickness of midsoles should be 2 to 3 cm.

There are hundreds of classifications of abnormal foot types, but most manufacturers mainly classify their running shoes into three designs: 1/ normal feet; 2/ high-arch, hypomobile feet; 3/ flat, hypermobile feet.

Normal feet – The ankle joint axis is in neutral position. The three arches of the feet are in proper positions. The joints and soft tissues of the feet are not overly tight or soft. The center of pressure of weight bearing does not deviate from the line of transmission. Normal feet can fit into any normal shoe types.

High-arch, hypomobile feet – Fewer people have high arches. An excessively elevated arch is also associated with tight muscles and joints. This affects the shock absorption ability of the feet which can cause many overuse injuries such as plantar fasciitis and different kinds of forefoot pain syndromes. Therefore, a high arch requires cushioned shoes with soft soles so as to provide adequate shock absorption.

Flat, hypermobile feet – One out of three people have flat feet to a certain degree. There are more detailed classifications, such as an overpronated navicular and/or calcaneus or tibialis posterior dysfunction. Support shoes are advised to be worn in many cases and they are usually marked with "support," "control," or "pronator" in addition to shoe size for easy identification. The midsole of support shoes are made up of two kinds of shock absorption material in different degrees of hardness. The inner part of the shoe is made of soft material while the outer part of the shoe is made of hard material. This helps to reduce the degree and speed of the pronation—the lowering of the longitudinal foot arch (Nigg, 1986). When we walk, the outer heel touches the ground first and the pressure from our body is transmitted from the outer side to the inner side, until the big toe curves and we step forward. A dual-density midsole thus reduces the speed of the pronation and overuse injuries such as plantar fasciitis, posterior tibialis tendinitis, or ITBFS (Kibler et al., 1991; Hintermann and Nigg, 1998), but if the symptoms are obvious, one should acquire specially designed insoles.

Other designs enhancing support and reducing overpronation are running shoes with built-in medial wedges which realign a more neutral

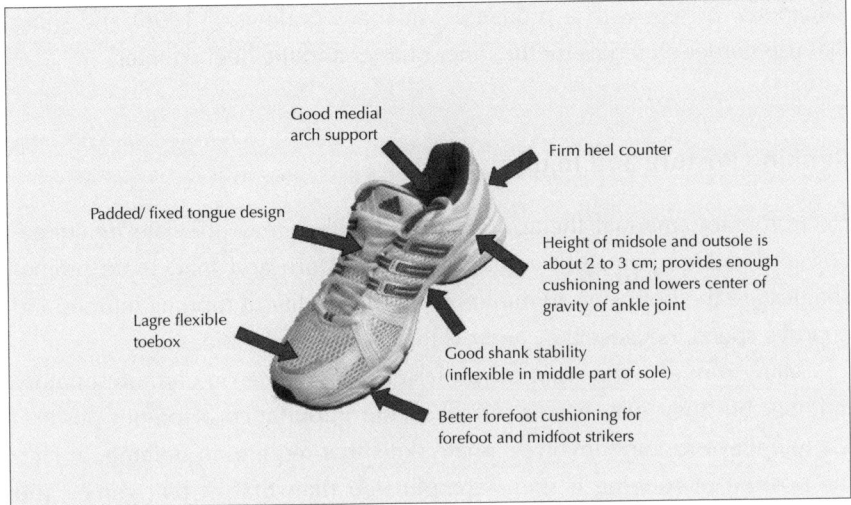

Good medial arch support

Firm heel counter

Padded/ fixed tongue design

Height of midsole and outsole is about 2 to 3 cm; provides enough cushioning and lowers center of gravity of ankle joint

Lagre flexible toebox

Good shank stability (inflexible in middle part of sole)

Better forefoot cushioning for forefoot and midfoot strikers

Fig 8 Common features of a good support shoes

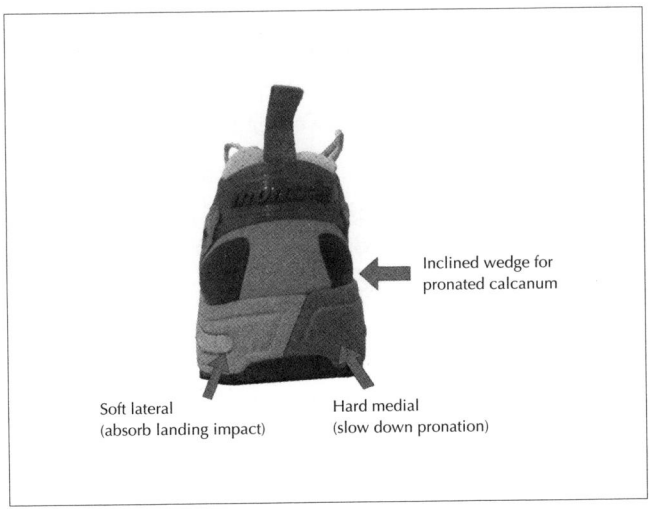

Inclined wedge for pronated calcanum

Soft lateral (absorb landing impact)

Hard medial (slow down pronation)

Fig 9 Rear veiw of a dual density midsole

calcaneus for feet with a pronated calcaneus (Valmassy, 1996) and shoes that use harder materials for the inner quarter and the heel counter.

Running Posture and Injury

Electrotherapy, manual therapy, and acupuncture may alleviate inflammation and reduce pain, but adjusting poor posture and inaccurate biomechanics are the best ways to minimize the possibility of running injuries and improve speed, because they address the root of the problem.

Many runners who want to run faster concentrate on cardiorespiratory training, but they may have overlooked the importance of proper posture. Many believe running involves innate skills that require no training. In fact, the posture of running is more complicated than that of ball games and swimming. However, it was only in the 1990s that systematic research on the pathological biomechanics of running appeared (Hintermann and Nigg, 1998; Novacheck, 1998). Our body moves vertically and linearly while walking and running. The spinal cord, hips, knees, and feet also move in a horizontal plane or spin coordinately in order to reduce nearly 75% of the vibrations that would otherwise be transmitted from the ground to the head. If a joint moves excessively or to an insufficient degree, the deviation will affect other joints and often lead to poor posture. Every time we go on a long run, our legs repeat the same movements thousands of times, resulting in various degenerating injuries.

Most common running injuries discussed in the previous paragraph usually occur in people with abnormal lower limb alignment and in those whose hip or knee muscles are not strong enough. The knee joint adducts and/or rotates internally when under pressure, causing the arch of the feet to collapse. This increases the pressure on the feet and both sides of the knee joint and its soft tissues. One can do a simple test in front of a mirror to see if the knee joint has the above problem when descending steps, running, or squatting. If the knee joint adducts or the arches of the feet collapse, it may be caused by abnormal lower limb alignment or weak muscles. Remedial training is very important when there is an obvious improper posture.

Demonstration of ideal running posture

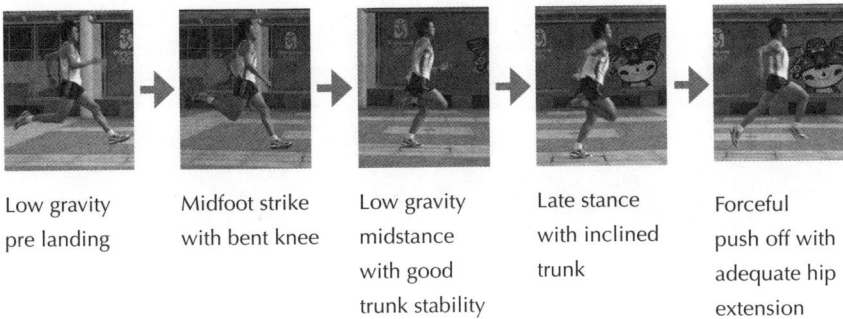

| Low gravity pre landing | Midfoot strike with bent knee | Low gravity midstance with good trunk stability | Late stance with inclined trunk | Forceful push off with adequate hip extension |

Demonstration of alternate leg bound

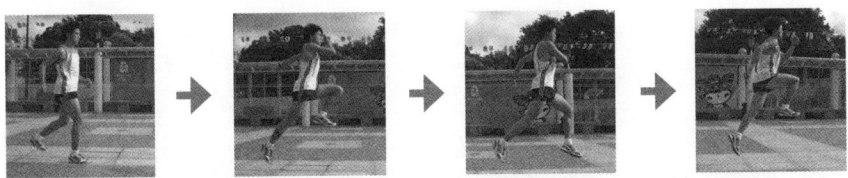

Alternate leg bound training improves whole lower-limb explosive power and reeducates a forceful push off with adequate hip extension.

Demonstration of high knee with extension

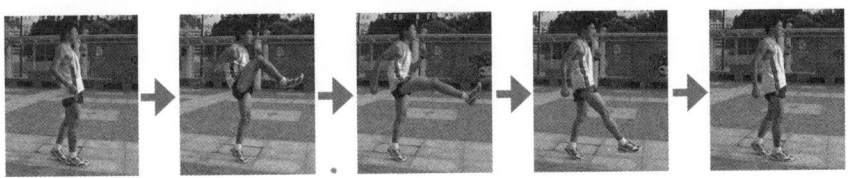

High knee with extension training practices a good form of swinging leg, this helps the runner to relax the unused muscle group.

Even if there is no significant deviation in your posture, you should practice core stabilization exercise so as to maintain a proper form.

Seated Row training

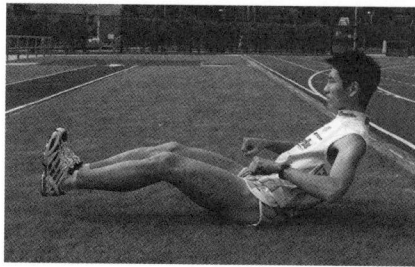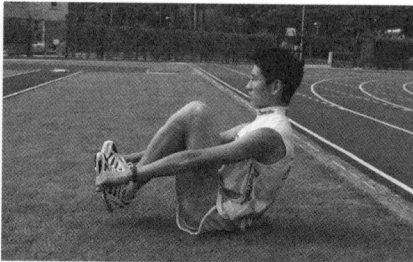

Bend the stomach while the leg muscle contracts. This improves the core stabilization and isolated coordination of legs.

Trunk Holding Exercise

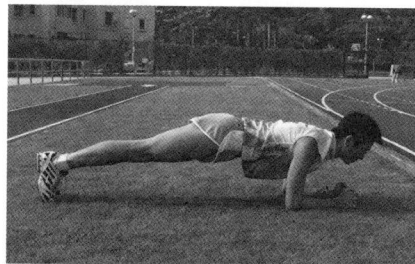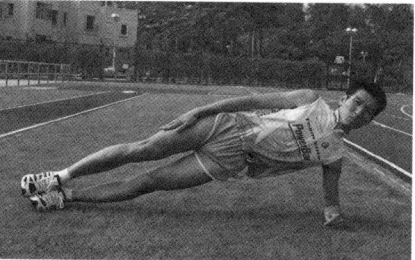

Maintain a proper form in a prone position on each side and hold for about 1 minute.

Summary

If runners want to have a better performance in the marathon, we hope that they undertand that it is not adequate to rely solely on cardiorespiratory training. Runners should also focus on other physical aspects and should learn about the basic concepts of injury treatment and prevention. Biomechanical analysis of running postures which aid in the prescription of therapeutic exercise is also important in daily routine training. Training plans should also be designed for gradual progression so that runners can enjoy the fun of running and improve without injuries.

References

1. Acevedo JI, Beskin JL. 1998. Complications of plantar fascia rupture associated with corticosteroid injection. *Foot Ankle Int* 19 (2): 91–97.
2. American College of Foot and Ankle Surgeons. 2001. The diagnosis and treatment of heel pain. *J Foot Ankle Surg* 40:329–40.
3. Böddeker R, Schäfer H, Haake M. 2001. Extracorporeal shockwave therapy (ESWT) in the treatment of plantar fasciitis—a biometrical review. *Clin Rheumatol* 20 (5): 324–30.
4. Bentley G and Dowd G. 1984. Concurrent concepts of etiology and treatment of chondromalacia patellae. *Clin Orthop* 189: 209–28.
5. Brukner P, Khan K. 2000. *Clinical sports medicine.* Sydney: McGrawHill.
6. Bynum EB, Barrack RL, Alexander AH. 1995. Open versus closed kinetic exercise after anterior cruciate ligament reconstruction. *Am J Sports Med* 23: 401–406.
7. Clarks, Ltd. Training Dept. 1989. *Manual of shoemaking.* 2nd ed. New York: Clarks, Ltd. Training Dept.
8. Cole C, Seto C, Gazewood J. 2005. Plantar Fasciitis: Evidence-Based Review of Diagnosis and Therapy. *Am Fam Physician* 72 (11): 2237–42.
9. Costa ML, Marshall T, Donell ST, Phillips H. 2004. Knee synovial cyst presenting as iliotibial band friction syndrome. *Knee* 11 (3): 247–48.
10. Cowan SM, Bennell KL, Hodges PW, Crossley KM, McConnell J. 2001. Delayed onset of electromyographic activity of vastus medialis obliquus relative to vastus lateralis in subjects with patellofemoral pain syndrome. *Arch Phys Med Rehabil* 82 (2): 183–89.
11. Cowan SM, Bennell KL, Hodges PW, Crossley KM, McConnell J. 2003. Simultaneous feedforward recruitment of the vasti in untrained postural tasks can be restored by physical therapy. *J Orthop Res* 21 (3): 553–58.
12. Cowan SM, Hodges PW, Bennell KL: 2001. Anticipatory activation of vastus lateralis and vastus medialis obliqus occurs simultaneously in voluntary heel and toe raises. *Phys Ther Sport* 2 (2): 71–79.
13. Cox AJ. 1990. Biomechanics of the patellofemoral joint. *Clin Biomech* 5:123–30, 1990.
14. Crawford F, Thomson C. 2003. Interventions for treating plantar heel pain. *Cochrane Database Syst Rev* (3):CD000416.
15. DiGiovanni BF, Nawoczenski DA, Lintal ME, Moore EA, Murray JC,Wilding

GE, et al. 2003. Tissue-specific plantar fascia stretching exercise enhances outcomes in patients with chronic heel pain. A prospective randomized study. *J Bone Joint Surg Am* 85-A (7): 1270–77.

16. DiMarcangelo MT, Yu TC. 1997. Diagnostic imaging of heel pain and plantar fasciitis. *Clin Podiatr Med Surg* 14 (2): 281–301.

17. Doucette SA and Child DD. 1996. The effect of open and closed chain exercise and knee joint position on patellar tracking in lateral patellar compression syndrome. *J Orthop Sports Phys Ther* 23 (2): 104–110.

18. Ferguson H, Raskowsky M, Blake RL, Denton JA. 1991. TL-61® versus Rohadur® orthoses in heel spur syndrome. *J Am Podiatr Med Assoc* 81 (8): 439–42.

19. Fredericson M, Powers CM. 2002. Practical Management of patellofemoral pain. *Clin J Sports Med* 12 (1): 36–38.

20. Fulkerson JP, Hungerford D. 1997. *Disorders of the patellofemoral joint* (3rd Ed.). Baltimore: Williams & Wilkins, 1–365.

21. Fulkerson JP, Shea KP. 1990. Current concepts review: disorder of patellofemoral alignment. *J Bone Joint Surg Am* 72 (9): 1424–29.

22. Gilleard W, McConnell J, Parsons D. 1998. The effect of patellar taping on the onset of vastus medialis obliquus and vastus lateralis muscle activity in persons with patellofemoral pain. *Phys Ther* 78 (1): 25–32.

23. Grabiner MD, Koh TJ, Draganich LF. 1994. Neuromechanics of the patellofemoral joint. *Med Sci Sports Exerc* 26 (1): 10–21.

24. Grelsamer RP, McConnell J. 1998. *The Patella: A Team Approach.* Gaithersburg, Maryland: Aspen.

25. Gross ML, Davlin LB, Evanski PM. 1991. Effectiveness of orthotic shoe inserts in the long-distance runner. *Am J Sports Med* 19 (4): 409–12.

26. Hanten WP and Schulthies SS. 1990. Exercise effect on electromyographic activity of the vastus medialis oblique and vastus lateralis muscles. *Phys Ther* 70 (9): 561–65.

27. Hintermann B, Nigg BM: 1998. Pronation in runners - implications for injuries. *Sports Med* 26 (3): 169–76.

28. Hodges P, Richardson CA. 1993a. An investigation into the effectiveness of hip adduction in the optimization of the vastus medialis oblique contraction. *Scand J Rehab Med* 25:57–62.

29. Hodges PW and Richardson CA. 1993b. The influence of isometric hip adduction on quadriceps femoris activity. *Scand J Rehabil Med* 25 (2): 57–62.

30. Hughston JC, Walsh WM, Puddu G. 1984. *Patellar Subluxation and Dislocation.*

Philadelphia: WB Saunders.

31. Hungerford DS, Barry M. 1979. Biomechanics of patellofemoral joint. *Clin Orthop* 144: 9–15.

32. Insall J. 1982. Current concepts review: patellar pain. *J Bone Joint Surg Am* 64 (1): 147–52.

33. Kibler WB, Goldberg C, Chandler TJ. 1991. Functional biomechanical deficits in running athletes with plantar fasciitis. *Am J Sports Med* 19 (1): 66–71.

34. Kirk KL, Kuklo T, Klemme W. 2000. Iliotibial band friction syndrome. *Orthopedics* 23 (11): 1209–14.

35. Lam PL, Ng GY. 2001. Activation of the quadriceps muscle during semisquatting with different hip and knee positions in patients with anterior knee pain. *Am J Phys Med Rehabil* 80 (11): 804–808.

36. McConnell J. 1986. The management of chondromalacia patellae: a long term solution. *Aust J Physiother* 32 (4): 215–23.

37. McConnell J. 1996. Management of patellofemoral problems. *Man Ther* 1 (2): 60–66.

38. Mercer RS, Rivett DA, Nelson RA. 1998. Stretching the Iliotibial Band: An Anatomical Perspective. *The NZ J of Physio* 5–7.

39. Miller JP, Sedory D, Croce RV. 1997. Vastus Medialis Oblique and Vastus Lateralis activity in patients with and without patellofemoral pain syndrome. *J Sports Rehab* 6:1–10.

40. Nemeth WC, Sanders BL. 1996. The lateral synovial recess of the knee: anatomy and role in chronic Iliotibial band friction syndrome. *Arthroscopy* 12 (5): 574–80.

41. Neptune RR, Wright IC, Van den Bogert AJ. 2000. The influence of orthotic devices and vastus medialis strength and timing on patellofemoral loads during running. *Clin Biomech* 15 (8): 611–18.

42. Nigg BM. 1986. *Biomechanics of running*. Champaign, IL: Human Kinetics Publishers.

43. Nigg BM. 2001. The role of impact forces and foot pronation: a new paradigm. *Clin J Sport Med* 11 (1): 2–9.

44. Novacheck TF. 1998. The biomechanics of running. Gait and Posture 7:77–95.

45. Orchard JW, Fricker PA, Abud AT, Mason BR. 1996. Biomechanics of Iliotibial Band Friction Syndrome in Runners. *Am J Sports Med* 24 (3): 375–79.

46. Schutzer SF, Ramsby GR, Fulkerson JP. 1986. The evaluation of patellofemoral pain using computerized tomography. A preliminary study. *Clin Orthop Relat*

Res 204:286–93.

47. Souza DR, Gross MT. 1991. Comparison of vastus medialis obliques: vastus lateralis muscle integrated electromyographic ratios between healthy subjects and patients with patellofemoral pain. *Phys Ther* 71 (4): 310–20.

48. Sykes K, Wong YM. 2003. Electrical activity of vastus medialis oblique muscle in straight leg raise exercise with different angles of hip rotation. *Physiotherapy* 89 (7): 423–30.

49. Taunton JE, Ryan MB, Clement DB, McKenzie DC, Lloyd-Smith DR, Zumbo BD. 2002. A retrospective case-control analysis of 2002 running injuries. *Br J Sports Med* 36 (2): 95–101.

50. Tepperman PS, Mazliah J, Naumann S, Delmore T. 1986. Effect of ankle position on isometric quadriceps strengthening. *Am J Phys Med* 65 (2): 69–75.

51. Thiranagama R. 1990. Nerve supply of the human vastus medialis muscle. *J Anat* 170:193–98.

52. Valmassy RL. 1996. *Clinical biomechanics of the lower extremities.* Missouri: Mosby, 8–57.

53. Van Mechelen W. 1992. Running injuries: a review of the epidemiological literature. *Sports Med* 14 (5): 320–35.

54. Voight M, Weider D. 1991. Comparative reflex response times of the vastus medialis and the vastus lateralis in normal subjects and subjects with extensor mechanism dysfunction. *Am J Sports Med* 10:131–37.

55. Wilk KE, Reinold MM. 2001. Principles of Patellofemoral Rehabilitation. Sports *Med Arthro Rev* 9:325–36.

56. Wise HH, Fiebert I, Kates JL. 1984. EMG biofeedback as treatment for patellofemoral pain syndrome. *J Orthop Sports Phys Ther* 6 (2): 95–103.

57. Witvrouw E, Sneyers C, Lysens R, Victor J, Bellemans J. 1996. Reflex response times of vastus medialis obliqus and vastus lateralis in normal subjects and in subjects with patellofemoral pain syndrome. *J Orthop Sports Phys Ther* 24 (3): 160–65.

58. Wit BD, Clerq DD, Aerts P. 2000. Biomechanical analysis of the stance phase during barefoot and shod running. *Journal of Biomechanics* 33 (3): 269–78.

59. Zachazewski JE, Magee DJ, Quillen WS. 1996. *Athletic Injuries & Rehabilitation.* Philadelphia: Saunders.

60. Zakaria D, Harburn KL, Kramer JF. 1997. Preferential activation of the vastus medialis oblique, vastus lateralis, and hip adductor muscles during isometric exercises in females. *J Orthop Sports Phys Ther* 26 (1): 23–28.

61. Wilk KE, Davies GJ, Mangine RE, Malone TR. 1998. Patellofemoral disorders: A classification system and clinical guidelines for non-operative rehabilitation. *J Orthop Sports Phys Ther* 28 (5): 310.
62. Cowan SM, Bennell KL, Hodges PW. 2002. Therapeutic patellar taping changes the timing of vasti muscle activation in people with patellofemoral pain syndrome. *Clin J Sport Med* 12 (6): 341.

Bibliography

- Bockrath K, Wooden C, Worrell T, Ingersoll CD, Farr J. "Effects of patella taping on patella position and perceived pain." *Med Sci Sports Exer* 25, no. 9 (1993): 989–92.

- Boucher JP, Cyr A, Lefebvre R, et al. "The vastus medialis obliquus (VMO) is more active at 90 degree of knee flexion." *Med Sci Sports Exer (Supp)* 24 (1992): S147.

- Brindle T, Nyland J, Ford K, Coppola A, Shapiro R. "Electromyographic comparison of standard and modified closed-chain isometric knee extension exercises." *J Strength Cond Res* 16, no. 1 (2002): 129–134.

- Cerny K. "Vastus medialis oblique/vastus lateralis muscle activity ratios for selected exercise in persons with and without patellofemoral pain syndrome." *Phys Ther* 75 (1995): 672–83.

- Clark DI, Downing N, Mitchell J, Coulson L, Syzpryt E, Doherty M. "Physiotherapy for anterior knee pain: a randomized controlled trail." *Ann Rheum Dis* 59, no. 9 (2000): 700–704.

- Cowan SM, Bennell KL, Crossley KM, Hodges PW, McConnell J. "Physical therapy alters recruitment of the vasti in patellofemoral pain syndrome." *Med Sci Sports Exer* 34, no. 12 (2002): 1879–85.

- Cowan SM, Bennell KL, Hodges PW. "Therapeutic patellar taping changes the timing of Vasti muscle activation in people with patellofemoral pain syndrome." *Clin J Sport Med* 12, no. 6 (2002): 339–47.

- Cowan SM, Hodges PW, Bennell KL, Crossley KM. "Altered vastii recruitment when people with patellofemoral pain syndrome complete a postural task." *Arch Phys Med Rehabil* 83, no. 7 (2002): 989–95.

- Earl JE, Schmitz RJ, Arnold BL. "Activation of the VMO and VL during dynamic mini-squat exercises with and without isometric hip adduction." *J Electromyogr Kinesiol* 11, no. 6 (2001): 381–86.

- Frederick EC. *Sport shoes and playing surfaces.* Champaign IL: Human Kinetics Publishers, 1984.

- Grabiner MD, Koh TJ, Von HL. "Effect of concomitant hip joint adduction and knee extension forces on quadriceps activation." *Eur J Exp Musculoskel Res* 1 (1993): 121–24.

- Herrington L, Payton CJ. "Effect of corrective taping of the patella on patients with patellofemoral pain." *Physiotherapy* 83 (1997): 566–72.

- Hertel J, Earl JE, Tsang KKW, Miller SJ. "Combining isometric knee extension exercises with hip adduction or abduction does not increase quadriceps EMG activity." *Br J Sports Med* 38, no.2 (2004): 210–13.

- Hodges PW, Bui BH. "A comparison of computer-based methods for the determination of onset of muscle contraction using electromyography." *Electroencephalogr Clin Neurophysiol* 101, no. 6 (1996): 511–19.

- Holmes SW Jr, Clancy WG Jr. "Clinical classification of patellofemoral pain and dysfunction." *J Orthop Sports Phys Ther* 28, no. 5 (1998): 299–306.

- Hung Y, Gross MT. "Effect of foot position on electromyographic activity of the vastus medialis oblique and vastus lateralis during lower-extremity weight bearing activities." *J Orthop Sports Phys Ther* 29, no. 2 (1999): 93–105.

- Karst GM, Jewett PD. "Electromyographic analysis of exercises proposed for differential activation of medial and lateral quadriceps femoris muscle components." *Phys Ther* 73 (1993): 286–95.

- Karst GM, Willett GM. "Onset timing of electromyographic activity in the vastus medialis oblique and vastus lateralis muscles in subjects with and without patellofemoral pain syndrome." *Phys Ther* 75, no. 9 (1995): 813–23.

- Kowall MG, Kolk G, Nuber GW, Cassisi JE, Stern SH. "Patellar taping in the treatment of patellofemoral pain: a prospective randomized study." *Am J Sports Med* 24, no. 1 (1996):61–66.

- Laprade J, Culham E, Brouwer B. "Comparison of five isometric exercises in the recruitment of vastus medialis oblique in persons with and without patellofemoral pain syndrome." *J Orthop Sports Phys Ther* 27, no. 3 (1998): 197–204.

- Larsen B, Andreasen E, Urfer A, Mickelson MR, Newhouse KE. "Patellar taping: a radiographic examination of the medial glide technique." *Am J Sports Med* 23, no. 4 (1995): 465–71.

- Lee H. "The role of Vastus Medialis Oblique in patellofemoral pain syndrome." *Crit Rev Phys Rehabil Med* 10 (1998): 257–63.

- LeVeau BF, Rogers C. "Selective training of the vastus medialis muscle using

EMG biofeedback." *Phys Ther* 60, no. 11 (1980):1410–15.

- Lohman EB, Harp TP. "A critical review of patellofemoral pain syndrome in rehabilitation." *Crit Rev Phys Rehabil Med* 14 (2002): 197–222.

- Lynch DM, Goforth WP, Martin JE, Odom RD, Preece CK, Kotter MW. "Conservative treatment of plantar fasciitis: a prospective study." *J Am Podiatr Med Assoc* 88, no. 8 (1998):375–80.

- Ng GY, Cheng JM. "The effects of patellar taping on pain and neuromuscular performance in subjects with patellofemoral pain syndrome." *Clin Rehabil* 16, no. 8 (2002): 821–27.

- Ng GYF, Man VY. "EMG analysis of vastus medialis obliquus and vastus lateralis during static knee extension with different hip and ankle position." *NZ J Physiother* 24 (1996):7–10.

- Ninos JC, Irrgang JJ, Burdett R, Weiss JR. "Electromyographic analysis of the squat performed in self-selected lower extremity neutral rotation and 30° of lower extremity turn-out from the self-selected neutral position." *J Orthop Sports Phys Ther* 25, no. 5 (1997): 307–15.

- Owing TM, Grabiner MD. "Motor control of the vastus medialis oblique and vastus lateralis muscles is disrupted during eccentric contractions on subjects with patellofemoral pain." *Am J Sports Med* 30 (2002): 483–88.

- Stiene HA, Brosky T, Reinking MF, Nyland J, Mason MB. "A comparison of closed kinetic chain and isokinetic joint isolation exercise in patients with patellofemoral dysfunction." *J Orthop Sports Phys Ther* 24, no. 3 (1996): 136–41.

- Subotnick SI. *Sports Medicine of the lower extremity.* 2nd ed. New York: Churchill Livingstone, 1999:113–85.

- Witvrouw E, Cambier D, Danneels L, Bellemans J, Werner S, Almqvist F, et al. "The effect of exercise regimens on reflex response time of the vasti muscles in patients with anterior knee pain: a prospective randomized intervention study." *Scand J Med Sci Sports* 13, no. 4 (2003): 251–58.

- Witvrouw E, Lysens R, Bellemans J, Peers K, Vanderstraeten G. "Open versus closed kinetic chain exercises for patellofemoral pain. A prospective, randomized study." *Am J Sports Med* 28, no. 5 (2000): 687–94.

SECTION IV

The Way Ahead

The Way Ahead

The Editors

Preparation for the Hong Kong Marathon

Hong Kong has done well with the marathon since 1997 and the Hong Kong Marathon has been growing from strength to strength. The annual international event has gained popularity and recognition over the years. It has attracted runners from all over the world, partly because of the increase in the total prize money to nearly one million Hong Kong dollars. The number of participants has also grown many times in this period, from slightly more than 1,000 runners in 1997 to more than 50,000 in 2009. These runners gather to compete in three different categories—a 10 km run, a 21 km half-marathon, and the 42 km marathon. In addition, the event is now a recognized tourist attraction for the city.

Arrangements, provisions, and supports for the marathon have achieved high scores in the conduct of the event. With the committed collaborative effort of all concerned parties, the Hong Kong marathon has become a world-class endurance race, seasoned with joy, personal achievement, organizational accomplishment, and considerable domestic and international media coverage. The event is safe and is as smooth as we want it to be. This is a result of contributions from organizing committee member organizations, including the Hong Kong Amateur Athletes Association, Home Affairs Bureau, Auxiliary Medical Service, Civil Aid Service, Food and Environmental Health Department, Environment Protection Department, Highways Department, Hong Kong Police, Hong Kong Convention and Exhibition Centre, Leisure and Cultural Services Department, Transport Department, Cross Harbour (Holdings) Ltd. for Cross Harbour Tunnel and Western Harbour Tunnel, Tsing Ma Bridge Management Ltd., and Hong Kong Tourism Board.

The organizing committee consistently pays close attention to the following matters while preparing for the event:

- event information and logistics
- police-escorted clock cars
- weather announcements, including air pollution
- traffic arrangements, including road closures and reopenings
- water stations, first-aid posts, refreshment distribution area
- runner traffic control before and after the race
- restricted areas to the general public
- media access
- baggage collection area
- crowd management and control at the starting and finish lines
- ambulance and first-aid routes, including suitable parking locations
- appointment of a medical director and a deputy from the AMS Medical Advisory Board
- time limits and strict adherence to those limits
- marketing and promotion

In 2008, a new and more leveled course was designated for the 10 km race. This new course allowed the half and full marathon runners more room to complete the race. Although Hong Kong's physical infrastructure is not designed for the marathon, the city is doing extremely well and has shown its ability to stage this international endurance race for such a large number of participants. The annual event is certainly a great challenge to all involved, including organizers, participants, and onlookers.

Training and Education of Runners

Health is a prime concern of daily living, and, therefore, there is a rising trend in exercise participation. People take up distance running such as the marathon to train for a stronger body and a healthier life. This endurance exercise improves cardiopulmonary function. Distance running is a very demanding exercise, both physically and mentally. Hence, this strenuous activity is not suitable for everyone. Intensive training poses great stress on the heart and lung functions, and it may trigger serious problems in runners with or without pre-existing diseases. Over-training may result in injuries to the body.

Thus, training for and education about long-distance running are very important to the participants, their families, and the organizers. These activities help the runners to improve and to avoid unnecessary bodily harm that might arise from intense endurance exercise. In addition, the resulting risk from the event will be less for the organizers, and fewer untoward incidents will occur. Marathon participants should follow a prescribed training program. Ideally, a coach should be engaged, particularly for more serious runners. Less experienced runners should train with experienced runners.

The Hong Kong marathon organizers have been staging talks by medical doctors at the information expo each year. Dissemination of information on pertinent issues, including training and tips, is also effected via the Internet. These educational activities supplement runners' training and preparation for the big event, resulting in a more safe and smooth race.

Publicity

The media are at times looking for controversial views and sensational statements, especially when unexpected or disastrous incidents take place. This phenomenon has become more apparent in Hong Kong during recent years. Hence, it is essential and advantageous for the marathon organizers to build a strong and close relationship with the media.

Press conferences are staged by the organizers to inform the public on issues related to the marathon. The media are kept well informed on the day of the race so that news about the event is reported immediately. At the same time, reporters will call on parties and individuals of concern to gather their views on the marathon and on specific incidents.

Safety

It has been found that air pollution in Los Angeles does not have any significant effect on the health of athletes. Inadequate training and preparation are the main causes for injuries and casualties in marathons. Hence, air pollution index (API) might not be the cause of the tragedy in the 2006 Hong Kong marathon but, rather, the pre-existing asthma and overestimation of self-stamina could be the cause. However, we must be aware that running in the controlled atmosphere of a gymnasium is completely different to running outdoors on the roads, where the climate, API, humidity, temperature, and other environmental factors have some influence on the runners' performance and the organizers' preparations.

For the safety of all runners, we often remind them to pay attention to their body conditions. Runners should listen to their bodies and make necessary adjustments in order to avoid untoward events. They should consult a doctor if they notice any unusual symptoms during training. Runners should reduce their speed or even stop running if they feel unwell at any time during the race.

A healthy mind is also very important. Runners should not focus too much on their results at the expense of their physical well-being. This is more important for individuals with chronic diseases such as high blood pressure, asthma, bronchitis, epilepsy, and for athletes over 45 years old, especially those who do not do regular exercise. Hence, runners should take note of their physical condition before, during, and after the race. Furthermore, they should eat correctly before the race and wear appropriate clothes and footwear; they are potential contributing factors to runners' safety during the marathon.

Listening to the Experts

Some doctors have suggested that organizers should limit marathon runners to athletes who have had body check-ups. However, a normal treadmill electrocardiogram (or other normal findings) may not be able to predict the performance of runners or prevent mishaps during an endurance race because most marathon runners collapse from electrolyte disturbances, exhaustion, or heat strokes.

Running a marathon is different from other sports because it requires special knowledge, gears, and preparations. Runners must have proper training and should know their own physical limitations. It is advisable to engage in a structured training program and, usually, a preparation period of six months is adequate.

Nonetheless, people with medical illnesses such as diabetes mellitus, asthma, heart disease, or musculoskeletal conditions are advised to consult their doctors before attempting the race. For those with diabetes or who take regular medications, the specific medications and any related information should be written down on the reverse side of the number plate to help the first-aid team recognize any pre-existing medical problems. Runners should also write down their body weight on the reverse side of the number plate to facilitate resuscitation and treatment in case of dehydration or overhydration.

The Physical Activity Readiness Questionnaire (PAR-Q) is a self-assessment questionnaire recommended to runners, particularly those embarking on endurance running for the first time.

Medical Supports

Experience accumulated from the events over the years has strengthened Hong Kong's position in this international endurance race, despite the untoward incidents in the 2006 marathon, in which one 53-year-old known asthmatic and a 32-year-old healthy male collapsed during the race. The first man died and became the first such statistic of this yearly international activity. Throughout the years, we have learned much and improved our performance. All kinds of supports and logistics are improving each time we organize the event in Hong Kong.

The Auxiliary Medical Service (AMS) has been providing first aid and medical supports to this international event over the years. Its first-aid team is better equipped as a result of more thorough data collection from the event and enhanced experience sharing of members on duty. The debriefing (Table 1) provides an opportunity for learning and improvement, most importantly through participatory input from members and officers deployed in the event. Suggestions are received from volunteer duty members and recommendations for improvement have been made in staffing, equipment procurement, supplies, signage, post location, patient flow, treatment records, communication, and hospital backup. As a result, automatic external defibrillators (AED) are now available in all first-aid posts.

Furthermore, since 2004, training and briefing sessions (Table 2) are conducted for officers and members who will be on duty during the marathon so that they are better trained to handle injuries and medical conditions encountered in the race. Training with infection control, contamination, and waste disposal in the first-aid stations are emphasized for the management of larges numbers of injured athletes. These have also been introduced in the training course.

Duty members are further supported by professional nurses and doctors at strategic locations along the course. Thus, with improvement of equipment and logistics, as well as qualified medical staff, the AMS team is able to handle cases effectively before they are sent to hospitals for further care. It is a joint effort and everybody has a specific role to play. Our cooperation, collaboration, and coercion are getting more on track, making the entire operation much more effective. All volunteers are committed to the best possible response and rescue in case of emergencies (or casualties).

Post-traumatic stress disorder (PTSD) among duty members was noted in the 2006 marathon. AMS immediately stepped up the Psycho First Aid, which was initiated in 2004 after the SARS endemic. A structure responsible for critical incident stress management (CISM) was considered under the Psychosocial Response Team Steering Committee. The committee has already conducted a training program on CISM for 35 selected officers and members, while there are a few hundred members in all districts who have undertaken the in-house Psycho First Aid course. The aim is to reduce the psychological impact after major events on AMS members.

Overall, the deployment of 400 AMS first-aid personnel was found to be sufficient to cover the marathon, even with the increase in runners to more than 50,000 in 2009. Moreover, water/sponging points were provided every 2.5 km, along with AMS first-aid posts. This provision is more generous than the requirements recommended by the International Association of Athletics Federations (IAAF). AMS is committed to continuing improvement in the training and equipment for major events held in our city.

Table 1 Issues Discussed at the Technical and Experience Sharing Session, 16 March 2007

1. What is your general impression from the marathon duty?
2. What are impressive cases you have handled or been involved with?
3. Are we appropriately staffed? Any suggestions for improvement?
4. Are the equipment and supplies adequate and suitable? Any suggestions for improvement?
5. Any issues that you would like to comment on?
6. What other improvements shall we make next year, in addition to what you have already mentioned above?
7. Will you help again next year?

Table 2 Items Discussed at the Briefing for AMS Officers Participating in the Standard Chartered Marathon, 26 February 2007

1. Number plate clothes (worn by runners)
2. Post and Map (starting line, finish line, and along the route)
3. Duty posts: where, when, and how to assemble
4. Role and relation with the officer-in-charge at first-aid posts (FAP)
5. Uniform number 3
6. Nurses' roles
7. Journal club
8. Basic life support and update
9. Reporting forms
10. What to bring along to the FAPs
11. Stand-down time
12. White form and blue form for duty records
13. Equipment, medical boxes
14. Liability
15. Reunion and wash-up meeting date: 16 March 2007
16. Experience sharing
17. Weather forecast on 4 March 2007 (7 days forecast from Hong Kong Observatory)
18. Personal equipment: torch, stethoscope, energy bar/water, hot soup, hand gel, hand warmer

Bibliography

Bibliography

Books and Monographs

方玉輝（編）（2008）。《馬拉松備戰攻略》。香港：和平圖書有限公司。

方玉輝（2009）。〈為參加馬拉松比賽作準備〉。《香港運動醫學及科學學會訊》第2期，第3頁。

美國心臟協會（2009）。《健康從業員基礎生命支持學生手冊》（Basic Life Support）。北京：人民衛生出版社。

陳啟明（編）（1995）。《運動醫學與科學》。香港：中文大學出版社。

傅浩堅、楊錫讓（編）（2003）。《運動健身的科學原理》。香港：商務印書館。

醫療輔助隊（2008）。《實用急救手冊》。香港：香港醫療輔助隊。

Bird W & Reynolds V. (2002). *Walking for health: the complete step-by-step guide to getting fit and feeling your best*. London: Carroll & Brown Publishers.

Chan KM & Chang JHT (Eds). (2008). *Golf for Health*. Hong Kong: Red Corporation Ltd.

Chan KM & Frontera W (Eds). (2006). *Sports medicine: Leader since 1928*. International Federation of Sports Medicine.

Fordyce B & Renssen M. (2003). *Marathon runner's handbook*. London: New Holland.

Frederick EC. (1984). Sport shoes and playing surfaces. Champaign IL: Human Kinetics Publishers.

Pedoe DT (Ed). (2000). *Marathon medicine*. London: the Royal Society of Medicine.

Subotnick S.I. (1999). *Sports Medicine of the lower extremity*. 2nd ed. New York: Churchill Livingstone.

St. John Ambulance, St. Andrew's Ambulance Association, & British Red Cross Society. (2002). *First Aid Manual* (8th Edition). London: Dorling Kindersley.

Papers

Billat V, Demarle A, Paiva M, & Koralsztein JP. 2002. Effect of training on the physiological factors of performance in elite marathon runners (males and females). *Int J Sports Med,* 23 (5): 336–41.

Bockrath K, Wooden C, Worrell T, Ingersoll CD, & Farr J. 1993. Effects of patella taping on patella position and perceived pain. *Med Sci Sports Exerc,* 25 (9): 989–92.

Boileau RA, Mayhew JL, Riner WF, & Lussier L. 1982. Physiological characteristics of elite middle and long distance runners. *Can J Appl Sport Sci,* 7 (3): 167–72.

Boucher JP, Cyr A, Lefebvre R, et al. 1992. The vastus medialis obliquus (VMO) is more active at 90 degree of knee flexion. *Med Sci Sports Ex* (Supp), 24: S147.

Brindle TJ, Nyland J, Ford K, Coppola A, & Shapiro R. 2002. Electromyographic comparison of standard and modified closed-chain isometric knee extension exercises. *J Strength Cond Res,* 16 (1): 129–134.

Butterworth DE, Nieman DC, Butler JV, & Herring JL. 1994. Food intake patterns of marathon runners. *Int J Sport Nutr*, 4 (1): 1–7.

Cantwell, JD. 1985. Cardiovascular aspects of running. *Clin Sports Med*, 4 (4): 627–40.

Cerny K. 1995. Vastus medialis oblique/vastus lateralis muscle activity ratios for selected exercise in persons with and without patellofemoral pain syndrome. *Phys Ther*, 75 (8): 672–83.

Cheuvront SN, Carter R, Deruisseau KC, & Moffatt RJ. 2005. Running performance differences between men and women: an update. *Sports Med*, 35 (12): 1017–24.

Cheuvront SN, & Haymes EM. 2005. Thermoregulation and marathon running: biological and environmental influences. *Sports Med*, 31 (10): 743–62.

Chorley JN, Cianca JC, Divine JG, & Hew TD. 2002. Baseline injury risk factors for runners starting a marathon training program. *Clin J Sport Med*, 12 (1): 18–23.

Clark D, Downing N, Mitchell J, Coulson, L, Syzpryt E, & Doherty P. 2002. Physiotherapy for anterior knee pain: a randomized controlled trial. *Ann Rheum Dis*, 59 (9): 700–704.

Cowan SM, Bennell KL, Crossley KM, Hodges PW, & McConnell J. 2002. Physical therapy alters recruitment of the vasti in patellofemoral pain syndrome. *Med Sci Sports Exerc*, 34 (12): 1879–85.

Cowan SM, Bennell KL, & Hodges PW. 2002. Therapeutic patellar taping changes the timing of Vasti muscle activation in people with patellofemoral pain syndrome. *Clin J Sport Med*, 12 (6): 339–47.

Cowan SM, Hodges PW, Bennell KL, & Crossley KM. 2002. Altered vastii recruitment when people with patellofemoral pain syndrome complete a postural task. *Arch Phys Med Rehabil*, 83 (7): 989–95.

Crouse B, & Beattie K. 1996. Marathon medical services: strategies to reduce runner morbidity. *Med Sci Sports Exerc*, 28 (9): 1093–96.

di Prampero PE, Atchou G, Bruckner JC, & Moia C. 1986. The energetics of endurance running. *Eur J Appl Physiol Occup Physiol*, 55 (3): 259–66.

Earl JE, Schmitz RJ, & Arnold BL. 2001. Activation of the VMO and VL during dynamic mini-squat exercises with and without isometric hip adduction. *J Electromyogr & Kinesiol*, 11 (6): 381–86.

Estok PJ, & Rudy EB. 1987. Marathon running: comparison of physical and psychosocial risks for men and women. *Res Nurs Health*, 10 (2): 79–85.

Fong B. 2006. Doctors and Voluntary Service in Doctors & Society. *Hong Kong Medical Journal*, 12 (3): 245–246.

Grabiner MD, Koh TJ, & Von Haefen L. 2004. Effect of concomitant hip joint adduction and knee extension forces on quadriceps activation. Eur J Exp Musculoskel Res, 1: 121–124.

Herrington L. 1998. The role of Vastus Medialis Oblique in patellofemoral pain syndrome. *Crit Review in Phys Rehab Med*, 10 (3): 257–263.

Herrington L, & Payton CJ. 1997. Effect of corrective taping of the patella on patients with patellofemoral pain. *Physiotherapy*, 83: 566–72.

Hertel J, Earl J, Tsang K, & Miller S. 2004. Combining isometric knee extension exercises with hip adduction or abduction does not increase quadriceps EMG activity. *Br J Sports Med*, 38 (2): 210–213.

Hodges PW, & Bui BH. 1996. A comparison of computer-based methods for the determination of onset of muscle contraction using electromyography. *Electroencephalogr Clin Neurophysiol*, 101 (6): 511–19.

Holmes SW Jr, & Clancy WG Jr. 1998. Clinical classification of patellofemoral pain and dysfunction. *J Orthop Sports Phys Ther*, 28 (5): 299–306.

Hung Y, & Gross MT. 1999. Effect of foot position on electromyographic activity of the vastus medialis oblique and vastus lateralis during lower-extemity weight bearing activities. *J Orthop Sports Phys Ther*, 29 (7): 93–105.

Karst GM, & Jewett PD. 1993. Electromyographic analysis of exercises proposed for differential activation of medial and lateral quadriceps femoris muscle components. *Phys Ther*, 73 (5): 286–295.

Karst GM, & Willett GM. 1995. Onset timing of electromyograhic activity in the vastus medialis oblique and vastus lateralis muscles in subjects with and without patellofemoral pain syndrome. *Phys Ther*, 75 (9): 813–823.

Kelly JC, & Godlonton JD. 1980. The 1980 Comrades Marathon. *S Afr Med J*, 58 (13): 509–10.

Kowall MG, Kolk G, Nuber GW, Cassisi JE, & Stern SH. 1996. Patellar taping in the treatment of patellofemoral pain: a prospective randomized study. *Am J Sports Med*, 24 (1): 61–66.

Laprade J, Culham E, & Brouwer B. 1998. Comparison of five isometric exercises in the recruitment of vastus medialis oblique in persons with and without patellofemoral pain syndrome. *J Orthop Sports Phys Ther*, 27 (3): 197–204.

Larsen B, Andreasen E, Urfer A, Mickelson MR, & Newhouse KE. 1995. Patellar taping: a radiographic examination of the medial glide technique. *Am J Sports Med*, 23 (4): 465–71.

LeVeau BF, & Rogers C. 1980. Selective training of the vastus medialis muscle using EMG biofeedback. *Phys Ther*, 60 (11): 1410–15.

Lohman EB, & Harp TP. 2002. A critical review of patellofemoral pain syndrome in rehabilitation. *Crit Review in Phys Rehab Med*, 14 (3&4): 197–222.

Lynch DM, Goforth WP, Martin JE, Odom RD, Preece CK, & Kotter MW. 1998. Conservative treatment of plantar fasciitis: a prospective study. *J Am Podiatr Med Assoc*, 88 (8): 375–80.

Macera CA, Pate RR, Powell KE, Jackson KL, Kendrick JS, & Craven TE. 1989. Predicting lower-extremity injuries among habitual runners. *Arch Intern Med*, 149 (11): 2565–68.

Maron MB, & Horvath SM. 1978. The marathon: a history and review of the literature. *Med Sci Sports*, 10 (2): 137–50.

Maughan RJ, Leiper JB, & Thompson J. 1985. Rectal temperature after marathon running. *Br J Sports Med*, 19 (4): 192–95.

Maughan RJ, & Shirreffs SM. 1997. Recovery from prolonged exercise: restoration of water and electrolyte balance. *J Sports Sci*, 15 (3): 297–303.

McLeavey BC, Corkery MB, & Cronin TE. 1984. The marathon runner: profile of health or vulnerable personality? *Ir Med J*, 77 (2): 37–39.

Myers KJ. Marathon running and vision. 1976. *J Am Optom Assoc*, 47 (4): 515–20.

Ng GY, & Cheng JM. 2002. The effects of patellar taping on pain and neuromuscular performance in subjects with patellofemoral pain syndrome. *Clin Rehabil*, 16 (8): 821–27.

Ng GYF, & Man VY. 1996. EMG analysis of vastus medialis obliquus and vastus lateralis during static knee extension with different hip and ankle position. *NZ J Physiotherapy*, 24: 7–10.

Ninos JC, Irrgang JJ, Burdett R, & Weiss JR. 1997. Electromyograhic analysis of the squat performed in self-selected lower extremity neutral rotation and 30° of lower extremity turn out from the self-selected neutral position. *J Orthop Sports Phys Ther*, 25 (5): 307–15.

Olivier LR, & Kriel JR. Health and marathon running. 1978. S Afr Med J, 53 (20): 778–79.

Owings TM, & Gradiner MD. 2002. Motor control of the Vastus medialis oblique and vastus lateralis muscles is disrupted during eccentric contractions on subjects with patellofemoral pain. *Am J Sports Med*, 30 (4): 483–87.

Parker Jones P, Davy KP, Desouza CA, & Tanaka H. 1999. Total blood volume in endurance-trained postmenopausal females: relation to exercise mode and maximal aerobic capacity. *Acta Physiol Scand*, 166 (4): 327–33.

Pastene J, Germain M, Allevard AM, Gharib C, & Lacour JR. 1996. Water balance during and after marathon running. *Eur J Appl Physiol Occup Physiol*, 73 (1–2): 49–55.

Platen P, & Schaar B. 2003. How to carry out a health-orientated marathon training programme for running and inline skating. *Eur J Cardiovasc Prev Rehabil*, 10 (4): 304–12.

Proceedings of the conference held before the 1984 London marathon. 1984. *Br J Sports Med*, 18 (4): 237–304.

Radford PF, & Ward-Smith AJ. 2003. British running performances in the eighteenth century. *J Sports Sci*, 21 (5): 429–38.

Richards D, Richards R, Schofield PJ, & Ross V. 1979. Biochemical and haematological changes in Sydney's the Sun City-to-Surf fun runners. *Med J Aust*, 2 (9): 449–53.

Roi GS, Giacometti M, & von Duvillard SP. Marathons in altitude. 1999. *Med Sci Sports Exerc*, 31 (5): 723–28.

Satterthwaite P, Norton R, Larmer P, & Robinson E. 1999. Risk factors for injuries and other health problems sustained in a marathon. *Br J Sports Med*, 33 (1): 22–26.

Schuchert A, Puschel K, Kupper W, Schafer H, & Bleifeld W. 1989. [Sudden heart death in a long distance runner during a marathon] [Article in German] *Z Kardiol*, 78 (4): 276–80.

Stiene HA, Brosky T, Reinking MF, Nyland J, & Mason MB. 1996. A comparison of closed kinetic chain and isokinetic joint isolation exercise in patients with patellofemoral dysfunction. *J Orthop Sports Phys Ther*, 24 (3): 136–41.

Utter AC, Kang J, Robertson RJ, Nieman DC, Chaloupka EC, Suminski RR, et al. 2002. Effect of carbohydrate ingestion on ratings of perceived exertion during a marathon. *Med Sci Sports Exerc*, 34 (11): 1779–84.

Weaving EA, Berro VE, & Kew MC. 1980. Heat stroke during a 'run for fun': A case report. *S Afr Med J*, 57 (18): 753–54.

Witvrouw E, Cambier D, Danneels L, Bellemans J, Werner S, Almqvist F, et al. 2003. The effect of exercise regimens on reflex response time of the vasti muscles in patients with anterior knee pain: a prospective randomized intervention study. *Scand J Med Sci Sports*, 13 (4): 251–58.

Witvrouw E, Lysens R, Bellemans J, Peers K, & Vanderstraeten G. 2000. Open versus closed kinetic chain exercises for patellofemoral pain. A prospective, randomized study. *Am J Sports Med*, 28 (5): 687–94.

Websites

Hong Kong Amateur Athletic Association. Standard Chartered Hong Kong Marathon. http://www.hkmarathon.com/marathon/eng/home/default.jsp

AIMS association. Association of International Marathons and Distance Races. http://www.aims-association.org/index.html

Hong Kong Amateur Athletic Associaion. Hong Kong Amateur Athletic Association. http://www.hkaaa.com/hkaaa/eindex.html

Hong Kong Association of Sports Medicine and Sports Science. Hong Kong Association of Sports Medicine and Sports Science. http://www.hkasmss.org.hk/

International Association of Athletics Federations. International Association of Athletics Federations. http://www.iaaf.org/

International Olympic Committee (IOC). The International Olympic Committee? http://www.olympic.org/

Amateur Athletic Union (AAU). Amateur Athletic Union of the USA. http://www.aausports.org/

United Kingdom Athletics 2010. UK Athletics. http://www.ukathletics.org/

US Track & Field. USATF - USA Track & Field. http://www.usatf.org/

Appendix

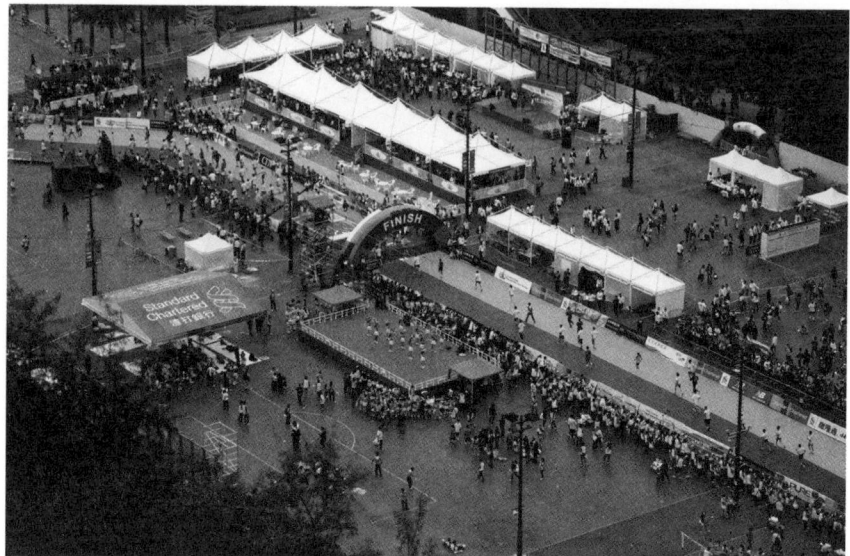

An overview of the finishing line at the Victoria Park (2009).

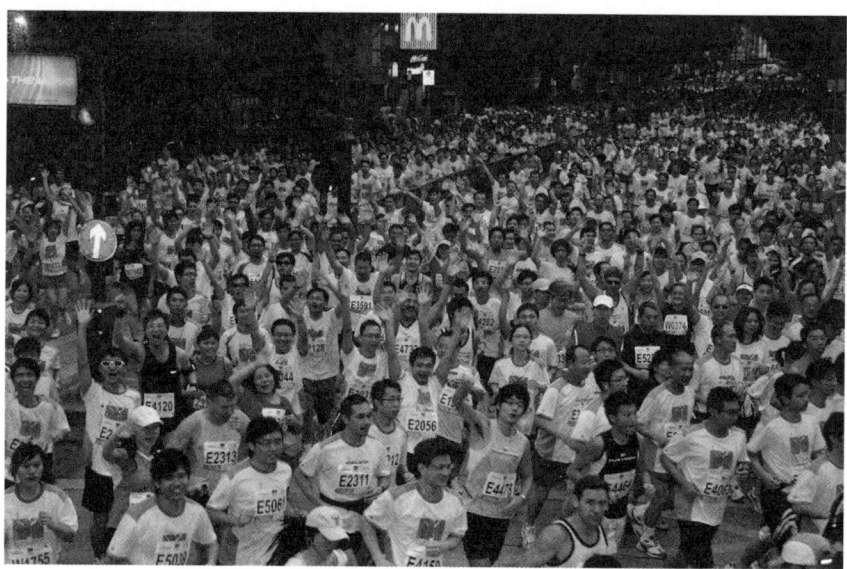

Half marathon runners at Tsim Sha Tsui (2009).

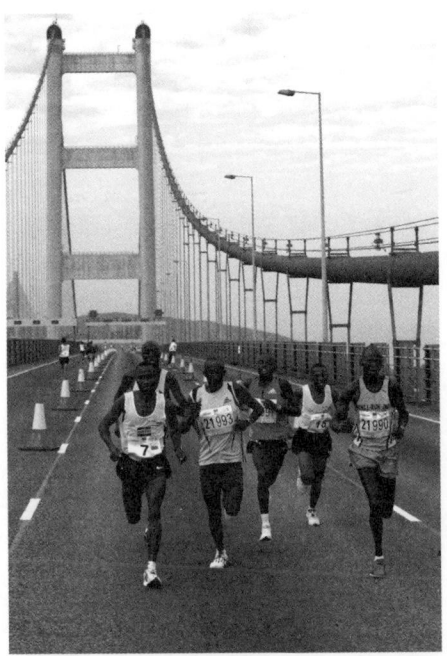

Elite runners, including Champion and first runner-up of Full Marathon Men at the Standard Chartered Hong Kong Marathon 2009 — Cyprian Kiogora Mwobi (left; #7) and John Chirchir Tubei (right; #21990), at Tsing Ma Bridge.

Fun facts of the Standard Chartered Hong Kong Marathon 2009:

70,290 bananas
80,600 chocolates & Energy Bars
57,525 pears
95,000 litres of water
50,000 litres of iso-Tone (sports drinks)
248 portable toilets
34 baggage trucks

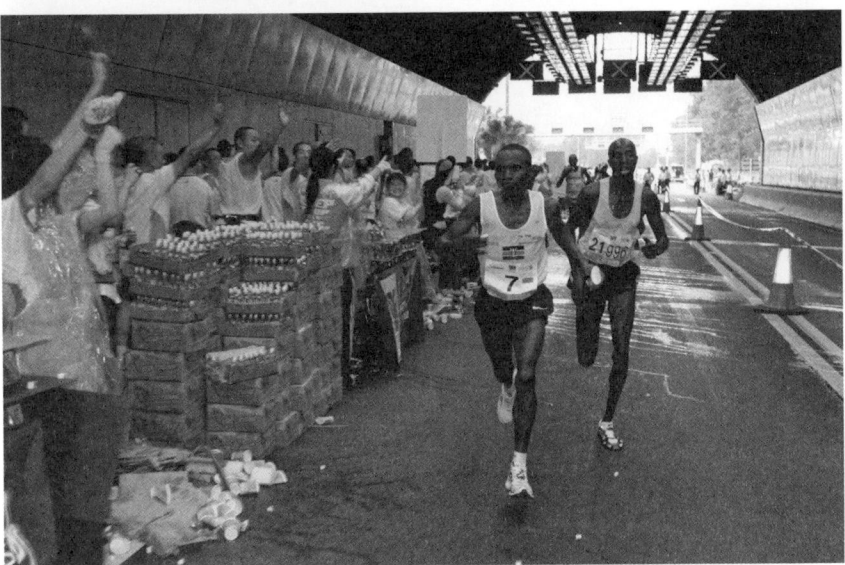

Champion of Standard Chartered Hong Kong Marathon 2009's Full Marathon Men — Cyprian Kiogora Mwobi (left) — from Kenya refilled water at a water station.

Photo on page 1 and above photos and fun facts courtesy of Standard Chartered Bank (Hong Kong) Ltd.

Acknowledgements

Dr. Ben Fong, Chief Editor

The Hong Kong Marathon: Challenges and Health has taken nearly three years to prepare. It all began with the Standard Chartered Hong Kong Marathon 2007, which marked the tenth anniversary of the event. After the event, a few of us suggested writing a book about the first ten years of providing first aid and medical coverage for this major international activity organized in Hong Kong annually.

Many thanks to all contributors in the preparation of this book, the scope of which has been broadened to include advice to the runners, media coverage, runners' experiences, injuries, nutrition, fluid balance, motivation, and physiotherapy. I wish to thank all twenty-one of my colleagues in writing the twenty-two chapters of the book. Most are professional associates, colleagues from the Auxiliary Medical Service (AMS) and the Chinese University of Hong Kong. Without their effort and input, this book would not be as comprehensive and informative as it is today.

I am very grateful for permission to use the data collected by the AMS. My thanks to Chief Staff Officer Dr. Chan Yiu Wing and Staff Officer Mr Lau Man Kwong of AMS for their kindness and assistance, and to Dr Chan particularly for his constant support and for writing the book's Foreword. The help from staff of the AMS Headquarters is also greatly appreciated. Moreover, I am very grateful to the members and officers engaged in the Sports Injuries course for their participation in the survey.

The help of Dr. Jonathan Wai, who has performed the tedious task of editing this book, is much appreciated as well. I also wish to thank Professor Chan Kai Ming, a colleague of mine and a good friend for over two decades, for his encouragement and advice in the preparation of this book from the beginning, and for writing the Preface. I am grateful to Professor Fok Tai Fai, Dean of the Medical Faculty at the University, for writing the commendation for our book. Dean Fok is a religious marathon runner himself, and has inspired many fellow colleagues and students to participate in the event.

My colleagues of the Chinese University Press have been instrumental in getting the book published. My special thanks go to Mr. Tse Wai Keung, Miss Rachel Pang and Mr. Luke Krawec for their professional advice and assistance.

Index